Medical **Ethics**
and **Law** THE CORE CURRICULUM

Commissioning Editor: Timothy Horne
Development Editor: Janice Urquhart
Project Manager: Andrew Palfreyman
Design Direction: Charles Gray

Medical **Ethics** and **Law** THE CORE CURRICULUM

SECOND EDITION

Tony Hope MA PhD MBBch FRCPsych MFPH
Professor of Medical Ethics, and Fellow of St Cross College,
University of Oxford, Oxford, UK, and Honorary Consultant
Psychiatrist

Julian Savulescu BMedSci MB BS MA PhD
Uehiro Chair in Practical Ethics and Director of the Oxford Uehiro
Centre for Practical Ethics, Faculty of Philosophy, University of
Oxford, Oxford, UK

Judith Hendrick BA LLM
Solicitor and Senior Lecturer in Law,
Oxford Brookes University,
Oxford, UK

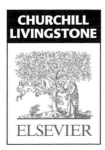

CHURCHILL
LIVINGSTONE

ELSEVIER

Edinburgh London New York Oxford Philadelphia St Louis Sydney Toronto 2008

CHURCHILL LIVINGSTONE
ELSEVIER

First edition 2003
Second edition 2008

ISBN: 9780443103377

British Library Cataloguing in Publication Data
A catalogue record for this book is available from the British Library

Library of Congress Cataloging in Publication Data
A catalog record for this book is available from the Library of Congress

Note
Knowledge and best practice in this field are constantly changing. As new research and experience broaden our knowledge, changes in practice, treatment and drug therapy may become necessary or appropriate. Readers are advised to check the most current information provided (i) on procedures featured or (ii) by the manufacturer of each product to be administered, to verify the recommended dose or formula, the method and duration of administration, and contraindications. It is the responsibility of the practitioner, relying on their own experience and knowledge of the patient, to make diagnoses, to determine dosages and the best treatment for each individual patient, and to take all appropriate safety precautions. To the fullest extent of the law, neither the Publisher nor the Authors assume any liability for any injury and/or damage to persons or property arising out or related to any use of the material contained in this book.

The Publisher

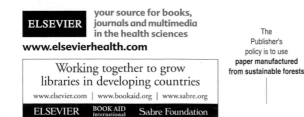

ELSEVIER your source for books, journals and multimedia in the health sciences
www.elsevierhealth.com

The Publisher's policy is to use paper manufactured from sustainable forests

Working together to grow libraries in developing countries
www.elsevier.com | www.bookaid.org | www.sabre.org
ELSEVIER BOOK AID International Sabre Foundation

Printed in China

PREFACE

Alfred North Whitehead famously said that European philosophy consists of a series of footnotes to Plato. If true, this might suggest that the subject of ethics, a branch after all of philosophy, develops slowly. Our experience in writing the second edition of this textbook of medical ethics and law suggests otherwise. We have been surprised by just how much has needed revising and updating. What we had naively assumed would be a small job has turned out to require rather a large number of long evenings and working weekends.

Since the first edition there have been many legal developments. The Mental Capacity Act 2005 has created for the first time in English law the possibility of proxy consent for adults who lack the capacity to consent for themselves. It has defined *best interests* for the first time in statute, as well as giving statutory provision for *advance decisions*. The law on confidentiality has developed as a result of the impact of the Human Rights Act, which enabled the supermodel, Naomi Campbell, to take Mirror Group Newspapers to court. The outcome needs to be taken into account when considering the law and medical confidentiality. The Human Tissue Act 2004, which was passed in the wake of various 'scandals' involving the removal and retention of body parts from children without parental consent, has revolutionized the law in this area. The regulation of medical research continues to change and develop.

Medical developments and social changes keep altering not only the legal but also the ethical contexts of clinical care. Political pressures to protect the public from those with mental disorder are in danger of leading to discriminatory legislation. The ethical discussion of the right balance between public protection and infringement of personal liberties is crucial here. Recent psychological research on human well-being provides a richer empirical context for the philosophical discussion of what is in patients' best interests. In this second edition we have not only updated the law but also added or developed the ethical discussions in many places. We have included a new final chapter that does some future gazing. Medical technologies may be used increasingly not only to treat disease but also to enhance human characteristics beyond the normal: characteristics such as intelligence and athletic ability. Should there be limitations on such uses, and, if so, in what ways?

Medical ethics and law are now firmly embedded in the curricula of medical schools. The ability to make clinical decisions on the basis of critical reasoning is a skill that is rightly presumed as necessary in today's doctors. Medical decisions involve not only scientific understanding but also ethical values and legal analysis. The belief that it is ethically right to act in one way rather than another should be based on good reasons: it is not enough to follow what doctors have always done, nor what experienced doctors now do.

This second edition aims to provide an up-to-date and clear account of medical ethics and law accessible to all medical students and doctors.

T.H.

J.S.

J.H.

ACKNOWLEDGEMENTS

The authors would like to thank the following for their help with this second edition through discussions and commenting on draft chapters: Janet Radcliffe Richards, Mike Parker, John McMillan, Roger Crisp, Anne Slowther, Jacinta Tan, Don Hill, Heather Bradshaw and Guy Kahane. We would also like to thank Janice Urquhart, Andrew Palfreyman and all their colleagues at Churchill Livingstone who helped to produce this second edition, and our copy-editor, Alex Balsdon.

PREFACE

CONTENTS

Part I
ETHICAL AND LEGAL BACK-GROUND

Reasoning about ethics

SCIENTIFIC REASONING IN CLINICAL MEDICINE: BEYOND THE APPRENTICESHIP MODEL

Much clinical education is apprenticeship. The apprentice learns at the master's side, copying and being coached and so becoming skilful. Apprenticeship is a powerful method of education and a good way of learning the old skills, many of which are valuable and important. But apprenticeship has two related limitations: it is conservative and it works by copying rather than reasoning. Apprenticeship, therefore, needs to be complemented by the opportunity to study, reason and discuss if medical education is to equip students for a lifetime's clinical practice. Critical skills must be developed alongside apprenticeship learning.

Critical skills are as important for the scientific aspects of medicine as they are for the ethical aspects. Evidence-based medicine emphasizes the importance of critical assessment: an intervention should be evaluated on the basis of evidence not tradition. Proponents of evidence-based medicine point to examples of useless and even harmful treatments being perpetuated because they were not critically evaluated. That is why it is important continually to scrutinize and develop the evidence concerning the efficacy of treatments.

Evidence-based medicine challenges the doctor to seek and to give reasons for the decisions that she and her patients make. In evaluating the evidence about the effects of an intervention many factors have to be taken into account: the methodological design; the size of the trial; the method of recruitment; the outcomes and the methods used to measure them. For the doctor who is helping the individual patient it is not sufficient simply to evaluate the quality and conclusions from the scientific trials. The doctor has to apply such evidence to the individual case. In doing this, questions arise as to the extent to which this patient does and does not resemble the people who took part in the trial – and judgement is needed in order to decide what features are important in assessing 'resemblance'. The doctor may also use implicit knowledge gained from experience that suggests that for this particular patient there are further factors that may be important in deciding on best treatment. And, of course, the patient may want to be involved in the decision – so the issue for the doctor may be more about how to help the patient make the decision than about what decision should be made. Indeed, evidence-based medicine is not value free. Sometimes the evidence about best treatment will depend on how you value different types of outcome and different side-effects. These are issues that different patients may value differently.

In thinking of the scientific assessment and justification of medical interventions a number of key points can be summarized as follows:

1. Most clinical situations and decisions require knowledge gained from scientific evaluation.
2. The fact that doctors 'traditionally' consider that X is the best treatment in these circumstances is not a good reason, and certainly not a sufficient reason, for offering X: the decision should be based on, or at least informed by, best evidence. The apprenticeship model of education whilst excellent for learning many clinical skills can mask the importance of independent scientific evaluation.
3. When a decision is made it is important to be able to give the reasons and the evidence for that decision.
4. There are structured approaches to assessing evidence and reasons for the scientific aspects of clinical decisions – methods that evidence-based medicine has highlighted as 'critical appraisal skills'.
5. Evidence may be more or less compelling in a particular set of circumstances. Clinical judgement will normally be needed in interpreting the evidence and relating it to the specific clinical decision and the specific patient.
6. Evidence is not value free because it will typically require some relative evaluation of different outcomes. Sometimes the evidence will be such that whatever values people hold, within reason, one specific intervention is clearly best in particular circumstances, but in many situations the balance of the different outcomes from different interventions might be evaluated differently by different patients.

ETHICAL REASONING IN CLINICAL MEDICINE

It is the argument of this book that ethical reasoning should be an integral part of modern medicine just as scientific reasoning should be. The following points concerning the roles of ethics mirror the points made above about science:

1. Many clinical situations, and decisions, involve a combination of factual concerns and ethical issues. Ethical values are part of many clinical decisions. Most of the rest of this book is about situations in which there are significant ethical aspects to decision-making.
2. The apprenticeship method of medical education can make doctors blind to these ethical components: the ethical and scientific components of the decisions are not separated or separately assessed but remain entwined within the notion of 'clinical decision-making' (see Box 1.1).
3. When a decision is made it is important to be able to give the reasons for the ethical aspects of that decision as well as for the scientific aspects.
4. Reasoning about ethics is not a random or purely introspective and intuitive process. There are good and bad reasons and a number of complementary ways of reasoning: what might be called 'critical appraisal skills in ethical reasoning'. These will be discussed as *tools of ethical reasoning* later in this chapter.
5. Judgement is needed in making final decisions – there is no ethical algorithm that can be applied without judgement.

Box 1.1 'Not clinically indicated'

Mr A is 82 years old. He can hardly walk because he becomes breathless on even mild exertion. The cause is aortic valve disease. The cardiac surgeon says: 'Surgery is not clinically indicated'.

This judgment 'not clinically indicated' sounds clear-cut and based on scientific evidence and experience. But what reasons might be given for the decision? Perhaps the chance of the patient dying perioperatively is so high as to make the operation worse than not doing the operation at all. But at this point two quite separate issues are in danger of being confused. One is scientific: what is his prognosis with and without surgery? How long is he likely to live, and in what condition, if he does not have surgery? If he does have surgery what are the chances of his dying peri-operatively, and if he survives the operation period what is his prognosis in terms of length and quality of life? These are exactly the kind of issues that evidence-based medicine seeks to answer.

The second issue involves values. For one patient the risk of perioperative death might be too great and he might want to continue in his present state. For another, surgery might be clearly the best solution: he finds his present condition almost worse than death. Surgery offers exactly what he wants: either (near) instant death, or improvement in his exercise tolerance.

So if by 'not clinically indicated' the surgeon meant that surgery was not in the patient's best interests, it would seem that the right thing to do is to discuss the situation with the patient. It cannot be assumed that a high risk of perioperative death makes surgery the worse option for all patients – it depends on how the patient values different outcomes.

But perhaps by 'not clinically indicated' the surgeon meant that given the limited resources of the NHS (or other health care system), and the limit to the number of operations that the system affords, this is not the kind of patient who should have surgery. Although the patient may benefit from surgery, other patients would benefit more and not all patients who would benefit can be given surgery. If this is what is meant then a quite different ethical analysis is needed: one that looks at the question of what is a just way of allocating resources.

In summary, the ethical aspects of clinical care and decision-making need to be explicit and reasons have to be given for the decisions taken. This is as true of the ethical as of the scientific aspects of clinical care. Society increasingly expects this from doctors as part of the general move towards transparent decision-making and the requirement that professionals should be able to account for and justify their decisions and actions. Doctors' reasoning about ethical aspects of care will need to be able to stand up to scrutiny – in a court if necessary – just as the scientific aspects of decision-making.

SCEPTICISM ABOUT ETHICS

We have emphasized the similarities between scientific and ethical evaluation in clinical care. But science and ethics are also different in important ways. Perhaps the most important is that science is about what is the case, whereas ethics is about how we ought to act, or think. 'Nature has no concern for the good or bad, right or wrong' (Blackburn 2001, p.114). Although in practice there are often areas of uncertainty about the scientific basis of clinical practice, and two doctors may disagree about which course of treatment will be the most effective, in theory at any rate, it should be possible to answer the question of which is the better treatment given agreement over the outcome measures and the relevant patient group. But the same may not be true of ethics. Two people may disagree over the morality of abortion and no amount of factual evidence will necessarily resolve their disagreement because the disagreement is over (moral) values not over empirical facts. This lack of a basis for ethical values in nature can lead to scepticism about ethics. If, in the end, ethical reasoning is based on personal or social values, then there are no ultimate ways of deciding whether your values are better than my values. Ethical values are mere opinion not objective fact. They are purely subjective or are relative to a particular culture. On this view your opinion is as good as my opinion, and if we disagree all we can say is: we beg to differ; end of story. On this view it seems that there is no point in our discussing ethical issues at all, except perhaps to identify false beliefs about the facts on which these are based.

This sceptical position is in our view based on a false assumption. This assumption is that if, in the end, there is no final natural (or divine) truth about ethics then there is no point to discussion, reasoning and argument about ethics. We believe that even if ethical values are based finally on our individual personal choices and commitments, or if they are based on social and cultural values, reasoning about ethics is still of crucial importance.

Consider first the view that ethical values are personal. Most of us do have standards of behaviour and an understanding of personal values. There may be no way of persuading the person who says: 'I don't think that the suffering of people other than me is of the slightest importance, and I don't think it matters whether I cause unnecessary suffering to others (other than that it might rebound on me)'. But from this it does not follow that reasoning about ethics is in general useless. It is unlikely that anyone who has chosen to enter the medical profession takes the view that the suffering of others is unimportant. Quite the contrary, most who enter the health professions have strong and complex views about what is right and are concerned to behave in ways that they consider ethically right. Most of us have standards of behaviour, and a concern for living in a morally good way. These standards 'can energize us to defend ourselves when those standards are belittled and threatened' (Blackburn 2001, p. 114). How do you come to examine your own moral standards and behaviour in specific circumstances, to develop them, and to question them to see whether they stand up? The answer is through subjecting them to rational enquiry. Such rational enquiry is helped by engaging with others in argument: trying to defend our own position. But if the counter-arguments are stronger, if there is a contradiction between what we thought our principles were and what we think is right in a specific situation, then we need to resolve that contradiction in one way or another. If we have certain moral views and standards then, at a personal level, ethical reasoning is important in order to test and develop them. And, of course, in discussion with another person we may come to a point where we disagree and take a fundamentally different view about a key issue. But this is only after argument and reasoning. There may be no final grounding of morality in nature, but from that it does not follow that our personal moral system should be irrational and arbitrary.

Rational analysis is important too if we focus on the social and cultural basis of morality. This is perhaps of particular importance to doctors because doctors practise within a highly socialized role. Society allows doctors a degree of personal freedom in making decisions and in their interactions with patients. But in giving doctors that freedom society expects them to be able to defend their decisions and actions with reasons. Through the legal system, and through guidelines from organizations such as the General Medical Council, society also provides specific ethical principles or concepts within which it expects doctors to work. Doctors must be able to show how their decisions and actions relate to the law and to relevant guidelines.

In summary, reasoning is important in coming to a view about what is the (morally) right thing to do. The importance of reasoning is not undermined by the point that there is no natural foundation for ethics. In any case, society increasingly expects doctors to be able to explain, giving the reasons, why they acted, or decided, in the way that they did; and this expectation applies as much to the ethical aspects of clinical practice as it does to the scientific aspects. It is important, therefore, that doctors are able to identify and reason about the ethical aspects of their work and to relate this to guidelines and law. This book aims to help doctors and medical students gain the knowledge and skills to do this.

THE ROLE OF EMOTION IN MORAL ARGUMENT

As will be clear from what we have said, throughout this book we stress the role of reason in ethical argument. Emotion, however, also plays a part, and this can arise in at least three ways:

1. A person's feelings and emotions may be of moral importance in a particular situation. The desire of a close family member to spend some time with a dying relative may provide grounds for extending the life of the patient in circumstances where otherwise such life-extending treatment would not be appropriate. More generally, patients' wishes are often of crucial significance in medical decisions, and such wishes may be based on the patient's feelings and emotions.
2. Our moral intuitions to particular cases play an important part in the process of moral reasoning (see below). When there is a mismatch between our theory and our intuitions in a particular case, then we may adjust either one or the other, or both. The key point in a rational ethics is that we must bring the two into line – not that a purely intellectual theory always trumps our responses to individual situations. Indeed, ethical reasoning often involves challenging a theoretical position by showing that it leads to conclusions in specific cases that few people would find intuitively acceptable. Emotions are often involved in such intuitive responses.
3. The ability to respond to, and have feelings towards, other people is important. Indeed, it is one of the most important aspects of our lives. A doctor who does not have such responses towards patients is unlikely to be able to help them in many situations. Communicating effectively,

and making the right decisions, often depends, in the medical setting, on appropriate emotional responses.

Emotional responses and moral intuitions, however, need to be subjected to rational analysis. An initial feeling of disgust (the 'yuk factor') may be irrational. The idea of using modern reproductive techniques to enable a 60-year old woman to conceive and give birth to a child may cause an initial feeling of outrage and moral repugnance. But in order to decide on the morality of such a use of these techniques it is necessary to think and not simply to react. Relevant considerations will include an analysis of how the best interests of the potential child can be understood (see p. 147), what additional reasons society has for interfering in the reproductive choices of women (and men), and whether there are grounds to justify a commonly held intuition that there is a moral difference between a man becoming a father at the age of 60, and a woman becoming a mother at the same age.

REFLECTIVE EQUILIBRIUM WITH DIALOGUE

Two caricatures of moral reasoning: the mathematical and the scientific models

All of us have gut reactions as to what we think is morally right in particular situations. Such reactions are a result of our previous experience, of our upbringing, perhaps on occasion of our genetic inheritance, and, in the case of medical decisions, of our apprenticeship learning. Such gut reactions need to be exposed to the crucible of rationality. But this raises the question of what is the relationship, within the context of rational argument, between our intuitive ethical responses to specific situations and our more general principles and theories.

There are two caricatures of moral reasoning. The first might be called the 'mathematical model' because it works from general theory to particular cases. According to this caricature, moral reasoning begins by examining the major moral theories and principles (see Chapter 2) and selecting that theory which, you believe, is right. This theory is then applied to individual situations in order to decide what it is right to do. For example, if you decide that utilitarianism (see Chapter 2) is the right moral theory, you can solve a dilemma in resource allocation by applying that theory. The problem with this 'mathematical model' is that moral theories are not taken on board once and for all. A problematic situation is a test of a moral theory and not simply to be solved from the perspective of that theory. This observation leads to the 'scientific model' of moral reasoning.

The 'scientific model' sees moral reasoning as moving from particular cases to general theories (although this is itself a caricature of the scientific process). According to this view, precedence is given to our moral intuitions in particular circumstances. If there is a clash between our moral theory and what we believe to be right in particular circumstances, then it is the theory that needs to be altered. Thus moral theories are, in effect, an organization or summary of our moral intuitions. The problem with this model is that it gives precedence to our intuitions, and effectively allows no reasoned or principled approach to ethics. Furthermore, our intuitions, or gut reactions, will come from our previous experience and upbringing. Rational morality requires that we test these gut reactions with reasons.

Reflective equilibrium

Reasoning about morality combines both the mathematical and the scientific models and requires a continual moving between our moral responses to specific situations and our moral theories. This process of moving between theory and individual situations is what Rawls (1972) has called 'reflective equilibrium'. Rawls coined this term in the setting of considerations of distributive justice: how should goods, such as money, be fairly distributed within a society? (see Chapter 13). He argued (Rawls 1972, p. 20) that in attempting to describe a fair distribution of, for example, wealth:

> " …we begin by describing it so that it represents generally shared and preferably weak conditions. We then see if these conditions are strong enough to yield a significant set of principles. If not we look for further premises equally reasonable. But if so, and these principles match our considered convictions of justice, so far well and good. But presumably there will be discrepancies. In this case we have a choice. We can either modify the account of the initial situation or we can revise our existing judgements, for even the judgements we take provisionally as fixed points are liable to revision. By going back and forth, sometimes altering the conditions of the contractual circumstances, at others withdrawing our judgement and conforming them to principle, I assume that eventually we shall find a description of the initial situation that both expresses reasonable conditions and yields principles which match our considered judgements duly pruned and adjusted. This state of affairs I refer to as reflective equilibrium.

Dialogue

In this process of reflective equilibrium we are attempting to ensure that our beliefs about what is right in various individual situations, and our theories, are consistent with each other. During the process both the theories and the beliefs can undergo revision. When there is lack of agreement, there is no algorithm, or automatic way, to tell us which or what we must change. That has to be a matter of judgement. This process of reflective equilibrium can be undertaken by an individual person, but dialogue – discussion with others – can help the process. Rawls emphasizes the importance of a group of competent people in the process of reflective equilibrium, that is, people capable and willing to engage in rational dialogue. Discussion of ethical issues is important for several reasons:

1. It helps us identify inconsistencies between our moral views; between our views in one situation and another; and between our theories and our intuitions.
2. It helps ensure that we are aware of the perspectives of different moral theories.
3. It helps ensure that we are aware of the perspectives of different people – and in the medical setting this can be particularly important.

In the remainder of this chapter we will outline various 'tools' of ethical reasoning and end with a discussion of the 'slippery slope argument' which is frequently used within ethical discussion. You will already use many of the 'tools' in discussions about ethical issues probably without bothering to name or classify the particular method of argument. You may want to skip the rest of this chapter and get straight on with reading about particular clinical settings (see Part 2). It can, however, be valuable when faced with an ethically problematic issue to consciously consider whether one or more of these tools might be particularly helpful. Thus, it can sometimes help to think explicitly about how different principles would apply to the situation: sometimes it is valuable to consider case comparisons; and sometimes ethical reasoning calls for conceptual analysis and clarification. We pick out seven tools of ethical reasoning that we find particularly helpful.

Tool 1: Distinguishing facts from values

In making medical decisions, particularly in difficult situations, it can be important to distinguish clearly between medical facts and moral evaluations.

It will typically be the case that rather different types of argument and evidence bear on the factual components compared to the evaluative components of a medical decision. Consider the following argument. Mr B has a persistently raised diastolic blood pressure of 105 mmHg. A blood pressure of this level is associated with a significantly increased risk of an earlier death over 20 years. Treatment, leading to a lowering of this blood pressure to less than 90 mmHg, will increase Mr B's likely lifespan. Therefore, the doctor should do what she can to persuade Mr B to take such treatment.

The key factual statements are: that Mr B's blood pressure is of a particular level; that such a level is associated with an increased mortality rate; and that lowering the pressure with treatment will reduce the risk of early death. The skills in assessing these statements are those of assessing empirical evidence – the skills of evidence-based medicine.

The key evaluative statements are that the increased mortality rate is 'significant', and that the facts justify trying to persuade Mr B to a certain course of action (to take the medication). The term 'significant' has two meanings, which can be confused. The first is a technical one in statistics, referring for example to the probability of obtaining the observed results if the null hypothesis is true. The second meaning is that of normal language, meaning that the results have some importance. It is the second meaning that incorporates values. Assessing these evaluative statements takes us into the realm of moral argument.

Tool 2: Clarifying the logical form of the argument

Reasoning must be logically sound. An argument is a set of reasons supporting a conclusion. A deductive, or logical, argument is a series of statements (called premises) that lead logically to a conclusion. A valid argument is one in which the conclusion follows as a matter of logical necessity from the premises. Box 1.2 summarizes some of the types and elements of formal logical arguments.

Box 1.2 Syllogisms: valid and invalid forms

A syllogism is the basic form of deductive argument. It is an argument that can be expressed in the form of two propositions, called premises, and a conclusion that results, as a matter of logic, from those premises. There are two main types of valid syllogism.

1. *Modus ponens* (in full: *modus ponendo ponens*)

A syllogism of the following form:

Premise 1 **(P1)**   If **p** then **q** (if statement **p** is true then statement **q** is true)

Premise 2 **(P2)**   **p** (i.e. statement **p** is true)

Conclusion **(C)**   **q** (therefore statement **q** is true)

An example:

P1   If a fetus is a person it is wrong to kill it.

P2   A fetus is a person.

C   It is wrong to kill a fetus.

2. *Modus tollens* (in full: *modus tollendo tollens*)

A syllogism of the following form:

Premise 1   If **p** then **q** (if statement **p** is true then statement **q** is true)

Premise 2   **Not q** (it is not the case that **q** is true; **q** is false)

Conclusion   **Not p** (therefore statement **p** is false)

Note: Not p is usually written as **–p** in formal logic.

An example:

P1   If a fetus is a person it is wrong to kill it.

P2   It is not wrong to kill a fetus.

C   A fetus is not a person.

Note: *Modus ponendo ponens* is medieval Latin meaning a method that, by affirming, affirms (by affirming **p** in **P2** it affirms **q** in **C**); and *modus tollendo tollens* means that by denying denies (by denying **q** in **P2**, it denies **p** in **C**).

An example of an invalid argument in the form of a syllogism

Premise 1   If **p** then **q** (if statement **p** is true then statement **q** is true)

Premise 2   **Not p** (i.e. statement **p** is false)

False conclusion   **Not q** (therefore statement **q** is false)

An example:

P1   If a fetus is a person it is wrong to kill it.

P2   A fetus is not a person.

C   It is not wrong to kill a fetus.

There might be reasons why it is wrong to kill a fetus other than its being a person.

Compare: If it is raining I will wear a coat. It is not raining. Therefore I will not wear a coat. This is an invalid argument: I might wear a coat because it is cold, although dry.

Iff: This is a shorthand, often employed in philosophical writing, for: '*if and only if*'. An example of its use is: 'A person is a minor in English law *iff* that person is under 18 years old'.

When testing our own arguments, or those of others, it can be helpful to summarize the argument in logical form. This enables the premises (often hidden assumptions) to be clearly identified – and examined – and will help expose any fallacy in the argument itself (Box 1.3).

Box 1.3 Some fallacies in argument (see Warburton 2000 for many further examples)

Ad hominem move
Shifting the argument from the point in question to an irrelevant aspect of the person who is making the argument.

Arguments from authority
Arguing that a statement or position or argument is true simply on the grounds that someone in authority has said that it is true.

Begging the question
An argument in which the conclusion, or the point that is in dispute, has already been assumed in the reasons given in favour of the conclusion. The argument is therefore a circular one.

But-there-is-always-someone-who-will-never-agree diversion (after Flew 1989, p. 23)
The fact that there are people who are not convinced by an argument, or set of reasons, does not in itself show that the argument is not valid.

Confusing necessary for sufficient conditions
A necessary condition for some state of affairs is one that is required, that is it has to be in place for that state of affairs to obtain. For example, it is a necessary condition for a doctor to be found liable in negligence for that doctor to have a relevant duty of care (see Chapter 4). However, this is not a sufficient condition, because other conditions are also required. Conversely, the absence of a train driver may be a sufficient condition for a train not to run, but it is not a necessary condition as a train may not run because it has broken down even though there is a driver present. Arguments are sometimes fallacious because they confuse necessary and sufficient conditions.

The intention-wasn't-bad-so-the-action-isn't-wrong fallacy
Judging people and judging acts or beliefs are two quite different things.

Motherhood statements
Bland statements that are used as rhetorical devices to gain agreement from others, often as a cloak to then gain agreement to more contentious statements without proper argument. For example: 'all humans are equal (so it would be wrong to withdraw treatment from a patient in a persistent unconscious state)'.

The no-true Scotsman move (after Flew 1989)
Someone says: 'No Scotsman would beat his wife to a shapeless pulp with a blunt instrument'. He is confronted with a falsifying instance: 'Mr Angus McSporran did just that". Instead of withdrawing, or at least qualifying, the too rash original claim our patriot insists: "Well, no true Scotsman would do such a thing!' (Flew 1989, p. 388)

What seems to be a statement of fact (an empirical claim) is made impervious to counter examples by adapting the meaning of the words so that the statement becomes true by definition and empty of any empirical content.

Overgeneralization
A fallacious argument which provides some examples that illustrate a point and uses those examples to conclude a much more general statement.

The ten-leaky-buckets tactic (after Flew 1989)
This is: '… presenting a series of severally unsound arguments as if their mere conjunction might render them collectively valid: something that needs to be distinguished carefully from the accumulation of evidence, where every item possesses some weight in its own right' (Flew 1989, p. 287).

Tool 3: Analysing concepts

An important component of valid reasoning is conceptual analysis. There are four types of conceptual analysis: providing a definition; elucidating a concept; making distinctions (splitting) and identifying similarities between two different concepts (lumping).

Philosophers are caricatured as replying to every question with the words 'it all depends on what you mean by…'. The fact is that it often does. Lack of clarity about the meanings or definitions of key concepts in an argument can be a rhetorical device to make an unsound argument persuasive. Consider the following argument:

> It is murder to kill another human being. A human fetus is a human being. Doctors who terminate a pregnancy (a euphemism for killing a human being) are murderers. They should be given life imprisonment, not an NHS salary.

A first stage in analysing this argument is to define key terms. The term 'murder' normally means an *unlawful* killing, and a 'murderer' is someone who has committed murder. In English law, killing a fetus is not normally murder (see Chapter 9). In the argument above the words 'murder' and 'murderer' are being used with a different meaning (perhaps to mean 'morally wrong killing') for rhetorical effect. The term 'human being' also needs to be defined.

Definition, however, is often only a first, and a rather small, step. In the example above, a definition of 'human being' may be readily agreed. What is at issue is not whether the fetus is a human being, but whether that fact alone provides a convincing reason as to why killing the fetus is, from a moral point of view, like killing, say, a 10-year-old child. In order to examine this issue it is necessary to go beyond definition and carry out some elucidation, or further analysis, of key concepts. In debates about termination of pregnancy, or embryo experiments, the concept of a 'person' has played a key role (see Chapter 9). This concept will need elucidating.

In addition to definition and elucidation, conceptual analysis may involve 'splitting' or 'lumping'. Splitting is the making of distinctions. In a discussion of the morality of euthanasia it is important to make distinctions between the different types of euthanasia (see Chapter 12). This is because the relevant ethical issues bear differently on these different types.

Lumping involves clarifying similarities between things that are usually considered to be quite different. For example, the argument might be made that there is no clear conceptual difference between withholding and withdrawing life-extending treatment on which to base a moral difference (see Chapter 12).

Tool 4: Reasoning from principles and theory

There are a number of principles relevant to many situations in medicine and which are endorsed as important by many moral theories (see Chapter 2). Four principles in particular have been identified (Beauchamp & Childress 2001, Gillon 1986). These are summarized in Box 1.4. When faced with an ethical problem in medical practice it can often be helpful to apply each of the four principles. This can help in clarifying the key moral issues that are relevant.

Reasoning using principles is often closely related to logically valid argument, with the principle or theory acting as one of the premises. However, the reasoning process is often more complex than this, involving a combination of logical argument and conceptual analysis.

Tool 5: Using case comparison

Perhaps the most powerful strategy in developing moral argument is the use of consistency. The underlying principle of consistency is that, if you conclude that you should make different decisions, or do different things, in two similar situations, then you must be able to point to a morally relevant difference between the two situations that accounts for the different decisions. Otherwise you are being inconsistent.

The method of case comparison is one use of the idea of consistency. It can be used as a method for deciding what it is right to do in a problematic situation. This method involves comparing the problematic case with cases that are more straightforward – or already decided. This contrasts with other methods of ethical analysis, such as applying an ethical principle or a particular moral theory. Case comparison is used extensively in legal decisions, where the legal position may be judged by comparing the case under examination with one that has already been decided (see Chapter 4). The key question is whether the two cases are sufficiently similar in the relevant ways for the earlier case to act as precedent for the later case.

Tool 6: Thought experiments

The cases used for case comparison, or for examining consistency, may be real or hypothetical, or even unrealistic. Philosophers frequently use imaginary cases in testing arguments and in examining concepts. These are called 'thought experiments' – like many scientific experiments, they are designed to test a theory. There are several examples of thought experiment in this book (e.g. the case of the connected violinist (see p. 141) and some of the imaginary cases in Chapter 12).

Some practically minded people, including doctors, are often sceptical of thought experiments because the cases do not describe real situations. Such scepticism can miss the purpose of the experiment. Suppose that person A justifies her view that withdrawing life-extending treatment is wrong by appealing to

Box 1.4 Four principles in medical ethics

1. Respect for patient autonomy (see also Chapter 3)

Autonomy (literally, self-rule) is the capacity to think, decide, and act on the basis of such thought and decision, freely and independently (Gillon 1986). Respect for patient autonomy requires health professionals (and others, including the patient's family) to help patients come to their own decisions (for example, by providing important information) and to respect and follow those decisions (even when the health professional believes that the decision is wrong).

2. Beneficence: the promotion of what is best for the patient (see also Chapter 3)

This principle emphasizes the moral importance of doing good to others, and in particular in the medical context, doing good to patients. Following this principle would entail doing what was best for the patient. This raises the question of who should be the judge of what is best for the patient. This principle is often interpreted as focusing on what an objective assessment by a relevant health professional would determine as being in the patient's best interests. The patient's own views are captured by the principle of respect for patient autonomy.

In most situations respecting the principle of beneficence and the principle of respect for patient autonomy will lead to the same conclusion, as most of the time patients want what is (objectively) in their best interests. The two principles conflict when a competent patient chooses a course of action that is not in his or her best interests.

3. Non-maleficence: avoiding harm

This principle is the other side of the coin of the principle of beneficence. It states that we should not harm patients. In most situations this principle adds nothing useful to the principle of beneficence. Most treatments have some (one hopes small) chance of doing more harm than good. It does not follow from this that such treatments should be avoided on the grounds that avoiding harming a patient should take priority over doing good. Rather, the potential goods and harms and their probabilities need to be weighed up at the same time to decide what overall is in the patient's best interests. The main reason for retaining the principle of non-maleficence is that it is generally thought that we have a *prima facie* duty not to harm anyone, whereas we owe a duty of beneficence to a limited number of people only.

4. Justice

Time and resources do not allow every patient to get the best possible treatment. Health professionals have to decide how much time to spend with different patients, and at various levels within a healthcare system, because of limited resources, decisions must be made about limitations on treatments that can be offered in various situations. The principle of justice emphasizes two points: first, that patients in similar situations should normally have access to the same health care and, second, that in determining what level of health care should be available for one set of patients we must take into account the effect of such a use of resources on other patients. In other words, we must try to distribute our limited resources (time, money, intensive care beds) fairly.

Reasoning about ethics

the general principle that intentional killing is always wrong. Person B might use a thought experiment to challenge this general principle. He might, for example, describe the situation of the trapped lorry driver (see Chapter 12, Box 12.4, Case 1). In this situation the driver will either burn to death with much suffering, or might be killed painlessly. The power of this thought experiment is that it provides a convincing example of when it would seem right, at least to many people, to kill. If you believe that it would be right to kill the trapped lorry driver then you need to modify your general principle that it is always wrong to kill. Your objection to withdrawing treatment will need to rest on a less general principle, and you will need either to give reasons that justify distinguishing, morally, between the two cases, or to change your position with regard to one of the situations. The fact that the case of the lorry driver is imaginary does not render it irrelevant as a test of the general principle.

Tool 7: Rational decision theory

We are often faced, in life, with making decisions in complex situations. We use many different strategies in coming to a decision and different people tend to use different strategies to differing extents. In some situations we may use a simple rule that is fairly easy to apply: 'buy the best', for example, for items we value and which are all comfortably within the size of our purse. In other situations we may search for the item we want, a washing machine for example, until we find one with the features that are satisfactory to us – not worrying about whether we might find a better machine if we went on looking. In still other situations our concern may be to avoid a particular outcome. We avoid this one risk, other considerations being of little importance to us.

Rational decision theory is none of these. It is a method derived from the systematic application of a *consequentialist* approach to decisions (see Chapter 2). If we apply rational decision theory then we will choose that option which maximizes the expected value (or utility), as we see it, of the outcome (for a more detailed discussion see Savulescu 1994).

Consider a simple example. I am offered the opportunity to take part in the following bet on the outcome of the throw of an unbiased die. If I throw a 1 or a 2 then I will win £15. If I throw any other number (a 3, 4, 5 or 6) then I must pay £10. Is it financially sensible to throw the die?

I have two options: either to refuse the offer and not to enter the gamble; or to enter the gamble and throw the die. If I take the first option and do not gamble then the expected 'value' of the outcome will be neither to win nor to lose any money: the financial expected value is £0.

If I take the second option and gamble, then there are two possible outcomes: to throw a 1 or 2 and win £15; or to throw a 3, 4, 5 or 6 and lose £10. Thus I have a one in three chance of winning £15 and a two in three chance of losing £10. Overall the expected value of taking part in the bet will be:

$$(1/3 \times £15) - (2/3 \times £10) = £5 - £6.67 = -£1.67.$$

The expected value if I join the gamble is −£1.67; the expected value of not joining the gamble is £0. As it is better not to lose anything than to lose £1.67, it is better (according to rational decision theory) not to bet.

What has this to do with ethics? In the above example the value of each outcome was calculated in terms of money. But the same general method can be applied whatever kind of evaluation we want: people's happiness for example, or some moral evaluation. The only two aspects that are formally necessary are that we can ascribe numerical (cardinal) values to the outcomes, and probabilities to their occurring given a choice of action. These two formal conditions are of course restrictive and rational decision theory cannot be applied if we can make no reasonable judgements on these two issues.

Let's go back to the above gamble. If what we are trying to do is to maximize our expected financial gain (and minimize our financial loss) then it is not rational, according to this approach, to take part in the gamble. But suppose that we are trying to maximize our expected pleasure, and suppose that we get pleasure from the gamble. Let us now work out what we should do if we want to maximize the expected value of our happiness. We will use a scale of happiness from (−10) to (+10), where 0 is neither happy nor sad, 10 is very happy indeed and −10 is very sad indeed.

Suppose that just taking part in the gamble gives me a pleasant thrill that I estimate as +1. Suppose that losing £10 makes me sad at a level I rate as −3. Suppose that I rate winning £15 at +4. How do the 'expected utilities' work out?

- If I don't enter the gamble my expected value will be 0.
- If I do gamble then two things can happen: either I win or I lose. If I win I will have gained the following happiness: +1 (for just gambling) + 4. That is a total of +5. If I lose my happiness will be: +1 (for just gambling) − 3. A total of − 2.

To work out the expected utility of gambling we multiply the total happiness for each of the possible outcomes by the probability of that outcome occurring and add them together. Thus:

$$[(+5) \times 1/3] + [-2 \times 2/3] = 5/3 - 4/3 = 1/3$$

The 'expected utility' of gambling is 1/3 units of happiness and that of not gambling is 0. Rational decision theory shows that if we want to maximize our expected happiness (on the values given above) we should gamble (even though the expected financial effect is a loss).

If we can ascribe both values and probabilities to the various possible outcomes of the various different choices that we might make, in a given situation, then rational decision theory can help us in coming to a decision.

Consider the medical example of attempting resuscitation. Mr Smith, a patient, is at risk of suffering a cardiac arrest. The question is: should resuscitation be attempted were he to have a cardiac arrest, or should he be given a 'do not attempt resuscitation' order? Suppose that the likely effects of resuscitation are as follows: there is a 10% (i.e. probability = 0.1) chance of successful resuscitation with a reasonable life afterwards; a 40% ($p = 0.4$) chance of successful resuscitation with a very poor life afterwards; and a 50% ($p = 0.5$) chance of immediate death. If no resuscitation were attempted he would certainly die immediately.

In order to use rational decision theory values must be given to these various possible outcomes. Let us give the value 0 for immediate death. For the sake of illustration we will give the value +5 for the 'reasonable life'; and the value −10 for the 'very poor life' (that is a value worse than death). Given these values we can calculate the 'expected utilities' of both attempting and not attempting resuscitation:

- The expected value (probability multiplied by value) of not attempting resuscitation is 0 (1 × 0).
- The expected value of attempting resuscitation is the sum of the various possible outcomes: (0.1 × 5) + (0.4 × − 10) + (0.5 × 0) = −3.5.

On the given assumptions of probabilities and values of the various outcomes not attempting resuscitation has greater expected utility than attempting resuscitation: resuscitation should not be attempted. Consequentialism can be applied to any dilemma about what we should do, no matter how complicated. But as the number of possible outcomes of each action grows, or there are many possible actions, decision-making is often made easier by constructing a branching tree of possible actions and outcomes.

This method of reasoning is only as good as the estimations of probabilities and values of the various outcomes. The values, in the example given, should ideally be those of the patient because it is his life and death that is at issue. One way of putting a value on the quality of life, a method used in calculating quality adjusted life years (QALYs) (see Chapter 13) is to employ 'time trade off'. Suppose you want to give a value to the quality of life were you to be in a particular health state (e.g. to become paralysed in both legs). Ask yourself this question: you have a choice between living 1 year in full health, and x years in the relevant health state (e.g. paraplegia). At what value of x are you unsure which you would prefer? Presumably you would prefer 1 year of healthy life to 1 year with paraplegia. But (perhaps) you would prefer 10 years of life with paraplegia to only 1 year of healthy life. If so, x lies somewhere between 1 and 10. At what value of x do you find it impossible to choose? Suppose the answer is 2 years. Then, according to the 'time trade off' approach, the quality of life with paraplegia is 0.5 (on a scale where 0 is death and 1 is full health). Using this method, the value to a particular outcome is given by the quality of life multiplied by the number of years of life in that state.

Rational decision theory allows for some uncertainty in the quantification of both probabilities and values of the outcomes as long as some limits can be put on these uncertainties. The expected utility of each possible decision can be worked out for the extreme values that are put on these quantities. In the example above, suppose that the chance of the very poor outcome is given as between 30% and 50% (and the chance of immediate death adjusted accordingly) and the value of the very poor outcome is given as between −7 and −12. Then, on the best scenario, the expected utility of carrying out resuscitation is: (0.1 × 5) + (0.3 × − 7) + (0) = −1.6.

Thus, even at its most favourable it would be better not to attempt resuscitation. Of course it might turn out that the best choice differs depending on which values, within the predicted range, you choose, in which case this method does not give a clear answer as to what to do. It may still be helpful because it will highlight which areas of uncertainty are crucial in coming to a decision and it may be possible to make a judgement as to the best guess for these areas of uncertainty.

THE SLIPPERY SLOPE ARGUMENT

The slippery slope argument is frequently used in moral discussion. It is important to judge when its use is valid. The core of the argument is that once you accept one particular position then it will be extremely difficult, or indeed impossible, not to accept more and more extreme positions. Thus, if you do not want to accept the more extreme positions you must not accept the original, less extreme position.

One example of the use of such an argument is against the practice of voluntary active euthanasia. Suppose, for example, that a proponent of such euthanasia gave an example of a situation when it seemed plausible to agree that euthanasia, in that situation, is acceptable. The case of mercy killing carried out by Dr Cox (see Chapter 12) could be such an example. The slippery slope argument might be used as providing grounds against such mercy killing, not on the grounds that it would be wrong as a matter of principle in this case, but on the grounds that allowing killing in this case would inevitably lead to allowing killing in situations where it would be wrong.

The main counter to the slippery slope argument is to claim that a barrier can be placed partway down the slope, or that there is a series of steps, so that in stepping on to the top we will not inevitably slide to the bottom.

There are two types of slippery slope argument: a logical type and an empirical type. We will consider each separately.

The logical type of slippery slope argument

The logical type of slippery slope argument can be seen as consisting of three steps:

- **Step 1** As a matter of logical connection, if you accept the (apparently reasonable) proposition, p, then you must also accept the closely related proposition, q. Similarly, if you accept q you must accept proposition r, and so on through propositions s, t, etc. The propositions p, q, r, s, t, etc., form a series of related propositions, such that adjacent propositions are more similar to each other than to those further apart in the series.
- **Step 2** This involves showing, or gaining agreement from the other side in the argument, that at some stage in this series the propositions become clearly unacceptable, or false.
- **Step 3** This involves applying formal logic (*modus tollens*; see Box 1.2) to conclude that, because one of the later propositions (proposition t, for example) is false, it follows that the first proposition (p) is false.

In summary, step 1 is to establish the premise *if p then t*. Step 2 is to establish the premise *t is false*. Step 3 is to point out that from these premises it follows, logically, that *p is false*.

The first step in the argument is what is special about slippery slopes. The crucial component in the argument is to establish a series of propositions such that for adjacent members of the series are so close that there can be no reasonable grounds for holding one proposition true (or false) and its adjacent proposition(s) false (or true).

Slippery slope arguments can have apparent force because many (perhaps most) of the concepts we use have a certain vagueness: if a concept applies to one object then the concept will still apply if there is a very small change in that object. There are two different ways of dealing with such vagueness from the logical point of view. The first is to deny that the concept has to be either completely true or completely false when applied to a particular object, that is, to claim that we cannot specify all its necessary conditions. For example, we may say, perhaps of someone aged 15 years, that she is partly a child and partly an adult – and that the same is true at 16 years, although she is then more of an adult and less of a child. The second way is to choose a point at which one concept ceases to apply. We stipulate, for example, that for many purposes a human is a child until the age of 18 years and then becomes an adult. The precise point, of course, is arbitrary.

These two ways of dealing with the logic of vague concepts are closely related to the two ways of dealing with the logical form of slippery slope argument. Consider the following example of such an argument:

Two people, A and B, agree that it would normally be wrong to terminate a pregnancy at 36 weeks' gestation. However, A believes that it is wrong to terminate pregnancy at any stage, whereas B believes that it is not wrong to terminate pregnancy at 10 weeks' gestation or less. Person A might start from the position agreed by B. He might argue that if it is wrong to terminate a pregnancy at 36 weeks, then it must be wrong to terminate a pregnancy at 35 weeks. The grounds for this assertion are that development is so slow that there is nothing that happens over a week that can make a crucial moral difference. Using a similar argument, if it is wrong to terminate a pregnancy at 35 weeks it is wrong to terminate it at 34 weeks. And so on until we are back at conception.

One response that could be made to this slippery slope argument is that terminating a pregnancy becomes increasingly problematic with age of gestation. At 10 weeks' gestation the wrong in terminating the pregnancy is so slight that the reasons that outweigh such wrong can also be quite slight – maternal wishes for almost any reason, for example. In contrast, the wrong of terminating a pregnancy at 36 weeks' gestation is considerable. There would have to be very good reasons to justify so doing: significant risk to the mother's life, for example. Between these two ages of gestation the weight of justification gradually changes.

The alternative approach is to draw a line at some age of gestation, such that prior to that age it is generally acceptable for termination to be carried out and after that age it is generally unacceptable. The precise drawing of the line is arbitrary; but it is not arbitrary that a line is drawn. In order to ensure clear policy (and clear laws) it is often sensible to draw precise lines even though the underlying concepts and moral values change more gradually.

The empirical form of slippery slope argument

The second form of slippery slope argument is empirical, not logical. An opponent of voluntary active euthanasia might argue that if we allow doctors to carry out such euthanasia, then, as a matter of fact, in the real world, this will lead to non-voluntary euthanasia (or beyond). Such an opponent might accept that there is no logical reason to slip from the one to the other, but in fact such slippage will occur. Therefore we should, as a matter of policy, not legitimize voluntary active euthanasia even if such euthanasia is, in itself, not wrong.

This empirical form of argument depends on making empirical assumptions about the world, and therefore raises the question of how compelling is the evidence for such assumptions. What will in fact happen is often likely to depend on how precisely the policy is worded. It may be possible to prevent slipping down the slope by putting up a barrier (as is done in abortion law with regard to 24 weeks' gestation; see Chapter 9); or by careful articulation of the circumstances under which an action is, or is not, legitimate (as might perhaps be done with euthanasia).

REFERENCES

Beauchamp T L, Childress J F 2001 Principles of biomedical ethics, 5th edn. Oxford University Press, New York

Blackburn S 2001 Ethics: A very shortintroduction. Oxford University Press, Oxford

Flew A 1989 An introduction to Western philosophy: ideas and arguments from Plato to Popper. Thames & Hudson, London

Gillon R 1986 Philosophical medical ethics. John Wiley, Chichester

Rawls J 1972 A theory of justice. Oxford University Press, Oxford

Savulescu J 1994 Treatment limitation decisions under uncertainty: the value of subsequent euthanasia. Bioethics 8:49–73

Warburton N 2000 Thinking from A to Z, 2nd edn. Routledge, London

FURTHER READING

Callahan S 1991 In good conscience: reason and emotion in moral decision making. Francisco: Harper Collins, San Francisco (currently out of print)

Many approaches to ethics emphasize rationality; emotion is seen as undesirable and irrational. This book, written by a philosophically minded psychologist, explores the positive and inevitable relationships between emotion and ethics.

Oakley J 1992 Morality and the emotions. Routledge, London

A more philosophical approach to the relationships between emotion and ethics than Callahan (1991).

Priest G 2000 Logic – a very short introduction. Oxford University Press, Oxford

An entertaining introduction to formal logic – but it gets into some pretty technical stuff.

Thomson A 1999 Critical reasoning in ethics. Routledge, London

A clear and thorough examination of thinking about ethics, with many examples.

Walton D 2005 Fundamentals of critical argumentation. Cambridge University Press, Cambridge

A slightly more technical approach to valid arguments.

Warburton N 2007 Thinking from A to Z, 3rd edn. Routledge, London

A useful source book of types of fallacy and of valid reasoning in a simple dictionary style.

Weston A 2001 A rulebook for arguments, 3rd edn. Hackett Publishing, Cambridge, MA

An engaging introduction to methods of valid argument and avoiding pitfalls.

Ethical and legal background

Ethical theories and perspectives

In the last chapter we argued the case for a rational approach to ethics and described a number of 'tools of reasoning'. One of the tools (tool 4) involved reasoning from principles and theory. We also discussed the interaction between higher level theories and ethical responses to specific situations and introduced the idea of 'reflective equilibrium' (see p. 9). But we did not say much about the different kinds of higher level theory. In this chapter we will outline some of the approaches that moral philosophers take to these higher level theories. Some of these theories have been developed over 2000 years and date back to the Ancient Greeks. Although moral philosophy is a great and ancient academic discipline, in most of the clinical situations that raise problematic ethical issues the key arguments will not require discussion of general ethical theory. But some readers may be interested in the kinds of issues that professional philosophers discuss and analyse in their exploration of general ethical theory. These ideas, which are the subject of this chapter, can be useful in ethical reasoning about practical matters, but for the most part they can be seen as underlying theory, providing a foundational basis for ethics rather than an ingredient of rational debate over day-to-day issues in practical medical ethics. These general ethical theories can perhaps be seen as analogous to general statistical theory, as opposed to the particular statistical tests that are used in assessing specific sets of data.

We will start with three different approaches or types of ethical theory: consequentialism; duty-based theories; and virtue theory. We will then outline two perspectives on ethics that have been influential in debates in medical ethics.

CONSEQUENTIALISM

Consequentialist theories of ethics focus on the question of what is the ethically right thing to do in a particular situation: they are concerned with the question of right action. The central tenet of consequentialism is that an action is right if, and only if, it promotes the best consequences. This can be put in a more practical form: out of all the possible actions in a given situation, the morally right action is that with the best foreseeable consequences.

According to consequentialist theories the only morally relevant features of an act are its (foreseeable) consequences. In contrast to duty-based theories (see p. 24), consequentialism holds that features such as a person's intention, or the fact that an act involves, for example, lying, are not in themselves morally relevant.

This does not necessarily mean that consequentialists are indifferent to lying, but for the consequentialist it is only the foreseeable consequences of lying that are morally important.

There is an ambiguity in the formulation presented above. Is the right action that which, as a matter of fact, leads to the best consequences, or is it that which the agent, at the time of acting, is justified in believing will lead to the best consequences? Most would argue that in applying consequentialist theories, and in judging whether someone has acted rightly or wrongly, it is the foreseeable consequences, taking into account the foreseeable probabilities, that are important.

Consequentialism is not in itself a specific ethical theory, but, rather, it defines a type of theory. It provides the structure for a set of ethical theories. In itself it cannot provide answers to questions about what we ought to do. This is because, as an ethical theory, it is incomplete. To be a complete ethical theory we need to know how to value, ethically, different consequences. If, as consequentialist theories tell us, we should act in order to promote the best consequences, we need a way of judging which of the possible consequences of our actions are the best. We will give examples of some answers to this question of how to evaluate, ethically, different consequences below. Before doing this, however, we will say a little more about consequentialist theories of ethics and how they differ from other types of ethical theory.

Let us, for the sake of exposition, contrast a consequentialist and a non-consequentialist duty-based theory (see below, p. 9), both of which put great value on parents being good parents to their children. Both theories, we shall suppose, agree as to what it is to be a good parent. The non-consequentialist duty-based theory says that, if we are parents, we have a moral duty to (try to) be *good* parents. The consequentialist theory is subtly different. Consequentialist theories hold that we should act in ways to bring about the best consequences – the best state of affairs. In this example the best state of affairs is judged to be that in which all parents are good parents. Suppose that I am wondering how I should live my life. One possibility, let us say, is to work extremely hard for an organization that is effective at promoting good parenting. Another possibility is that I work less hard but have much more time with my children and will myself be a better parent. Suppose that if I work hard for the organization the result will be that, overall, more parents will be good parents than if I work less hard; but that if I work less hard I will be a better parent to my own children. Put in a rather extreme way in order to hammer home the point: if I work hard (option 1) I will be a lousy parent but I will have a great impact on others and overall more parents will be good parents. If I work less hard (option 2) I will be a very good parent myself, but I will have little impact in increasing good parenting in others.

According to a consequentialist theory that values good parenting I should choose option 1 and act to bring about the best consequences. A non-consequentialist duty-based theory, on the other hand, might say that my duty to be a good parent to my children outweighs the general good achieved by my working hard, and that I should choose option 2.

Utilitarianism: an example of a consequentialist theory of ethics

Consequentialism is not by itself a specific ethical theory because it does not tell us what aspects of the consequences are morally important. Specific consequentialist theories do just this. The best known specific consequentialist theory is utilitarianism – or we should say theories because there are at least three different versions of utilitarianism: hedonic, preference and ideal.

Hedonic utilitarianism

According to classical hedonic utilitarianism, the best consequences are those in which (human) happiness is maximized. In 1863, John Stuart Mill (1987, Chapter 2, p. 278 of reference cited) wrote of utilitarianism: 'The creed which accepts as the foundation of morals, Utility, or the Greatest Happiness Principle, holds that actions are right in proportion as they tend to promote happiness, wrong as they tend to produce the reverse of happiness'.

Mill went on to write: 'By happiness is intended pleasure, and the absence of pain; by unhappiness, pain, and the privation of pleasure'. Thus, overall, 'utility' is the balance of pleasure over pain.

Preference utilitarianism

Utilitarians such as R M Hare and Peter Singer define human well-being as: 'the obtaining to a high or at least reasonable degree of a quality of life which on the whole a person wants, or prefers to have' (Hare 1998). For these utilitarians we should act on the whole to bring about the maximum amount, not of human happiness, but of humans realizing their preferences.

Ideal utilitarianism

According to ideal utilitarians such as G E Moore, what matters is not mere happiness or getting what we want, but doing worthwhile things.

" [C]ertain things are good or bad for people, whether or not these people want to have the good things or avoid the bad things. The good things might include moral goodness, rational activity, the development of one's abilities, having children and being a good parent, knowledge and the awareness of true beauty. The bad things might include being betrayed, manipulated, slandered, deceived, being deprived of liberty and dignity, and enjoying either sadistic pleasure, or aesthetic pleasure in what is in fact ugly (Parfit 1984, p. 499)

Each of these theories has its strengths and weaknesses as an account of what is good for people. Derek Parfit has argued that what is good is a combination of all three of these elements.

DUTY-BASED MORAL THEORIES

There are ethical theories that consider aspects other than consequences as relevant to ethics. Many of these focus on duties. Moral theories that emphasize duties are sometimes called 'deontological' (from the Greek *deon*, duty). We will use the term 'duty-based' theories. The key belief of duty-based ethical theories is that there are certain acts that are wrong in themselves, independent of their foreseeable consequences. Such acts may be morally unacceptable even if they are carried out in order to pursue ends that are morally admirable. According to such theories, the question of which action is right is not answered by looking at the consequences of the possible actions but by looking at the nature of the actions themselves. For example, one duty might be that we should not tell lies to one another. According to a duty-based theory it may be wrong to tell a lie even if the consequences of doing so would be better than the consequences of telling the truth.

The concept of *duty-based theory* (like that of *consequentialism*) defines a type of ethical theory – it is not a specific theory. In order to guide action the duties that are morally relevant must be specified. These duties in practice are often phrased as prohibitions, like the Ten Commandments. Duties often cited are: keeping promises; not lying; not betraying; not violating various rights of others (rights such as not to be killed, injured, imprisoned, threatened, tortured, coerced, robbed); and not imposing certain sacrifices on someone as a means to an end (Davis 1991). Most of Western morality in recent times has been dominated by Judeo-Christian morality, which is duty based. In moral philosophy, Christian morality is only one morality amongst many.

According to consequentialist theories there will usually be one right act in any given situation. In contrast, for duty-based theories there will usually be many right acts. The list of duties – mainly prohibitions – will define some acts as wrong; but any act that is not wrong is one possible right act.

Types of duty-based theory

One of the main issues for duty-based theories is what should happen when two or more duties conflict. What should one do, for example, if the only way not to betray someone is by lying? According to some theories there is one single rule from which all others are derived. The famous German philosopher, Immanuel Kant, adopts such an approach (see below). Others try to rank the principles or duties into a hierarchy, such that if there is conflict then that which is highest in the hierarchy should be followed. Still other theories accept that we have a range of duties, and when they conflict in a particular situation one has to make a judgement in order to decide the most important duty in that specific situation. The theory of *prima facie* duties (see below) is of this type.

Kant's moral theory

Immanuel Kant (1724–1804) aimed to develop maxims that would tell us what we ought to do (Kant 1998; O'Neill 1991, pp. 176–177). His minimal assumption was that a moral principle has to be a principle for all people. This idea leads to the 'categorical imperative'.

Kant distinguished two kinds of imperative, hypothetical and categorical. A hypothetical imperative is of the form: 'Do this in order to achieve that'. A categorical imperative is one that expresses a command that is not conditional on any further purpose. It is of the form: 'Do this'. Kant sought to identify what categorical imperative would be agreed by a hypothetical community of rational people. If he could identify such an imperative, then that would provide the foundation for a morality derived from pure reason. The categorical imperative that he identified he formulated in a number of ways, and it is not clear that they are all equivalent. The best known of these is: 'Act only on that maxim which you can at the same time will that it should become a universal law'. A second formulation is: 'So act as to treat humanity, whether in your own person or in that of any other, never solely as a means but always as an end'. This second formulation, with the idea that people should be treated as 'ends in themselves', has been influential in political philosophy. It stresses the liberal principle that people should not have their individual freedom compromised for some other end, in particular for the good of society more generally.

Kant believed that his categorical imperative could be used to derive the specific moral duties that make up a complete ethical framework. For example, he derived a duty to keep promises as follows. Suppose we are considering breaking our promise. We could not will that promise-breaking would be a universal law, for that would result in a breakdown of the trust that is needed for promises to mean anything at all.

Modern duty-based theories

Rawls is one modern philosopher whose theory shares many characteristics with Kant's. Rawls (1972) sought to provide an account of distributive justice (the question of how money and other goods should be distributed between people in a society). The way in which Rawls approached this question was by considering which society we would choose behind a 'veil of ignorance' (see p. 207). He sought to develop a theory about what is right from those principles that would be chosen by rational people. Kant's and Rawls' approaches differ in one important way: Kant tried to determine his ethics with regard to what rational people would consistently choose regardless of their individual desires, preferences, or goals; Rawls, on the other hand, imagines that the rational people are making choices, behind the veil of ignorance, based on their goals and preferences.

Prima facie duties

W D Ross (Dancy 1991, Ross 1930) developed a duty-based approach to ethics that has influenced the 'four-principle' approach to medical ethics (see p. 15). Ross believed that, although the consequences of one's actions are morally important, other things matter as well. Examples of these other things that matter morally are: help others when you can; foster your own talents; treat others fairly; keep your promises; and show gratitude. Ross's approach has a number of features that are not shared by many other duty-based theories. First, he gives considerable weight to consequences. Second, he calls the various duties '*prima facie* duties'. By this he means that in any specific situation, where there is a clash between different duties, we have to decide in the light of the circumstances whether it is morally more important to follow one duty or another. Deciding where the balance lies is, inescapably, a matter of judgement. There is no general ranking of the duties. Third, Ross did not believe that we know the truth of a moral principle or duty by understanding and thinking about the principle in abstract: we know a principle only by discovering its truth in a particular situation.

VIRTUE ETHICS

For over a century the major focus for discussions of ethical theory has been centred on the *ethics of action* – that is on answering the question of what is the morally right way to act in various situations. This is the main focus also of this book which, on the whole, is concerned with ethical and legal accounts of how doctors should act in a variety of situations. For some, including Aristotle, *virtue ethics* contributes to this *ethics of action*. But the *ethics of action*, and the related issue of moral decision-making (how we should make decisions about what is the right thing to do in a variety of situations), represent only one aspect of ethics, or the moral life. There are at least three aspects of ethical theory: the ethics of action; the ethics of character; and the ethics of motives and attitudes (for example, see Adams 2006). Although related to each other they are not the same. Many readers of this book may be at least as much interested in the question of how they might develop good moral character as they are in how they might act rightly. For them, the ethics of virtue will be of particular interest.

The central focus of virtue ethics is the character of the person. In the context of medical ethics, virtue ethics is concerned with the characteristics of a good doctor (or other health professional). Box 2.1 compares duty-based ethics, consequentialism and virtue ethics. Virtue ethics was first developed by Aristotle in the fourth century BC (Aristotle 1976). In Aristotle's view the right act is that

---

Box 2.1 A comparison of duty-based ethics, consequentialism and virtue ethics (adapted from Hursthouse 1991)

Duty-based ethics

1. An action is right if, and only if, it is in accord with a moral rule or principle.
2. A moral rule is one that:
   - is laid on us by God
   - is laid on us by reason
   - would be chosen by all rational beings.

The theory thus depends critically on the concept of rationality (or alternatively on understanding God's will).

Consequentialism

1. An action is right if, and only if, it promotes the best consequences.
2. An account must be given of how different states of affair (consequences) can be morally evaluated and ranked.

The theory thus depends critically on the concepts used to evaluate states of affairs (such as happiness in the case of hedonic utilitarianism).

Virtue ethics

1a. An action is right if, and only if, it is what a virtuous agent would do in the circumstances.
1b. A virtuous person is one who exercises the virtues.
2. A virtue is a character trait a human being needs in order to flourish.

The theory thus depends critically on the concept of human flourishing.

which a virtuous person would do in the circumstances, and a virtuous person is a person who exhibits the virtues. The virtues are those characteristics that will ensure that those endowed with them will have the best life overall. The best life, for Aristotle, is that associated with *eudemonia*, often translated as *flourishing*. This flourishing can perhaps be seen as a kind of deep happiness, which is less connected with the pleasures than is the concept of happiness, or well-being, used to underpin utilitarianism. In one sense Aristotle's theory could be seen as a selfish theory, as it depends ultimately on self-interest – maximizing one's personal *eudemonia*. However, many of the virtues are not selfish at all in the ordinary sense, for example kindness, generosity. For Aristotle, being kind and generous to others contributes to one's own flourishing – virtue is its own reward. There is some psychological evidence to support this idea (Haidt 2006).

Virtue theory, like consequentialism and duty-based theories, articulates a type of moral theory, but it is not a specific moral theory. In order to have moral content the virtues (and vices) must be specified. There is an indeterminate number of specific virtue theories just as there is an indeterminate number of specific duty-based, or consequentialist, theories.

Virtue ethics in clinical practice – the example of abortion

A standard form of the discussion on abortion is underpinned by the following antiabortion argument (see Chapter 9):

- Premise 1: Killing a person is wrong.
- Premise 2: A fetus is a person.
- Conclusion: Killing a fetus is wrong.

Most discussions about the morality of abortion focus on the issue of whether a fetus is a person. Virtue ethics, according to Hursthouse, opposes this general approach. The question of whether abortion is right or wrong, according to virtue ethics, should not depend on an esoteric metaphysical fact about personhood, but on familiar biological facts. From the perspective of virtue theory the question is not about the status of the fetus but about how the biological facts figure 'in the practical reasoning, actions and passions, thoughts and reactions, of the virtuous and the non-virtuous?' (Hursthouse 1991, p. 229 in 1997 reference).

Virtue theory tends to describe acts using many different terms (i.e. the different virtues or vices). In this way it provides a richer vocabulary than is found in many ethical discussions. An act (e.g. undergoing an abortion during a planned pregnancy because the birth will interfere with a summer holiday) might be described not so much as either right (permissible) or wrong, but as 'callous' or 'light-minded'. Assuming that on the specific virtue theory these are considered vices rather than virtues, the implication is that it would be wrong to undergo an abortion for such reasons, but not wrong in the same way (and perhaps not to the same degree) as an act that is cruel.

PERSPECTIVES

We have outlined the three major types of ethical theory that are dominant in Anglo-American philosophy. There are two broad perspectives on ethics that are relevant to current medical ethics: *communitarianism* and *feminism*. What might be seen as a third perspective, the *ethics of care*, we have classified under *feminism*. These are not high-level theories; rather they emphasize particular issues and aspects of ethics, which is why we call them 'perspectives'. They have developed, in part, as a critical response to much modern medical ethics (and, indeed, other forms of practical ethics), taking issue with what from these perspectives is seen as an undue emphasis on some issues or approaches, and a neglect of others.

Communitarianism

Much of modern medical ethics has focused on individual rights and individual autonomy. This perspective has led to a reaction – communitarianism. One of the central tenets of individualism is that each person should be allowed to pursue his or her own life's goals without interference. The only significant limit to this is that such freedom should not interfere with a similar freedom for others. From the public standpoint there is no evaluation of different preferences held by citizens.

Communitarianism, in contrast, emphasizes our individual responsibilities as part of a community, together with the responsibilities of communities themselves to care for their vulnerable members. At the theoretical level, communitarianism is at odds with liberalism in that it holds a conception of the common good that is held at public level. This common good, instead of adjusting itself to people's preferences, as is the case with liberalism, provides a standard by which those individual preferences are evaluated. On this view the public pursuit of shared ends can take precedence over the claim of individuals to pursue their own conceptions of the good. Thus, according to communitarianism, there is a primary idea of an agreed way of life for the community. This provides a standard by which different values can be ranked and a reason for the state to use measures (for example, subsidy for some activities) to promote those activities that promote the community's values.

This has practical implications for medical ethics. Consider the issue of volunteering to take part in medical research. Individualism emphasizes the idea that patients have a right to decide this matter for themselves. It tends to address the issue not of what the person ought to do, but of what other people can or cannot legitimately force him to do. From the point of view of communitarianism, however, the most salient feature might be that, as a community, we stand to gain a great deal from good medical research, and that because of this each of us might have a *prima facie* moral duty to participate in such research. The community's resources might therefore be used to promote such participation. The communitarian approach to the allocation of medical resources would emphasize the importance of reaching consensus at the public level on what are the goals of health care. Thus we have to work not at the level of individuals but at the level of consensus within communities (Zwart 1999).

As can be seen from this example, a communitarian perspective may lead to specifying particular moral duties or might lead to valuing certain types of consequence. It is not an alternative to the general types of ethical theory described above, but a perspective that can inform the values of specific ethical theories.

A feminist approach to ethics

One central modern issue for feminist ethics is the question of whether there is a specifically female ethic. There have been two contradictory feminist

Ethical and legal background

responses to this question. The first is to argue that there is an essential difference between female and male ethics and values. This response has been strongly influenced by the work of Gilligan (1982), who claimed, on the basis of experiment, that boys and girls tend to think about ethical issues in significantly different ways. To put it baldly, girls tend to approach a dilemma by suggesting that the right thing to do is to discuss the situation with the key people involved and try to find an agreed way of proceeding. Boys tend to approach solving the dilemma on the basis of principles, using these principles to decide what is the right thing to do.

The second response has been to deny that there is an essential difference between a male and a female approach. According to this response, however, there is an approach to ethics informed by those experiences (typically domestic) that are traditionally associated with women's positions in society. Conversely, there is an approach informed by those experiences (typically in the public sphere) traditionally associated with men's positions in society.

What both responses share is a preference for the 'female' approach to ethics, whether or not it originates in an essential difference between men and women.

The feminist perspective is distinctive in a number of ways. First, it is suspicious of simplifying the specific situation so as to focus on what are traditionally seen as the essential moral features. This simplification will often remove factors that are important in thinking about the ethical issues. This is because many of the important factors, from the feminist perspective, involve details of the people involved and their relationships, and the details of exactly what interactions people have had. Second, feminism is sceptical of applying principles in the abstract. Again, the details are important. Third, if only the bare essential outline is given, the assumption is that we can then decide what is the right thing to do (e.g. switch off the ventilator). The feminist perspective is likely to emphasize that the right thing to do will often be to discuss the issues with the key people involved, rather than rush into a decision. The right action may emerge from discussion: the key people may come to some kind of consensus. In its application to medical ethics feminism has tended to provide criticism of the approach that relies on brief summaries of the situation and the application of a theoretical standpoint and clear reasoning.

These characteristics of feminist medical ethics overlap with other perspectives. In particular there are three other perspectives that share many of these features of feminism. These are: narrative ethics, which emphasizes the details of cases – what have come to be known as 'thick cases' rather than 'thin cases'; communitarian ethics (see above), which emphasizes the importance of discussion and coming to a negotiated agreement; and the 'ethics of care'.

The 'ethics of care' is a strand in feminist ethics that has developed a life of its own. This approach has been developed particularly by Joan Tronto. It shares some features with virtue ethics in that it approaches many issues in medical (and nursing) ethics from the point of view of what a caring person would do. Tronto (1994) identifies four virtues of caring: attentiveness, for example to people's needs; responsibility; competence and responsiveness. In a practical situation this approach suggests that one asks what each of these virtues requires one to do, rather than asking what is the right final act.

REFERENCES

Adams R M A 2006 Theory of virtue. Oxford University Press, Oxford

Aristotle 1976 The ethics of Aristotle: the Nicomachean ethics. Translated by J A K Thomson, revised by H Tredennick. Penguin, Harmondsworth (many other translations exist)

Dancy J 1991 An ethic of *prima facie* duties. In: Singer P (ed.) A companion to ethics. Blackwell, Oxford, p. 219–229

Davis N 1991 Contemporary deontology. In: Singer P (ed.) A companion to ethics. Blackwell, Oxford, p. 205–218

Gilligan C 1982 In a different voice: psychological theory and women's development. Harvard University Press, Cambridge, MA.

Haidt J 2006 The happiness hypothesis. Heinemann, London

Hare R M 1998 Essays on religion and education. Clarendon Press, Oxford

Hursthouse R 1991 Virtue theory and abortion. Philosophy and Public Affairs 20:223–246 (reprinted in Crisp R, Slote M (eds) 1997 Virtue ethics. Oxford University Press, Oxford, p. 217–238)

Kant I 1998 Groundwork of the metaphysics of morals. Translated and edited by M Gregor. Cambridge University Press, Cambridge

Mill J S 1863 Utilitarianism. In: Ryan A (ed.) 1987 Utilitarianism and other essays (J S Mill and J Bentham). Penguin, Harmondsworth, p. 272–338

O'Neil O 1991 Kantian ethics. In: Singer P (ed.) A companion to ethics. Blackwell, Oxford, p. 175–185

Parfit D 1984 Reasons and persons. Oxford University Press, Oxford

Rawls J 1972 A theory of justice. Oxford University Press, Oxford

Ross W D 1930 The right and the good. Oxford University Press, Oxford

Tronto J 1994 Moral boundaries: political argument for an ethic of care. Routledge, London

Zwart H 1999 All you need is health: liberal and communitarian views on the allocation of health care resources. In: Parker M (ed.) Ethics and community in the health care professions. Routledge, London, p. 30–46

FURTHER READING: ETHICAL THEORY

General

Benn P 1997 Ethics. Taylor & Francis, London
A clear introduction to ethics.

Copp D 2006 The Oxford handbook of ethical theory. Oxford University Press, Oxford
A collection of specially written essays from experts in the fields. Each essay takes an approach either to normative ethics (such as virtue ethics) or to meta-ethics (such as moral relativism).

Frey R, Wellman R, Heath C (eds) 2003 A companion to bioethics. Blackwell Companions to Philosophy. Blackwell, Oxford

LaFollete H (ed.) 2003 The Oxford handbook of practical ethics. Oxford University Press, Oxford

MacIntyre A 2006 A short history of ethics. Routledge, London
Originally published in 1966, this classic work provides an impressive and sophisticated overview of the history of ethics from Ancient Greece to recent times.

Norman R 1998 The moral philosophers, 2nd edn. Oxford University Press, Oxford
Another good introduction to ethics organized around key people in the history of ethics.

Oderberg D S 2000 Applied ethics: a non-consequentialist approach. Blackwell, Cambridge

Rachels J 1995 The elements of moral philosophy, 2nd edn. McGraw-Hill, New York
An excellent introduction to moral philosophy.

Singer P (ed.) 1991 A companion to ethics. Blackwell, Oxford
Another good collection of essays on a wide variety of ethical theories.

Encyclopaedias

There are several good encyclopaedias of ethics that provide good introductions to a particular topic, with good reference lists. Examples are:

Becker L C (ed.) 1992 Encyclopedia of ethics. Garland, New York

Chadwick R F, Callahan D, Singer P (eds) 1997 Encyclopedia of applied ethics. Elsevier, London (three volumes)

Edwards P (ed.) 2005 The encyclopedia of philosophy. Macmillan, Farmingham Hills (ten volumes)

Utilitarianism

Crisp R 1997 Mill on utilitarianism. Routledge, London

A clear and wide-ranging book that provides a useful and up-to-date analysis of utilitarianism.

Ryan A (ed.) 1987 Utilitarianism and other essays (J S Mill and J Bentham). Penguin, Harmondsworth

Key essays by the founders of utilitarianism, Jeremy Bentham and John Stuart Mill, including Mill's classic essay.

Duty-based theories

Three chapters in A companion to ethics edited by Peter Singer provide clear and fairly detailed accounts of various deontological approaches to ethics:

Dancy J 1991 An ethic of *prima facie* duties. In: Singer P (ed.) A companion to ethics. Blackwell, Oxford, p. 219–229

Davis N 1991 Contemporary deontology. In: Singer P (ed.) A companion to ethics. Blackwell, Oxford, p. 205–218

O'Neil O 1991 Kantian ethics. In: Singer P (ed.) A companion to ethics. Blackwell, Oxford, p. 175–185

The most accessible of Kant's own writings on ethics is:

Kant I 1998 Groundwork of the metaphysics of morals. Translated and edited by M Gregor. Cambridge University Press, Cambridge

Virtue ethics

Crisp R, Slote M (eds) 1997 Virtue ethics. Oxford University Press, Oxford

A good collection of journal articles in virtue ethics including some in medical ethics.

Communitarianism

Parker M 1999 Ethics and community in the health care professions. Routledge, London

This book provides various communitarian perspectives applied to a range of healthcare issues.

Feminism

Gilligan C 1982 In a different voice: psychological theory and women's development. Harvard University Press, Cambridge, MA

This classic book, which argues on the basis of some empirical data that females approach ethical thinking in a different way from males, has provided much of a spur to the development of feminist ethics.

Grimshaw J 1991 The idea of a female ethics. In: Singer P, (ed.), A companion to ethics. Blackwell, Oxford, p. 491–499

This is a brief, clear and balanced account of feminist ethics in general.

Mahowald M B 2006 Bioethics and women: across the life span. Oxford University Press, Oxford

Noddings N 1978 Caring: a feminine approach to ethics and education. University of California Press, Berkeley, CA

Another classic work in the development of feminist ethics and in the ethics of caring.

FURTHER READING: GENERAL MEDICAL ETHICS

Collections of key articles

Arras J D, Steinbock B 1999 Ethical issues in modern medicine, 5th edn. Mayfield, Toronto

Beauchamp T, Walters L (eds) Contemporary issues in bioethics, 5th edn. Wadsworth, Belmont, CA

Freeman M (ed.) 2001 Ethics and medical decision-making. Ashgate, Aldershot

Kuhse H, Singer P (eds) 1998 A companion to bioethics. Blackwell, Oxford

Kuhse H, Singer P (eds) 1999 Bioethics: an anthology. Blackwell, Oxford

General books on medical ethics

Ashcroft R, Lucassen A, Parker M, Verkerk M, Widdershoven G 2005 Case analysis in clinical ethics. Cambridge University Press, Cambridge

A single case from the area of clinical genetics is analysed in detail by 11 authors, each from a different ethical perspective. This book demonstrates how different approaches to medical ethics lead to different analyses.

Ashcroft R, Draper H, Dawson A, McMillan J (eds) 2007 Principles of health care ethics, 2nd edn. John Wiley, Chichester

An enormous single-volume collection of specially written chapters covering a wide range of medical ethics explored from many perspectives.

Beauchamp T L, Childress J F 2001 Principles of biomedical ethics, 5th edn. Oxford University Press, New York

A well-established, detailed and well-written textbook of medical ethics organized around the four-principle approach.

British Medical Association, Sommerville A 1993 Medical ethics today: its practice and philosophy. BMJ Publishing Group, London

More medical in its orientation than most textbooks of medical ethics.

Campbell A, Gillett G, Jones G 2005 Medical ethics, 4th edn. Oxford University Press, Melbourne

Accessible and relatively small textbook written by a team of philosophers and doctors.

Caplan A, McCartney J J, Sisti D A 2004 Health, disease and illness. Georgetown University Press, Washington, DC

Frances D, Silvers L, Rhodes R 2006 The Blackwell guide to medical ethics. Blackwell, Oxford

Gillon R 1986 Philosophical medical ethics. John Wiley, Chichester

A more medically accessible and shorter account than Beauchamp & Childress.

Glannon W 2005 Biomedical ethics. Oxford University Press, Oxford

Glover J 1977 Causing death and saving lives. Penguin, London

Although this is about end-of-life issues, it is a good introduction to philosophical thinking applied to the medical setting.

Harris J 1985 The value of life. Routledge & Kegan Paul, London

Hope T 2004 Medical ethics: a very short introduction. Oxford University Press, Oxford

Intended as an introduction, each chapter makes an argument for a particular ethical position concerning an issue in medical ethics.

Kerridge I, Lowe M, McPhee J 1998 Ethics and law for the health professions. Social Science Press, Katoomba, Australia

A good overview of medical ethics and law from an Australian perspective.

Parker M, Dickenson D 2001 The Cambridge medical ethics workbook. Cambridge University Press, Cambridge

This provides many cases taken from health care across several European countries, together with in-depth analysis of the cases. A combination of textbook and case book.

Rhodes R, Francis L P, Silvers A 2007 The Blackwell guide to medical ethics. Blackwell, Oxford

Selgelid M, Battin M P, Smith C B 2006 Ethics and infectious disease. Blackwell, Oxford

Singer P 1993 Practical ethics, 2nd edn. Cambridge University Press, New York

A racy and readable examination of some of the philosophical issues underpinning medical ethics.

Steinbock B 2007 The Oxford handbook of bioethics. Oxford University Press, Oxford

Encyclopaedias of Bioethics

Murray T, Mehlman M J 2000 Encyclopedia of ethical, legal and policy issues in biotechnology. John Wiley, New York

Reich W T 1995 Encyclopedia of bioethics, Macmillan, New York

Case Books in Medical Ethics

Pence G E 1994 Classic cases in medical ethics, 2nd edn. McGraw-Hill, New York

Pence G E 1998 Classic works in medical ethics: core philosophical readings. McGraw-Hill, Boston

Strong C, Ackerman T F 1989 A casebook of medical ethics. Oxford University Press, New York

Veatch R M 1977 Case studies in medical ethics. Harvard University Press, Cambridge, MA

Three core concepts in medical ethics: best interests, autonomy and rights

BEST INTERESTS

The value of patients' best interests is at the heart of medicine. It forms the core of the doctor–patient relationship (see Chapter 5) and is the legal standard for the treatment of patients who lack the capacity to take part in their own medical decisions (see Chapter 6). What is meant, however, by 'best interests', and how they can be determined and pursued, is often problematic, as all parents know. The philosophical discussion relevant to 'best interests' has been conducted mainly in terms of the concept of 'well-being'. There are three theoretical approaches to well-being.

Mental state theory

According to this theory well-being is defined in terms of mental states. At its simplest (hedonism) it is the view that happiness or pleasure is the only intrinsic good, and unhappiness or pain the only intrinsic bad. The theory can be enriched (and complicated) by allowing a greater plurality of states of mind as contributing to well-being, although this raises the problem of which mental states these should be.

Objections to mental state theories

1. There are things that contribute to, or detract from, our well-being that are not mental states or experiences. For example, if we are deceived but do not know it, it could be argued that this takes away from our well-being even if it does not affect our mental state.
2. Nozick (1974, p. 42) asks us to imagine a machine (the 'experience machine') with electrodes that can be implanted into our brains to provide any set of experiences, including the experience (but not the actuality) of 'writing a great novel, or making a friend, or reading an interesting book. All the time you would be floating in a tank, with electrodes attached to your brain'. Even if we choose those mental states that we most want, few of us, Nozick believes, would choose to live our life connected to such a

machine. This is because we also want to do certain things, and we want to be a certain way, to be a certain sort of person (Nozick 1974, p. 43). (While this example was constructed as a hypothetical case, deep brain stimulation is now being employed to alter mood in depressed people.)

Desire fulfilment theories

According to desire fulfilment theories, well-being consists in having one's desires fulfilled. It is plausible that to maximize a person's well-being we ought to give the person what they want. If desire fulfilment theories are to provide a plausible account of well-being, it is necessary to restrict the relevant set of desires: '…when the gods wish to punish us they answer our prayers' (Wilde 1895). On one view only those desires pertaining to life as a whole count as relevant in the analysis of well-being. These are desires that relate to a person's life plan.

Objections to desire fulfilment theories

Suppose that I desire something – a particular thing, or an entire 'life plan'. It seems quite reasonable to ask the question, 'Is that something good for me?', i.e. does it contribute to my well-being? It seems coherent to claim that there can be a conflict between what a person most desires and what is good for that person. Indeed, an individual may well be trying to decide what end to pursue – what to desire – and in order to help answer this wants to know what would contribute most to his well-being. According to desire fulfilment theories of well-being, such concerns are empty.

Objective list theories

There is a long history, going back to Aristotle, of a concept of happiness that is multidimensional and, more importantly, where the dimensions are determined not by each individual but are seen as intrinsic to the concept. The term in English usually used for this concept of happiness is 'flourishing'. Such theories are more generally known as 'objective list theories'.

According to objective list theories of well-being, certain things can be good or bad for a person and can contribute to her well-being, whether or not they are desired and whether or not they lead to a 'pleasurable' mental state. Examples of the kind of thing that have been given as intrinsically good in this way are engaging in deep personal relationships, rational activity and the development of one's abilities. Examples of things that are bad might include being betrayed or deceived, or gaining pleasure from cruelty (see quote on p. 24, Chapter 2).

Objections to objective list theories

1. A major problem with objective list theories is that it is difficult to give an account of why one thing is good, and thus contributes to well-being, whereas another thing is bad. Are we supposed to know what is good and what is bad by some kind of special (moral) intuition?

2. In contrast to both of the other theories it is difficult to explain why, according to objective list theory, we would be motivated to pursue our well-being.

Composite theories

Each of the three theories of well-being outlined above seems to identify something of importance, but none seems adequate. Because of this, we might opt for a composite theory in which well-being is seen as requiring aspects of all the theories. Whatever its theoretical weaknesses, a composite theory has some practical implications for medical practice. The main implication is that, when considering what is in a patient's best interests, particularly when these are not clear, it may be relevant to consider the aspects of well-being that are highlighted by each of the three theories.

Case example: Alzheimer's disease

Mr D has always valued academic and artistic pursuits and it is important to him that he be remembered as someone with an intellect. 'If I develop Alzheimer's disease allow me to die if given the chance', he says. Mr D subsequently develops Alzheimer's disease. He becomes quite severely affected. He no longer recognizes his family, but remains physically fit. He is looked after in a nursing home and appears to be able to enjoy a simple life: flowers, food, TV. Mr D gets a chest infection. This could be treated, probably effectively, with antibiotics. Without curative treatment he could be kept comfortable and would probably soon die.

What is in Mr D's best interests: to treat or not to treat? According to mental state theory, Mr D's mental state, as far as can be judged, is mainly positive. His best interests on this analysis would be served by treating his pneumonia and extending his simple but generally pleasurable life.

On a desire fulfilment theory the question is which desires are to be followed. It is unclear whether in his current state he is able to form desires of the kind that are crucial to best interests. If such desires, in order to underpin best interests, require some rational consideration, then the important desires are those that he formed before the onset of dementia. These desires will be particularly important if they are formed around a life plan. If such desires are considered to be more important than his current mental state, the best interests of Mr D would be served by following his previous wishes. This would involve keeping him comfortable but not treating his chest infection.

An objective list theory does not give an unequivocal answer to what is in Mr D's best interests. On most lists – although not all – the pursuit of worthwhile life goals would normally take precedence over very simple pleasures. But that is not the choice that faces the carers of Mr D. The question is whether it is in Mr D's best interests to be dead, given that he can enjoy only these simple pleasures. It would be a dangerous presumption for health professionals to decide not to provide non-invasive treatment, such as oral antibiotics, for Mr D, on the grounds of an objective account of his well-being, without consideration of what his values might formerly have been (Dresser 1995, Dworkin 1993, Hope 1996).

Measuring well-being

The psychological study of human happiness and flourishing has burgeoned in recent years under the broad term of 'positive psychology' (Carr 2004, Huppert et al 2005, Layard 2006, Nettle 2005, Snyder & Lopez 2005). This scientific study has required psychologists (and economists) to develop methods for the measurement of well-being. There are three fundamentally different concepts that psychologists measure:

1. Happiness as a subjective experience. On this view at any moment each of us is experiencing a particular level of happiness or unhappiness. This is the approach of *quantitative hedonism* and is a measure based on the *mental state theory* (see above).
2. Happiness as a judgement that each of us can make about our feelings and life experiences. This might be called the *life satisfaction approach*. This measurement is not the same as any of the three philosophical concepts outlined above, although it might be seen as a form of global desire fulfilment theory, the desire being for how our lives should go as a whole.
3. Happiness as a multidimensional concept covering many aspects of what we might judge to be the various components of a happy and fulfilled life. This is sometimes called the 'flourishing approach' and is an example of an *objective list* theory.

Quantitative hedonism – the 'smiley' approach

Kahneman and his colleagues (see Kahneman & Riis 2005), building on Bentham's idea of a calculus of happiness, call the basic unit of measurement *moment utility* (happiness at each particular moment in time). This is measured most clearly by asking people to give a quantitative measure as to how happy they feel at this moment on some suitably defined scale. Total happiness over any particular period of time is simply the integral of these *moment utilities*. Kahneman calls this integral *experienced well-being*.

It is difficult to measure happiness in this way because it requires rather frequent measurements. One can try to overcome this technical problem by asking people to give a single average measure over a period of time (e.g. over the previous 24 hours). In practice, however, when people are asked to give a single measure of happiness over time they do not so much remember (and integrate) the *moment utilities* as evaluate, or make a judgement about, their overall well-being – what Kahneman calls *evaluated well-being*. These evaluations can be rather peculiar – in fact downright illogical. In one experiment Kahneman asked participants to dip their hands in painfully cold water. Participants reported that 60 seconds in very cold water was worse than 60 seconds in very cold water followed by 30 seconds in slightly warmer (but still painful) water. This is one instance of a general finding that in evaluating a painful past experience people give most weight to the peak pain and to the level of pain at the end of the experience. Because of this illogicality Kahneman thought until recently that measures of *evaluated well-being* are simply flawed measures of *experienced well-being* (what he thinks of as 'objective happiness').

Life satisfaction and evaluated well-being

There are grounds, however, for preferring *evaluated well-being* over *experienced well-being*. Consider a life of lotus-eating pleasure – the Land of Cockaigne. Would my life overall be as happy if it were spent exclusively in eating strawberries and cream, watching episodes of *Sex and the City*, and enjoying carnal pleasures? Such pleasures might pall, and overall there might be higher levels of *experienced well-being* in a life that included the challenges, say, of writing this textbook and seeing clients with psychological problems. But this could be wrong. The lotus-eating existence might well produce more well-being as measured by the integration of momentary utilities and yet I might still reasonably judge that my life would be more satisfactory, and preferable, and happier if I spent time pursuing goals that I value. Such a judgement would not be unreasonable, let alone illogical.

An analogy might be made with judging the quality of a detective novel. A novel that has been a good read until near the end can be seriously discredited by a poor solution. The quality of the whole work is not simply the addition of the quality page by page. Periods of our lives might be seen in the same way: our well-being is not simply the piecemeal adding up of well-being over each minute.

Kahneman himself now sees *evaluated well-being* as a valid measure in its own right and not simply as a flawed approximation to *experienced well-being*.

For both practical and theoretical reasons, therefore, many measures of well-being are essentially evaluations of people's own satisfaction with life over longer or shorter periods of time (see Carr 2004).

Flourishing

'Flourishing' is the term used most frequently by psychologists who, influenced by Aristotle, are developing an 'objective list' approach to the measurement of well-being. Unlike *quantitative hedonism* and the *life satisfaction approach* the measurement of *flourishing* includes marked value judgements that are imposed by the experimenter on the participant. One example of a scale for measuring well-being based on this approach is that of Ryff (1989, Ryff & Keyes 1995).

The legal approach to best interests

A doctor's general duty is to treat patients in their best interests, although a competent patient (a patient with the capacity to give or withhold consent) can refuse the treatment offered (see Chapter 6). The concept of best interests (at least for patients who are aged 16 years and over) is now governed by the Mental Capacity Act 2005 (MCA) which provides detailed guidance on how the concept should be determined (Box 3.1). In addition there are several principles (as part of the MCA) that must be taken into account by doctors (and more generally by all carers) in healthcare settings:

- A patient (if 16 years or older) must be assumed to have capacity unless there is evidence to the contrary.
- A patient must be given as much support as is reasonable to help him or her make decisions.

Box 3.1   Patients' best interests

The Mental Capacity Act 2005 (MCA)

Section four (s.4) of the MCA states how a person's best interests are to be determined and there is further detailed guidance in the Code of Practice that supplements the Act. The intention behind s.4 is to set out the common factors that must always be taken into account by anyone (e.g. a doctor) who needs to decide what is in the best interests of another person (e.g. a patient) who lacks capacity. Some of the most important points are:

- s.4(1): the principle of equal consideration, i.e. that no-one can assume a person cannot make a decision just because of their age, disability or how they look. (Note, however, that the Act applies only to patients aged 16 years and over.)
- s.4(3): the duty to consider whether the person is likely to regain capacity to make the decision in question; if so to put off the decision until then.
- s.4(4): permitting and encouraging participation, i.e. ensure that the person is involved in the decision-making process to the fullest possible extent.

One of the section's key provisions is s.4(6), which requires decisions-makers (e.g. doctors) to take into account the following specific factors when deciding what is in a person's best interests. These are:

1. his past and present wishes and feelings (including any written statements)
2. his beliefs and values that would be likely to influence his decisions
3. other factors that the patient would be likely to consider, were he able to do so (e.g. altruistic motives).

Also worth noting is s.4(7), which for the first time establishes the right for family members, partners, carers and other relevant people to be consulted on decisions affecting a person who lacks capacity. Again, the primary purpose in consulting relatives is to obtain evidence concerning the above three issues (see also Chapter 6).

The General Medical Council's guidelines on the concept of patients' best interests

'Best interests' principle

In deciding what options may reasonably be considered as being in the best interests of a patient who lacks capacity to decide, you should take into account:

- options for treatment or investigation that are clinically indicated
- any evidence of the patient's previously expressed preferences, including an advance statement
- your own and the healthcare team's knowledge of the patient's background, such as cultural, religious or employment considerations
- views about the patient's preferences given by a third party who may have other knowledge of the patient, for example the patient's partner, family, carer, tutor-dative (Scotland) or a person with parental responsibility
- which option least restricts the patient's future choices, where more than one option (including non-treatment) seems reasonable in the patient's best interest.

- No-one with capacity should be stopped from making a decision just because someone else thinks it is an unwise decision.
- If a patient lacks capacity to make the relevant (healthcare) decisions, then the doctor should act, and make decisions, in the patient's best interests.
- In making decisions, or acting, on behalf of a patient who lacks capacity, every effort must be made to ensure that the patient's freedom and rights are limited as little as possible.

It is worth noting that the legal concept of best interests is centred primarily around respecting and promoting patients' autonomy (see below) – the 'best interests' of a patient who lacks capacity is to do what that patient would choose were he or she (magically) to gain capacity. In terms of the theories described above of well-being, the legal concept of best interests is most closely allied to the 'desire fulfilment theory'.

AUTONOMY

The principle of respect for patient autonomy (see Chapter 1) has had an enormous effect in changing attitudes to the doctor–patient relationship over the past 30 years. It has been used to criticize medical paternalism, and has informed the development of 'patient-centred' medicine. It has led to ever-increasing standards in providing patients with information, and to the development of the concept of *informed* consent (see Chapter 6). Some definitions of autonomy are given in Box 3.2.

Liberty and freedom

The liberal tradition has placed great emphasis on the moral and political importance of freedom for the individual and, in particular, freedom from the interference of others. This has been expressed by Berlin (1969, p. lx) as follows:

> " … those who have ever valued liberty for its own sake believed that to be free to choose, and not to be chosen for, is an inalienable ingredient in what makes human beings human; and that this underlies … the … demand … to

---

Box 3.2 Some explanations, or definitions, of autonomy in recent philosophical writings

1. 'I am autonomous if I rule me, and no one else rules I' (Joel Feinberg, quoted in Dworkin 1988, p. 5).
2. 'To regard himself as autonomous … a person must see himself as sovereign in deciding what to believe and in weighing competing reasons for action' (Scanlon T, in Dworkin 1988, p. 5).
3. 'It is apparent that …"autonomy" is used in an exceedingly broad fashion. It is sometimes used as an equivalent of liberty …, sometimes as equivalent to self-rule or sovereignty, sometimes as identical with freedom of the will … It is identified with qualities of self-assertion, with critical reflection, with freedom from obligation, with absence of external causation, with knowledge of one's own interests … It is related to actions, to beliefs, to reasons for acting, to rules, to the will of other persons, to thoughts and to principles' (Dworkin 1988, p. 6).

be accorded an area … in which one is one's own master, a 'negative' area in which a man is not obliged to account for his activities to any man so far as this is compatible with the existence of organised society.

This freedom includes freedom from unwanted interference even if the interference is for the good of the person who suffers it. Mill, writing in 1859, argued against paternalism, and in favour of liberty. He wrote:

" … the only purpose for which power can be rightfully exercised over any member of a civilised community, against his will, is to prevent harm to others. His own good, either physical or moral, is not a sufficient warrant. He cannot rightfully be compelled to do or forbear … because, in the opinion of others, to do so would not be wise, or even right (Mill 1859, Chapter 1).

In modern medicine this freedom from unwanted interference is protected by the law relating to consent (see Chapter 6). A competent adult patient has the legal right to refuse any – even life-saving – treatment. On those occasions when a competent adult patient is refusing treatment that is, objectively, good for her, a conflict arises between respecting the patient's wishes, and doing what is best for the patient. This is widely seen as a conflict between the principle of respect for patient autonomy and the principle of beneficence (see Chapter 1). However, the concept of autonomy is not straightforward, and respecting what a patient says (e.g. her refusal of treatment) and respecting her autonomy may, on occasions, be in conflict (see below). Many political liberals, such as Berlin (1958), generally favour respecting what a person says. It is too easy and dangerous, they believe, for a repressive political regime, or for powerful people, to impose their will on the grounds that their will coincides with what the other person really wants, despite his saying to the contrary.

Some aspects of autonomy

One key issue in the analysis of autonomy is what conditions need to be met for a person's decisions and actions to be autonomous, i.e. truly their own. Three aspects have been the focus of recent analysis:

1. *To be autonomous one must make evaluations.* The ideal of the autonomous person is the person who forms desires for how her life is to go (life plans) and can act on those desires (Young 1986). In order to create such a life plan for ourselves we need to make evaluations, in particular about what kind of life we think we should live, or that we think might be best for us.
2. *Evaluations should be rational.* In the ideal of autonomy day-to-day decisions should be rational, i.e. consistent with the person's life plans. There are three key components of an autonomous evaluation:
   - It is based on a correct understanding of the relevant facts.
   - The information is evaluated without making a relevant error of logic.
   - The person has been able to imagine what the relevant states of affairs will be like, i.e. the likely states of affairs for the various choice options.

These three components provide the philosophical underpinning to the idea of capacity to consent (see Chapter 6). If a desire, or choice, is not based on a rational evaluation then it is not autonomous. This is one reason why respecting a person's autonomy is not always the same as respecting their choice.

3. *Desires higher in the hierarchy should be respected.* A person may have a simultaneous conflict in desires. For example, a person addicted to alcohol may simultaneously desire alcohol and desire not to have the desire for alcohol. The desire for alcohol is a 'first-order' desire and the desire not to desire alcohol is a 'second-order' desire. Some (e.g. Dworkin 1988) have argued that respecting autonomy implies respecting the higher (second-order) desire on the grounds that it is the one that is part of the life plan.

Advance directives and autonomy

In one study, pregnant women were asked about their views with regard to the use of anaesthesia to avoid pain during labour. Preferences changed during labour. In broad terms the women were more likely to want to suffer the pain and avoid the anaesthesia before, and indeed after, labour than during labour, when they were experiencing the pain (Christensen-Szalanski 1984).

When desires shift in these ways two interpretations of autonomy are possible. On the one hand, one can say that the desire for analgesia while experiencing, for example, the pain of labour is not the autonomous desire – it is equivalent to Odysseus' desire while listening to the Sirens' song (Lattimore 1965). On the other hand, it can be argued that the desire to avoid analgesia, when not in labour, does not properly take into account just how bad the pain will be. On this second interpretation, the prior evaluation was not rational because it was based on insufficient imagination of the future state of affairs.

When faced with situations where patients' desires fluctuate, doctors may need to decide what, given the patient's general values, is most important overall. In the case of pain during labour, where the analgesia poses little risk to the mother or fetus, it is likely to be in favour of analgesia at the time when the mother asks for it.

Can one autonomously choose to delegate choice?

In his essay *On Liberty*, Mill (1859) considered the question: Should a liberal society allow people to sell themselves into slavery? He concluded that this would be contrary to the idea of liberty. In medical practice patients quite frequently want the doctor to make decisions, and may even request that they themselves are not given relevant information. Is this a case of a patient autonomously relinquishing autonomy?

The answer depends on why the patient has chosen to delegate choices. Consider the 'happy follower'. This person is happy being one of the herd. She passively does as others do. She lets her friends and family decide for her. If this 'happy follower' has never deliberately chosen to lead such a life, if there has been no conscious planning, then such a life would not be autonomous. However, if she has deliberately chosen to lead such a passive life, and for good reasons, then this life is part of her life plan and is autonomous. The good

THREE CORE CONCEPTS IN MEDICAL ETHICS

reasons for choosing such a life plan might be that she finds choice burdensome, that she is not very good at choosing for herself, and that she usually enjoys going along with the choices of her friends.

On this analysis, a patient who asks the doctor to choose for him may be acting autonomously if he has good reasons: he trusts the doctor's judgement; finds making choices about his own health difficult; and believes that the doctor's experience about how patients react to different situations is likely to predict his own responses correctly.

RIGHTS

A competent adult patient has a *right* to refuse any treatment. We could say that a patient has a *right* to the best available treatment. Doctors, too, have rights. It is often claimed that a doctor – an obstetrician, for example – has a right to refuse to carry out a termination of pregnancy on grounds of conscientious objection, although there are varying views about the nature and extent of this right (Savulescu 2006). In wider society claims about rights are frequently made. We hear of animal rights and the rights of the disabled.

We talk of both legal rights and moral rights. The two are often linked, in that a moral right forms the basis for a legal right. The Declaration of Human Rights, for example, seeks to establish moral rights that can then be enforced through legal process involving the Court of Human Rights. These moral rights also form the basis for the Human Rights Act (see Chapter 4).

What are rights?

Rights impose moral (and legal) constraints on collective social goals. If a person has a right, it gives him a special advantage – a safeguard so that his right is respected even if the overall social good is thereby diminished. Sumner (2000) explains rights in the following way. He says that there is a part of our moral thinking that is concerned with the promotion of collective social goals. Such thinking is particularly evident in consequentialist moral theories such as utilitarianism, but is also found in duty-based approaches to morality. For example, we may have a duty to bring about some social good. In health care we may consider that bringing about the best health, either for an individual patient or in the setting of public health, is a major ethical duty. However, the ethical duty to bring about a desirable goal may be trumped by the moral requirement to respect an individual's rights. For example, an individual's right to refuse treatment might trump the doctor's duty to treat in the best interests of the patient. Similarly, we might believe that there are circumstances when a person has a right to treatment. Someone injured in a road accident, for example, might be considered to have a right to treatment even if the resources needed could be better spent in terms of social goals.

Rights have been politically important in protecting minority groups and those who might be the victims of more powerful groups. In employment law, for example, they help to ensure that certain groups cannot be unfairly discriminated against.

> **Box 3.3** Types of right
>
> **Claim rights**
> The subject of the right has a claim against another person or people (who are the object of the right). A patient may have a claim right arising from the doctor's duty of care; for example, the patient may be able to claim a certain level of medical care. Contracts normally establish certain claim rights. If I have entered into a contract to sell my house to another for a certain price then I may have a right to claim the money agreed. Outside the legal sphere, claim rights may arise from a promise. If I have promised to lend you a book then you have a moral claim against me for the loan of that book.
>
> **Liberty rights**
> Liberty rights give rights of action to the subject rather than the object of the right. The law may give to someone a liberty, or privilege, for example to seek private medical insurance. Liberties are generally protected by what has been called a 'protective perimeter' of duties imposed on others not to frustrate those liberties. These others are the objects of the right. Property rights usually confer liberty rights (for example the liberty right to use the things you own).
>
> **Powers**
> Many rights provide people with powers to do things. A claim right usually gives the person who holds the right the power to waive the claim, and a property right would include the power to give the property to another.
>
> **Immunities**
> Liberty rights normally give people immunities, that is, they give to the right holder a protection from certain actions of others. My liberty to belong to a political party provides me with immunity from my employer seeking to forbid this.

Types of rights

There are several types of right that are sometimes distinguished (Box 3.3).

Are rights absolute?

Rights need not be absolute. One could say that any particular right has a certain strength. Strength in this sense means the degree to which it stands up to other ethical claims. Thus, if a right had no strength in the light of consequentialist moral claims it would become redundant and the ethical theory would be purely consequentialist. If, on the other hand, a right had infinite strength it would mean that the right was absolute. In Sumner's words (Sumner 2000): 'rights raise thresholds against considerations of social utility but these thresholds are seldom insurmountable', i.e. the rights are seldom absolute. Rights might clash not only with some ethical theory, but also with other rights. Even the most ardent supporter of rights would not be able to claim that two rights were absolute if there were possible situations in which they could conflict.

REFERENCES

Berlin I 1958 Two concepts of liberty. Republished in Berlin I 1969 Four essays on liberty. Oxford University Press, Oxford

Berlin I 1969 Four essays on liberty; introduction. Oxford University Press, Oxford

Carr A 2004 Positive psychology: the science of happiness and human strengths. Brunner-Routledge, Hove

Christensen-Szalanski J J J 1984 Discount functions and the measurement of patients' values Women's decisions during childbirth. Medical Decision Making 4:47–58

Dresser R S 1995 Dworkin on dementia: elegant theory, questionable policy. Hastings Center Report 25:(6):32–38

Dworkin G 1988 The theory and practice of autonomy. Cambridge University Press, Cambridge

Dworkin R 1993 Life's dominion. Harper Collins, London

Hope T 1996 Advance directives (editorial). Journal of Medical Ethics 22:67–68

Huppert F, Baylis N, Keverne B (eds) 2005 The science of well-being. Oxford University Press, Oxford

Kahneman D, Riis J 2005 Living, and thinking about it: two perspectives on life. In: Huppert F, Baylis N, Keverne B (eds) The science of well-being. Oxford University Press, Oxford, p. 285–304

Lattimore R 1965 The odyssey of Homer. Harper & Row, New York

Layard R 2006 Happiness: lessons from a new science. Penguin, London

Mill J S 1859 On liberty. Many modern editions, including. Penguin Books, Harmondsworth, 1982

Nettle D 2005 Happiness: the science behind your smile. Oxford University Press, Oxford

Nozick R 1974 Anarchy, state and utopia. Blackwell, Oxford

Ryff C 1989 Happiness is everything, or is it? Explorations on the meanings of psychological well-being. Journal of Personality and Social Psychology 57:1069–1081

Ryff C, Keyes C 1995 The structure of psychological well-being revisited. Journal of Personality and Social Psychology 69:719–727

Savulescu J 2006 Against medical conscientious objection. British Medical Journal 332:294–297

Snyder C, Lopez S (eds) 2005 Handbook of positive psychology. Oxford University Press, New York

Sumner L W 2000 Rights. In: LaFollette H (ed.) The Blackwell guide to ethical theory. Blackwell, Oxford, p. 288–305

Wilde O 1895 An ideal husband, Act 2 (quote from The Complete Works of Oscar Wilde, New Edition 1966, reprinted 1968 Collins, London, p. 506)

Young R 1986 Personal autonomy: beyond negative and positive liberty. Croom Helm, London

FURTHER READING

Rights

Two good short accounts are:
Almond B 1991 Rights. In: Singer P (ed.) A companion to ethics. Blackwell, Oxford, p. 259–269

Sumner L W 2000 Rights. In: LaFollette H (ed.) The Blackwell guide to ethical theory. Blackwell, Oxford, p. 288–305

A more extended analysis can be found in:
Thomson J J 1990 The realm of rights. Harvard University Press, London

Two classic texts on rights in a political context are:
Berlin I 1969 Four essays on liberty; introduction. Oxford University Press, Oxford

Mill J S 1859 On liberty. Many modern editions, including: Penguin Books, Harmondsworth, 1982

Well-being

Crisp R 1997 Mill on utilitarianism. Routledge, London

Three core concepts in medical ethics

This provides a discussion of well-being in the context of utilitarianism.

Griffin J 1986 Well being. Oxford University Press, Oxford

A detailed philosophical analysis of the concept of well-being.

Kahneman D, Diener E, Schwarz N 1999 Well-being: the foundations of hedonic psychology. Russell Sage Foundation, New York

An excellent overview of the psychological determinants of happiness.

Nussbaum M C, Sen A (eds) 1993 The quality of life. Clarendon Press, Oxford

A collection of essays from a variety of disciplines.

Parfit D 1984 Reasons and persons. Oxford University Press, Oxford

Appendix I is one of the best introductions to what constitutes well-being from a philosophical perspective. This is one of the most influential books in ethics.

Autonomy

Dworkin G 1988 The theory and practice of autonomy. Cambridge University Press, Cambridge

A detailed philosophical analysis of the concept of autonomy.

Savulescu J 2007 Autonomy, the good life and controversial choices. In: Rhodes R (ed.) The Blackwell guide to medical ethics. Blackwell, Oxford, p. 17–37

Discussions of several issues relevant to medicine in the context of the concepts of autonomy and liberalism.

Spriggs M 2005 Autonomy and patients' decisions. Rowan & Littlefield, Lanham, MD

An excellent account of different approaches to autonomy in the setting of medicine.

An introduction to law

4

England and Wales share a single legal system; Scotland's system is different both in having a different structure of courts (see below) and in having its own parliament. Some statutes (see below) apply only to England and Wales, and others only to Scotland. For these reasons there are differences between Scottish law and the law in England and Wales, and some of these differences have an impact on medical law. Northern Ireland has a separate system again, with its own appeal court. For the most part this book describes law that applies to England and Wales. We have, however, attempted to outline the approach taken by Scottish law when this differs significantly from English law in its application to medical practice.

There are two principal sources of law. The most obvious is when a law is passed by Parliament. Such laws are called *Acts of Parliament* or *statutes*. Parliament typically passes about 50 laws each year. Much English law, however, has originated not from Acts of Parliament, but has built up on the basis of court decisions over the past nine centuries. Such law is called *case law*. The term *common law* can be used synonymously with case law. This is how we will use the term in this book (although it also has other meanings).

THE MAIN TYPES OF LAW

One way of dividing the law is into *common (or case) law* on the one hand and *statute law* on the other. The crime of theft is defined by the Theft Act 1968, and is therefore part of statute law. Murder, on the other hand, is a common law crime as there is no statutory definition.

Another, and quite different, division is between *public law* and *private law* (also called *civil law*) (Box 4.1). Both public law and private law are made up of both statute law and case law. Public law involves the state or government; private law is concerned with disputes between private individuals and businesses. The largest part of public law (see Box 4.1) is criminal law. Thus the division between public and private law is largely that between *criminal law* and *civil law*. The differences between these two key aspects of law are summarized in Box 4.2.

THE PLACE OF PRECEDENT IN ENGLISH LAW

Central to case law is the idea of judicial precedent. This means that court decisions must, where relevant, follow previous decisions. Once a case has been heard there is a judgment. That judgment not only gives the court's decisions, but also

Box 4.1 Public law and private law

Types of public law

1. *Criminal law.* This determines the kinds of behaviour that are forbidden (by the State) at risk of punishment. It is normally the State that prosecutes the person who is thought to have committed the crime, and not the victim(s) of the crime. The victim(s) can bring a private prosecution, but the State can intervene and take over.
2. *Constitutional law.* This controls the method of government. If a dispute arises, for example over who can vote, or who can become a Member of Parliament, then it is constitutional law that is involved.
3. *Administrative law.* This controls how public bodies such as local councils, government departments or ministers should operate.

Some types of private law (civil law)

1. *Law of contract.* An agreement between two or more persons that is legally binding.
2. *Law of tort.* The word *tort* comes from the French, meaning a wrong. A tort is a civil (not criminal) wrong other than a breach of contract or trust. In the case of contracts and trusts the parties agree the terms; it is a breach of those terms by one of the parties that constitutes the wrong which may be addressed. A tort is a duty fixed by law that affects all persons – it does not arise from a prior agreement. Torts cover negligence, nuisance, trespass and defamation. The most important of these in medical practice are negligence and battery (a part of the tort of trespass).
3. *Law of property.* This covers legal rights to property of all types.
4. *Family law.* This covers the law relating to marriage, divorce and the responsibilities of parents to children.
5. *Welfare law.* This is concerned with the rights of individuals to obtain State benefits, and the rights and duties that arise with regard to housing and employment.

the reasons for those decisions and the principles on which they are based. It is these legal principles that create a 'binding precedent' and which future judges must follow (subject to certain caveats) if that previous decision was made in a court higher in the hierarchy than the court in which the current case is being heard (Box 4.3). A binding precedent must normally be followed even if the judge does not agree with it. A precedent may be 'persuasive' but not binding. A persuasive precedent is not binding on the court, but it is one that the judge is persuaded should be followed. Such precedents may originate, for example, from courts lower in the hierarchy, or from decisions of the courts in other countries that use a common law system, notably Canada, Australia and New Zealand.

The doctrine of precedent only came to be applied in Scotland in the 19th century. The doctrine recognizes the hierarchy of the Scottish courts (see Box 4.3). Decisions in English courts may form persuasive precedents in Scottish courts. The House of Lords is the highest UK court for civil cases in the Scottish (as well as in the English and Welsh) court system.

STATUTE LAW (ACTS OF PARLIAMENT)

Statute law is made by Parliament. In the case of major pieces of legislation there is frequently a consultation period prior to consideration by Parliament.

Box 4.2 Distinctions between criminal and civil cases (Martin 1997, based on Fig. 1.2)

Criminal cases

Purpose To maintain law and order and protect society

Person originating the case The State (through the police and Crown Prosecution Service)

Legal name of person bringing the case Prosecutor

Legal name of person against whom the case is brought Defendant

Courts involved See Box 4.3

Standard of proof Beyond reasonable doubt

Person(s) making the decision Magistrates or jury

Decision Guilty or not guilty

Sanction if guilty Punishment

Powers of court Prison, fine, probation, discharge, community service order, etc.

Civil cases

Purpose To uphold the rights of individuals

Person originating the case The individual whose rights have been affected

Legal name of person bringing the case Claimant (formerly plaintiff)

Legal name of person against whom the case is brought Defendant

Courts involve See Box 4.3

Standard of proof Balance of probabilities

Person(s) making the decision Judge or panel of judges (very occasionally a jury)

Decision Liable or not liable

Sanction if liable Usually compensation (damages)

Powers of court Usually an award of damages, but also injunction, etc.

Typically the relevant government minister produces a consultative document known as a *Green Paper*. Comments on this paper are sought from relevant people and institutions, and changes are made to the original proposals in the light of these comments. This results in the publication of a *White Paper*, which contains firm proposals for the new law to be considered by Parliament.

Not every statute passed in the UK Parliament applies to Scotland. Acts passed since 1707 (the Union of the Parliaments) apply to Scotland unless there is a specific statement to the contrary. Conversely, some Acts apply only to Scotland. These have the word 'Scotland' in brackets in the title. Examples of such Acts are: National Health Service (Scotland) Act 1978, Mental Health (Care and Treatment) (Scotland) Act 2003, and The Adults with Incapacity (Scotland) Act 2000.

THE TORT OF NEGLIGENCE

The single most common reason for doctors to be taken to court is because they are being sued for negligence. In order for a doctor to be found liable in negligence the claimant (see Box 4.2) would need to prove three things:

1. That the doctor owed a *duty of care* to the relevant patient.
2. That the doctor was *in breach of the appropriate standard of care* imposed by the law.
3. That the *breach in the duty of care caused the patient harm* meriting compensation.

Box 4.3 The hierarchy of courts (from highest to lowest)

England and Wales

Criminal cases
European Court of Human Rights
House of Lords
Court of Appeal (Criminal Division)
Crown Court
Magistrates' Court

Civil cases
European Court of Justice (with regard only to EC law); European Court of Human Rights
House of Lords
Court of Appeal (Civil Division)
The Divisional Courts (two or three judges hear each case)
High Court (which has three divisions: Queen's Bench; Chancery; Family)
County Court
Magistrates' Court

Scotland
The judicial system in Scotland is also based on a division between civil and criminal law.

Civil cases
In civil cases the highest UK court is the *House of Lords*. Two of the Law Lords are Scottish in origin and experience, although there is no binding rule that a Scottish Law Lord must sit on a Scottish case. The next most senior court is the *Court of Session*, which consists of an *Inner House* and an *Outer House*. The Inner House primarily hears appeals. The Outer House hears new cases. Only occasionally will there be a jury in the Outer House. The lowest civil courts are the *Sheriff Courts*. These courts hear a very large number of cases. They correspond most closely to the English county courts.

Criminal cases
The House of Lords does not hear criminal cases from Scotland. The highest Scottish criminal court is the *High Court of Judiciary*. In addition to sitting as a court of first instance, the High Court acts as an appeal court for the lower criminal courts. The *Sheriff Court* deals with the more serious summary cases (i.e. literally cases involving a 'summons', and in practice those cases heard without a jury) and can deal with all but the most serious indictable offences as well (literally cases involving an indictment, which is a formal document containing the alleged offence). In the latter case the sheriff sits with a jury. In Scotland, the case against the accused is brought by (prosecuted by) local 'procurators', called the Procurator Fiscal (as opposed to the Crown Prosecution Service, which prosecutes all cases in England and Wales).

The lowest criminal courts are the *district courts*. These are presided over by a magistrate. These courts deal with a wide variety of petty crime and minor offences. There are, in addition, specialist courts. For example, cases involving children under 16 years of age who are alleged to have committed a crime, or who for other reasons might be 'in need of compulsory measures of care', are dealt with at special *Children's Hearings*. The main statutory provisions relevant to such hearings are in the Children (Scotland) Act 1995 (see Chapter 10).

Duty of care

A duty of care is an obligation on one party to take care to prevent harm being suffered by another. Generally doctors owe a duty of care to their patients. A hospital Trust would normally owe a duty of care to a patient of a doctor employed by that Trust. If a person comes into the casualty department of a hospital and the casualty doctor is informed of this, then normally both the hospital Trust and the doctor would owe a duty of care to that person.

Outside a hospital or a doctor's surgery, for example at the scene of an accident, a doctor would not normally owe a duty of care if he did not attempt to help. In other words, doctors are not legally obliged to act as 'good Samaritans'. However, once a doctor stops and either says that she is a doctor, or starts to act as though she is a doctor, she has taken on a duty of care to that patient. This means that she is now potentially liable in negligence. However, a general practitioner, who is within his geographical practice area does normally owe a duty of care to a person in need of medical help (for example, if the GP is at the scene of an accident). This is a result of the GP's contract with the health authority.

Standard of care – the Bolam test and its aftermath

In most cases of negligence the key issue is whether the doctor was in breach of the standard of care. The test in English law is whether the doctor fell below 'the standard of the ordinary skilled man exercising and professing to have that special skill. A man need not possess the highest expert skill at the risk of being found negligent. It is a well established law that it is sufficient if he exercises the ordinary skill of an ordinary man exercising that particular art' (Bolam v Friern Hospital Management Committee [1957]). See Box 4.4.

Where the profession is divided as to what is the appropriate management (as was the case in Bolam) the doctor will not be found negligent simply because the procedure adopted was not approved by the majority of the profession. In the Bolam case the judge said: 'A doctor is not guilty [sic] of negligence if he has acted in accordance with a practice accepted as proper by a responsible body of medical men skilled in that particular art'. This is known as the Bolam test. Thus a doctor will not be found negligent if the court is satisfied that there is a responsible body of medical opinion that would consider that the doctor had acted properly. That responsible body need not be the majority of the profession. The courts, however, do not simply accept what a group of doctors says is acceptable practice. In the case of Hills v Potter [1984], the judge said: 'In every case the court must be satisfied that the standard contended for on their behalf accords with that upheld by a substantial body of medical opinion …'. Other terms have been employed in other judgments. The judge in Bolam talked not only about a responsible body but also, elsewhere in his judgment, of a reasonable body of opinion. In other judgments the term respectable body has been used. Essentially, therefore, the effect of the Bolam test is that it is difficult to establish that a doctor has breached the duty of care.

Box 4.4 The Bolam case (Bolam v Friern Hospital Management Committee [1957])

Electroconvulsive treatment (ECT) is now used mainly in the treatment of severe depressive illness. It is carried out under general anaesthetic with the use of a muscle relaxant. The muscle relaxant is important, because ECT causes powerful contractions of skeletal muscle and, without relaxant, this can result in torn muscles and fractured bones. In the 1950s muscle relaxants were less well established than they are now. The majority of doctors used such relaxants during the administration of ECT, but the relaxants were not without potential risks. Bolam was given ECT without the use of muscle relaxants and without restraining his limbs. As a result he suffered a fractured hip from the contraction induced by the ECT.

The legal question was whether the doctors had acted negligently. The evidence before the court was that, although most doctors with expertise in this area would use either relaxants or limb restraint, there was a body of medical opinion that supported the method used for Bolam.

The case established that a doctor is not negligent if he or she acts in accordance with a responsible body of medical opinion, even if that opinion is in the minority. This is known as the *Bolam test*. The interpretation of what counts as a responsible body has been developed in subsequent cases (see text).

However, following the important case of Bolitho v City & Hackney Health Authority [1998] the law's approach is less clearcut. In that case one of the Law Lords said:

> … the court has to be satisfied that the exponents of the body of opinion relied upon can demonstrate that such opinion has a logical basis. In particular in cases involving, as they so often do, the weighing of risks against benefits, the judge before accepting a body of opinion as being responsible, reasonable or respectable, will need to be satisfied that, in forming their views, the experts have directed their minds to the question of comparative risks and benefits and have reached a defensible conclusion on the matter … In the vast majority of cases the fact that distinguished experts in the field are of a particular opinion will demonstrate the reasonableness of that opinion … But if, in a rare case, it can be demonstrated that the professional opinion is not capable of withstanding logical analysis, the judge is entitled to hold that the body of opinion is not reasonable or responsible.

Many legal commentators interpreted the Bolitho decision as representing a radical departure from the courts' traditional deferential approach to doctors. But others were more sceptical and doubted that the courts would play a more active role in reviewing medical decisions and setting the legal standard of care. An analysis of post-Bolitho case law (e.g. Hanson v Airedale Hospital NHS Trust [2003], French v Thames Valley Strategic Health Authority [2005]) does, however, reveal that judges are much more willing than in the past to scrutinize medical experts even though it will 'very seldom be right' for a judge to regard competent medical experts' views as unreasonable (per Siber J in M (A Child by his Mother) v Blackpool Victoria Hospital NHS Trust [2003]). In others words, although the Bolam test will usually prevail, it is no longer impregnable.

One important issue that has been clarified by the courts is that the Bolam test (as modified by Bolitho) has now been comprehensively applied, i.e. to the provision of information (see Chapter 6), to diagnosis and to treatment (see Lewis 2006).

Although clinical judgement will in all probability continue to be endorsed by the courts, the case of Bolitho is important because it shows that, in principle, English courts have determined that they should play a role in reviewing medical decisions and setting the legal standard of care.

The breach of the duty of care caused the patient harm

In order to show negligence the patient must prove that, on the balance of probabilities, the harm resulted from the breach in the duty of care. In one case (Barnett v Chelsea and Kensington Hospital Management [1968]), for example, three night watchmen came to the casualty department of a hospital with abdominal pains after drinking tea. The doctor told them to go and see their own doctors, without examining them. One man died after leaving the hospital from what was later discovered to be arsenic poisoning. The court found that the casualty doctor owed a duty of care to the patient, and that he had been in breach of the appropriate standard of care. However, the expert evidence was that even had the casualty doctor acted properly he would not have been able to save the man's life. The harm (of death) was therefore found not to have been caused by the breach in the duty of care, and so neither the hospital nor the doctor was negligent.

Case law on causation has consistently revealed how difficult a hurdle this element is for any potential claimant to overcome. Thus, it is rare for cases to be as simple as the Barnett case above where failure to treat a patient made no difference because he would have died anyway (i.e. his death was not caused by the negligence). In practice most causation cases are far more complex. The aetiology of medical conditions is often unclear, so that it is uncertain whether the injury was 'caused' by the defendant's action (or inaction) or by some other cause (or even multiple causes). Often, too, the situation will be further complicated by the presence of an underlying illness or other pre-existing vulnerability.

One typical situation is where what the patient has been deprived of (for example, through a missed or delayed diagnosis) is the chance of treatment, and what is uncertain is whether the prognosis would have been substantially different had the diagnosis not been missed (see on this Gregg v Scott [2005]). Yet, despite the difficulties of proving causation, several legal commentators (e.g. Mason & Laurie 2006) have suggested that the courts seem increasingly willing to bend causation rules to achieve what they see as a just outcome. This is perhaps why in some cases (albeit rarely), even if it cannot be shown that the harm was caused by a breach in the defendant's standard of care, damages may be awarded. In Chester v Afshar [2004] the House of Lords held that a patient was entitled to damages because she had not been warned about a risk of injury that in fact occurred (although not due to any negligence in how the operation was performed). As a result of that failure she underwent surgery (which she would not have had at that particular time had she been properly informed).

In Scottish law liability in negligence rests on the principle of 'delict' or 'reparation' rather than tort. A key Scottish case was that of Hunter v Hanley

[1955], which predates the Bolam case in England (see above) and which established that a doctor's conduct, in the setting of negligence, should be judged against the normal and usual practice of his profession. In practice the law regarding negligence in Scotland is similar, although not identical, to that in England and Wales.

Reform of the law of negligence

The law of negligence has long been criticized as a system of compensation. The most common criticisms are that the law is too complex, unfair, slow and costly. It also fosters a climate of blame and confrontation that undermines the doctor–patient relationship and discourages the reporting of errors (see also Department of Health 2003).

The response to these criticisms is the NHS Redress Act 2006. Under the Act patients would no longer have to go to court to get compensation, care or an investigation when something goes wrong. They would instead be entitled to receive a more consistent, speedy and appropriate response to their claims of negligence. Currently it is proposed to limit claims to an upper limit of £20 000 (although this may increase). Interestingly the new redress scheme is designed to give claimants an alternative to litigation rather than replace court proceedings.

TRESPASS TO THE PERSON

There are three forms of trespass: trespass to the person, trespass to goods and trespass to land. The most important of these for health professionals is trespass to the person. Trespass to the person can consist of assault, battery or false imprisonment. It is the first two that concern us here. Assault is when a person threatens, or attempts, physically to injure another person, and the other person has reasonable fear that the threat will be carried out. Battery occurs when the act goes beyond a threat and the person is touched, without consent. Battery can also occur if the touching is indirect, as, for example, if a person throws an object at another and hits her.

Assault and battery are both potentially criminal offences, but they can also give rise to civil actions (in the tort of trespass to the person). In the setting of medical practice it is the tort (i.e. civil action; see Box 4.1) of battery that is of most significance. If a surgeon, for example, removes a patient's uterus, for justifiable medical reasons but without the consent of the patient, the surgeon may be successfully sued for battery (and the patient may be awarded damages). It is very unlikely that criminal proceedings would be taken against the doctor, unless she was trying to harm the patient or was grossly negligent.

The tort of battery is of considerable importance in medical practice. It establishes that a doctor can touch a patient only with that patient's consent, unless the patient lacks capacity to give or withhold consent. Because examination, investigations and many treatments involve the doctor touching a patient, this requirement means that a patient can in general refuse medical help and treatment, even if this results in considerable harm or death. This issue is discussed in detail in Chapter 6.

4

The European Court of Justice (also called the Court of Justice of the European Communities)

This is the judicial branch of the European Union. It reviews the legality of the acts of the Commission and the Council of Members of the European Union, for example concerning issues involving disputes over trade or environment. Rulings made by the Court are binding on the member states, including both England and Wales, and Scotland (see Box 4.3). The Court is located in Luxembourg.

The European Court of Human Rights

The purpose of this court, which is located in Strasbourg, is to protect rights set out in the European Convention on Human Rights. It does not deal with any other set of issues. The Convention and the Court are established under the Council of Europe (not to be confused with the European Union). Individuals can take cases to the Court, usually against the state (country) of that individual. The court has no legal power to enforce its decisions (in contrast to the European Court of Justice). However, most states that belong to the Council of Europe (currently 46 members) would follow its rulings. The ultimate sanction available to the Council of Europe would be to expel the offending member state. However, an important development in English law is the Human Rights Act 1998.

The Human Rights Act 1998 (HRA)

The Human Rights Act 1998 came into force in October 2000. The Act makes the rights and freedoms that are set out in the European Convention of Human Rights (ECHR) admissible, and potentially enforceable, in English (and Scottish) courts. This means that it is unlawful for a public authority to act in a way that is incompatible with a Convention right. Some predicted that the HRA would have enormous impact on medical law. In fact, its effect has been modest. The Act has been used successfully to ensure that procedural safeguards are in place to protect patients' rights. In Glass v UK [2004], for example, the ECHR held that treating a child against its parents' wishes was a breach of the child's right to respect for its private and family life under Article 8(1).

Three of the Rights in particular may be relevant to clinical practice.

The right to life (Article 2 of the Convention)

According to this Article everyone's right to life shall be protected by law, and no one shall be deprived of their life intentionally. The European Court has interpreted this as placing a positive obligation to protect life, and not simply as guaranteeing the negative obligation not to take life. This might have implications for the allocation of resources because it might allow a patient to take legal action if denied expensive treatment that could save life (for example, expensive chemotherapy). Individual patients or their relatives might be able to challenge the withdrawal or withholding of life-prolonging

An introduction to law

treatment. The courts, however, ruled that there was no breach of Article 2 either in a case involving the withdrawing of artificial nutrition and hydration in two patients in persistent vegetative state (NHS Trust A v M and NHS Trust B v H [2001]), or in another case involving excluding the resuscitation of a 19-month-old child who was dying (A National Health Trust v D [2000]).

The prohibition of torture (Article 3 of the Convention)

This Article states that 'No one shall be subjected to torture or to inhuman or degrading treatment or punishment'. It is well established through decisions of the European Court that there is an obligation to provide adequate medical treatment for patients who are detained (for example, in prison or in a psychiatric hospital). This Article may also be interpreted as implying that experimental medical treatment could amount to inhuman treatment, in which case it could have implications for clinical research. Furthermore, it could be relevant to the provision of information in the context of consent to treatment and research. In a key case, Diane Pretty, who suffered from motor neuron disease, argued that, when the time came, her husband should be able to assist her suicide. The European Court, however, confirmed the House of Lords' ruling, that Section 2 of the Suicide Act 1961, which makes assisting suicide a crime, is not incompatible with Article 3 (Pretty v United Kingdom [2002]).

Right to respect for private and family life (Article 8 of the Convention)

This Article states that 'Everyone has the right to respect for his private and family life, his home and his correspondence'. Whether this will set a standard for confidentiality that is different from that already set by the law and the General Medical Council is unclear. The leading case on breach of confidence is now Campbell v MGN [2004]. Here the House of Lords emphasized that the protection of confidential information is about respecting the autonomy and dignity of individuals. The court also emphasized that the right to respect for private and family life under Article 8 should be regarded as underpinning the law's protection of confidentiality.

UNDERSTANDING LEGAL REFERENCES AND REPORTS

Cases

Doctors are used to the system of citing references in terms of author, date, title of article, journal (or book), volume number and page numbers. References to legal cases can appear puzzling, and even daunting. The most authoritative legal reports are those produced by the Incorporated Council of Law Reporting, and published as a general series known as the *Law Reports*. There are four series of reports depending on the type of case and the court: Appeal Cases (AC), Chancery Division (Ch), Queen's Bench (QB) and Family Division (Fam). These Law Reports are referenced by name of case, year, the law report series abbreviation and the starting page. For example, the reference to the House of Lords hearing of the 'Gillick' case (see Chapter 10) is: **Gillick v West Norfolk and Wisbech AHA [1986] AC 112.**

The two parties concerned in the action were Mrs Gillick and the West Norfolk and Wisbech Area Health Authority, and this provides the name of the case. The 'v' stands for the Latin *versus*, i.e. against. Sometimes a case arises not because one party is suing the other, but because one party wants a court ruling on some issue, or an injunction to prevent something from happening. A hospital may, for example, in unusual circumstances, want a court to determine whether a treatment can be imposed on a patient. Typically, in such instances, the person who is the subject of the case is referred to by an upper-case single letter of the alphabet, and the name of the case will include a brief description. For example, the case name might be: **Re B (A minor) (Wardship: Medical Treatment)**.

The Incorporated Council of Law Reporting also produces *Weekly Law Reports* (WLR). These are available more quickly than the Law Reports themselves and are generally more readily available. In most years there are several volumes (typically four). Unlike with most medical journals, the volume number starts at 1 at the beginning of each year. A case is referenced by name of case, year, volume, WLR, and starting page. The reference for the House of Lords hearing of the Gillick case in the Weekly Law Reports has the same title as for the Law Reports and the reference: [1985] 2 WLR 413. The earlier year, 1985 as opposed to 1986, reflects the earlier reporting in the Weekly Law Reports.

In addition to these 'official' reports there are also commercially produced reports. The most important of these is the *All England Law Reports* (All ER) available weekly. The reference system is similar to that of the Weekly Law Reports, and the reference to Gillick is: [1985] 3 All ER 402. There are many other commercially produced reports that can be cited, usually focusing on particular areas of law, such as Cox's Criminal Law Cases (Cox CC). Each court hearing of a case is the subject of a different law report and will have different references.

When a specific part of a judgment is being quoted, the reference may give the page of the report where the quotation appears, for example: 1 All ER 533 at 550. Thus the quotation is taken from page 550, but the first page of the report is page 533.

Sometimes a reference includes an abbreviation of the court in which the case was heard. For example, reference to the Gillick case may be written: [1985] 3 All ER 402 (HL). The (HL) tells you that the case was heard in the House of Lords. The abbreviation (CA) refers to the Court of Appeal. Another form of citation that is increasingly used is the so-called *neutral citation*, e.g. [2004] EWCA Civ, 123. The figure in square brackets is the year of the case. EWCA is an abbreviation for the England and Wales, Court of Appeal. 'Civ' refers to 'civil' (as opposed to criminal). The last figure (123) is the number for the case (i.e. case 123) – a number given to the case by the court itself. This method of citation does not, therefore, depend on the particular report of the case in a particular law report.

Statutes

Statutes are Acts of Parliaments. The most authoritative publication of statutes is the *Public General Acts*, duplicated in the *Law Reports Statutes,* which are published by the Incorporated Council of Law Reporting. These are both arranged chronologically. HM Stationery Office publishes statutes by subject as *Statutes in Force*, and a similar arrangement is used in *Halsbury's Statutes of England*.

REFERENCES

A National Health Trust v D [2000] 2 FLR 677

Barnett v Chelsea and Kensington Hospital Management Committee [1968] 1 All ER 1068

Bolam v Friern Hospital Management Committee [1957] 1 WLR 582

Bolitho v City and Hackney HA [1997] 4 All ER 771 HL

Campbell v MGN [2004] UKHL 22

Chester v Afshar [2004] UKHL 41

Department of Health 2003 Making amends: a consultation paper setting out proposals for reforming the approach to clinical negligence in the NHS. Online. Available:http://www.dh.gov.uk

French v Thames Valley Strategic health Authority [2005] EWHC 459

Glass v UK 2004 Maternal instinct vs. medical opinion. Child and Family Law Quarterly 16:(3):339–354

Gregg v Scott [2005] UKHL 2

Hanson v Airedale Hospital NHS Trust [2003] CLY 2989 (QBD)

Hills v Potter [1984] 1 WLR 641

Hunter v Hanley [1955] SC 200

Lewis C 2006 Clinical negligence a practical guide. 6th edn. Tottel, Haywards Heath

M, Re (A Child by his Mother) v Blackpool Victoria Hospital NHS Trust [2003] EWHC 1744

Martin J 1997 The English legal system. Hodder & Stoughton, London

Mason J K, Laurie GT 2006 Mason & McCall Smith's law and medical ethics. 7th edn. Oxford University Press, Oxford

NHS Trust A v M and NHS Trust B v H [2001] 2 WLR

Pretty v United Kingdom (Application No. 2346/002) [2002] 2 FLR 45

FURTHER READING

Branthwaite M 2000 Law for doctors: principles and practicalities. Royal Society of Medicine Press, London
A short practical account of English law by a barrister who was an anaesthetist.

Hendrick J 1997 Law and ethics in health care. Thornes, Cheltenham
The main focus is English healthcare law, although ethical issues are also discussed. Relevant to nurses as well as doctors.

Herring J 2006 Medical law and ethics. Oxford University Press, Oxford
A clear, accessible reference book on medical law.

Kennedy I, Grubb A 2000 Medical law, 3rd edn. Butterworths, London
The most detailed sourcebook of English healthcare law, providing extensive extracts from judgments. For reference only (over 2000 pages, much in small type).

Lewis C 2006 Clinical negligence a practical guide. 6th edn. Tottel, Haywards Heath
A comprehensive practical guide through the complex legal and procedural aspects of negligence law.

Martin J 1997 The English legal system. Hodder & Stoughton, London
A good general introduction to English law.

Mason J K, Laurie G T 2006 Mason & McCall Smith's law and medical ethics. 7th edn. Oxford University Press, Oxford
A well established book that focuses more on law than ethics.

McHale J, Fox M 2007 Health care law: test and materials. Sweet and Maxwell, London
Similar to Stauch, Wheat and Tingle, but almost double the length (at 1204 pages).

Montgomery J 2003 Health care law, 2nd edn. Oxford University Press, Oxford
Another good, clear account accessible to doctors.

Skene L 1998 Law and medical practice. Butterworths, Sydney
An overview of Australian medical law.

Stauch M, Wheat K, Tingle J 2006 Text, cases and materials on medical law, 3rd edn. Routledge, Abingdon
Draws together a wide range of material from statutes, judgments and academic commentaries (700 pages).

Doctors, patients and professions

WHAT IS A PROFESSION?

Medicine is not, of course, the oldest profession. That accolade belongs to religion, although other candidates have been suggested. There is no very precise meaning to the term profession. Sometimes it is used in distinction to a craft (such as furniture making), and sometimes in distinction to amateur (a professional as opposed to an amateur cricketer, for example). A number of features that typically characterize a profession, including medicine, are listed in Box 5.1.

THE GENERAL MEDICAL COUNCIL AND ITS CODES OF CONDUCT

The General Medical Council (GMC) is the professional body for doctors in the UK. It has the duty to ensure that those who are allowed to practise medicine (registered medical practitioners) are fit to do so. As part of this duty it provides guidelines (Box 5.2) for doctors as to what is good practice, and it has a quasijudicial process to decide whether a doctor is in breach of those guidelines. The main power of the GMC is to determine who can and who cannot practise medicine in the UK. Its ultimate sanction is to 'strike a doctor off the register' if he or she is found to be in breach of the Council's standards of practice, with the result that the doctor cannot practise medicine in the UK. This sanction can be temporary or permanent. In addition, the GMC stipulates, in general terms, the syllabus for medical training (General Medical Council 1993) and carries out regular visits to medical schools to ensure that students are receiving the appropriate education and assessment. Medical ethics and law are part of the 'core curriculum' for medical student education.

Doctors need to take the GMC's guidelines seriously for three reasons. First, the guidelines represent the considered opinion of the professional body on what it is ethically right for doctors to do in various situations with regard to their professional work. Second, the GMC has the power to prevent a doctor from continuing to practise medicine. Third, although the GMC is not part of the legal system, the courts take its standards into account (see Chapter 7).

Medical students, particularly once they are involved in seeing patients, would be expected to behave to the same standards, for example with regard to medical confidentiality, as doctors. The standards of behaviour expected

Box 5.1   Some features that are typical of professions (based on Bayles 1988)

1. A commitment to serve the public good and provide an important public service.
2. A great deal of generalized and systematized knowledge is required in order to practise the specific profession. Becoming a professional often requires extensive training, usually in the form of a higher degree.
3. The standards in carrying out professional work are set by the profession and there is an important element of self-regulation. These standards normally include ethical components. Increasingly, at least in the UK, there is state regulation in addition to self-regulation.
4. A certification or licensing procedure that determines who can be part of the specific profession. This goes hand-in-hand with those in the profession having a monopoly on being able (lawfully) to carry out the work of that profession.
5. The existence of a professional body that takes on a number of these aspects of a profession, for example setting professional standards, overseeing disciplinary mechanisms to ensure that those in the profession maintain those standards, determining the content for training to become professional, and carrying out a certification or licensing procedure.

Box 5.2   The General Medical Council's duties of a doctor (published as booklets by the Council and also available at http://www.gmc-uk.org)

These duties constitute the central statements concerning professional behaviour and medical ethics for doctors produced by the General Medical Council (GMC). Doctors in breach of these guidelines may face disciplinary action by the GMC (see text). The courts take notice of these guidelines, which are frequently updated. There are four booklets, as follows.

Good medical practice
This states: '... we as a profession have a duty to maintain a good standard of practice and care and to show respect for human life'. One of the principles is: 'make the care of your patient your first concern'. The booklet goes on to emphasize: respect for patients and their views, the importance of keeping up-to-date, working effectively with colleagues, and probity in professional practice, for example when there are conflicts of interest.

Seeking patients' consent: the ethical considerations
This focuses on issues of patient consent, covering such issues as the provision of information, ensuring that patients give consent voluntarily, what to do when patients lack capacity to give consent, and the criteria for establishing the 'best interests' of patients.

Confidentiality: protecting and providing information
This focuses on the importance of confidentiality for maintaining trust between doctor and patient (see Chapter 7).

Serious communicable diseases
This covers consent, confidentiality, research, and injuries to healthcare workers, all within the context of communicable diseases.

of medical students may be higher than those expected of students generally, because medical schools must ensure that their graduates behave in a way appropriate to the professional standards of the medical profession.

THE DOCTOR–PATIENT RELATIONSHIP

For those few years before qualifying, clinical students can observe how different doctors form relationships with their patients within the consultation. After qualifying, there is rarely a chance for a doctor to observe any consultation except her own. If doctors are to subject their consultation style to critical analysis, and develop the types of relationships with their patients that they think are right, then it is helpful to think about the different possible models of doctor–patient relationship.

Case example

Mrs P has a malignant breast lump. Good data suggest that with this kind of breast cancer, the 5-year survival rate following mastectomy is 90%. The 5-year survival rate following lumpectomy is about 75%. Without treatment, the 5-year survival rate is less than 20%. Mrs P's surgeon, Mr S, believes that mastectomy followed by breast implant is the treatment of choice. Mrs P wants lumpectomy. A friend of hers had a breast implant and it moved to the lateral side of her chest. Mrs P argues that quality of life is important, and not simply quantity of life.

Four models of the doctor–patient relationship

Emanuel & Emanuel (1992) proposed four models of the doctor–patient relationship. These can be represented as four points on a spectrum, and are summarized in Table 5.1. Each model is based on particular views of the medical consultation, the values of well-being and autonomy, and the nature of ethical dialogue.

The paternalistic (traditional or priestly) model

A paternalistic relationship derives from the idea of the relationship between a father and his child. The idea is that a father tries to do what is best for his child principally as he, the father, sees it. A good father may override the child's own wishes or choices for the child's own good.

The paternalistic model of doctor–patient relationship sees the doctor as making the main decisions about health care. In making the decisions the doctor has only the best interests of the patient at heart. The doctor, on this model, is seen as being in a better position than the patient to decide what is in the patient's best interests. The doctor can decide what is best for the patient from knowledge of the medical facts alone. The doctor's role in the consultation is to reach a diagnosis and to plan management. There is little or no discussion of what the patient's views and values are. Criticisms of this model include:

1. It adopts too narrow a meaning of 'well-being' or of the best interests of a patient. Such best interests are not determined by the medical facts alone but may differ depending on the patient's own values – her views of what are the most important things to her.

Doctors, patients and professions

Table 5.1 Four models of the doctor–patient relationship (based on Emanuel and Emanuel 1992)

	Informative	Interpretative	Deliberative	Paternalistic
Patient values	Defined, fixed, and known to the patient	Inchoate and conflicting, requiring elucidation	Open to development and revision through moral discussion	Objective and shared by the physician and patient
Doctor's obligation	Providing relevant factual information and implementing patient's selected intervention	Elucidating and interpreting relevant patient values as well as informing the patient and implementing the patient's selected intervention	Articulating and persuading the patient of the most admirable values as well as informing the patient and implementing their selected intervention	Promoting the patient's well-being, independent of their current preferences
Conception of patient's autonomy	Choice of, and control over, medical care	Self-understanding relevant to medical care	Moral self-development relevant to medical care	Assenting to objective values
Conception of doctor's role	Competent technical expert	Counsellor or adviser	Friend or teacher	Guardian

2. It tends to conflate factual claims and value judgements (see Chapter 2). The idea of something's being 'medically, or clinically, indicated' sounds as though it is purely a factual issue, whereas it often includes values. Thus, in the case of Mrs P above, it may be claimed that mastectomy is 'clinically indicated'. This phrase is a piece of rhetoric that tends to hide the values that go into making the decision.

3. It does not take into account values other than the patient's well-being, and in particular the valuing of patient autonomy (see Chapter 3).

The advantage of the paternalistic model is that it emphasizes the importance of the best interests and well-being of the patient. It draws attention to a doctor's duty to do what is best for the patient, and not to do what is best for the doctor, or for society more broadly. The paternalistic model works best in clinical situations where it is unlikely that any set of patient values would make a difference to the treatment, and where the illness interferes with the patient's ability to take part in the decision-making process. A patient with acute appendicitis is an example. Patients who have trust in their doctor, and who do not particularly want to have to think about the details of their condition and its management, and who see making decisions as a burden, may be particularly satisfied with this model of the doctor–patient relationship.

The informative (consumer or engineering) model

This model is at the opposite end of the spectrum from the paternalistic model. It is based on the analogy between patient and consumer. The doctor's role is to provide the patient with all the medical facts relevant to deciding on the management of the condition. The patient then decides what she wants. Finally, the doctor carries out that part of the management plan that requires his technical or clinical skills.

What this model has in common with the paternalistic model is that there is little discussion between doctor and patient over what is the best decision, and little if any overt acknowledgement of the patient's (or the doctor's) values. In the case of the paternalistic model this is because the doctor can decide the best treatment without knowledge of the patient's own values; in the case of the informative model this is because all the patient requires of the doctor are the medical facts.

The informative model derives from one view of the principle of respecting patient autonomy, whereas the paternalistic model emphasizes the principle of beneficence. There are several criticisms of the informative model:

1. It provides insufficient support for the patient in coming to a decision about management.
2. More sophisticated views of respect for patient autonomy emphasize the value of discussion (see Chapter 3).
3. Patients may come to bad decisions – bad even on their own valuation – because they may make mistakes. Discussion with the doctor will help to minimize this risk, particularly as doctors are likely to have experience of the longer-term issues that have been important to other patients in similar situations.
4. It treats the doctor as technician and does not sufficiently respect his autonomy.

The advantage of the model is that it allows patients to choose their own management on the basis of good information, but without the intrusion of the doctor's values or interests. In many other walks of life this is the model that we generally prefer. In matters such as buying a house, or deciding on investments, we generally expect the experts to provide the important information and to carry out the client's wishes.

The interpretative (interpretive) model

The interpretative model and the deliberative model (see below) are both reactions to what is seen as unsatisfactory in the two previous models. If the four models are placed on a spectrum, the paternalistic and informative models are at either end and the interpretative and deliberative models are between them, the interpretative model being closer to the informative model than is the deliberative model.

According to the interpretative model it is often helpful for the patient to discuss decisions about management with the doctor. The doctor may enable the patient to clarify her values and help her make the decision that is most in keeping with those values. Furthermore, the facts that the patient may need to know cannot necessarily be determined unless the doctor knows something about the patient's values. The doctor may also play a useful role in helping the patient to understand the implications of the different possible management decisions.

If Mr S, the surgeon in the above case example, believes that Mrs P is making the wrong decision it would be appropriate, on the interpretative model, for him to discuss this further. Such further discussion would be aimed at ensuring that Mrs P had thought clearly about the implications of choosing lumpectomy – in particular the implications of a reduced chance of long-term survival. Mr S might also, on this model, challenge Mrs P's negative view of breast implants, based on a single anecdote. It might be appropriate, too, for Mr P to tell Mrs S what treatment he would advise, as long as he gave the reasons for such advice.

The strength of the interpretative model is that it addresses some of the problems with the informative model, in particular by giving the patient more support in reaching a decision.

Various forms of *patient-centred* medicine, and patient-centred consultation style, have been developed over recent years (Makoul et al 1995). These began as a reaction to the paternalistic model, and tend to range from the informative to the interpretative models. Models of shared decision-making (Edwards & Elwyn 2001) have developed more recently and are partly a reaction to the informative model, which is seen as leaving the patient too unsupported. Shared decision-making therefore emphasizes the role of the doctor, as well as the patient, in making decisions. When there is disagreement there is negotiation and the possibility of the doctor trying to persuade the patient. However, most models of shared decision-making would envisage, in the end, that the patient's view should prevail, as long as the patient has been properly informed and as long as the doctor has made clear why he disagrees with the patient's decision.

With the increasingly prominent nature of evidence-based medicine, some models of shared decision-making focus on the issue of how patients can be helped to understand, and make use of, good-quality information in coming to healthcare decisions. Evidence-based patient choice (Edwards & Elwyn 2001, Hope 1996) is one such model. This model is closer to the interpretative model than to the deliberative model of the doctor–patient relationship.

The deliberative model

The deliberative model shares many of the properties of the interpretive model but differs in one important respect. In the deliberative model the doctor not only helps the patient to clarify her values, but may also discuss, and challenge, those values. According to the deliberative model the doctor should be prepared to try to persuade the patient to alter values if the doctor thinks that these are not right, just as a teacher or friend might seek to challenge values. This model can be derived from a concept of respect for patient autonomy that sees an element of moral development as part of promoting autonomy.

According to the deliberative model, it might be right for the surgeon, Mr S, to challenge some of Mrs P's values. The doctor may believe that Mrs P is undervaluing the importance of maximizing chance of survival. He may also believe that she would be likely to change her values were she to have lumpectomy and, 3 years later, develop metastases. For both of these reasons Mr S might seek to change Mrs P's current values.

Values might also be at stake when the doctor believes that a patient, or a relative, is overvaluing or undervaluing aspects of health care that impinge on others. Suppose that Mrs P has dependent children. In refusing the treatment that gives her the best chance of long-term survival, Mrs P may not be doing what would be best for her children. The doctor may believe that her values are wrong, and on the deliberative model it may be appropriate for him to challenge those values.

In neither the deliberative nor the interpretative models is it envisaged that the doctor is overbearing in challenging a patient's decisions or values. In the end it is for the patient to decide. The main point at issue between the models is whether a doctor should stick to helping a patient to understand and think through the issues, trying to persuade only when the patient appears to be making the wrong decision given the patient's own values (the interpretative model), or whether it is appropriate in some circumstances to try to persuade the patient to change her own values (the deliberative model).

REFERENCES

Bayles M D 1988 The professions. In: Callahan J C (ed.) Ethical issues in professional life. Oxford University Press, New York, p. 27–30

Edwards A, Elwyn G 2001 Evidence-based patient choice: inevitable or impossible? Oxford University Press, Oxford

Emanuel E J, Emanuel L L 1992 Four models of the physician–patient relationship. Journal of the American Medical Association 267:2221–2226

General Medical Council 1993 Tomorrow's doctors. GMC, London(update available online:http://www.gmc-uk.org)

Hope T 1996 Evidence-based patient choice. Kings Fund, London

Makoul G, Arnson P, Schofield T 1995 Health promotion in primary care: physician–patient communication and decision making about prescribed medications. Social Science and Medicine 315:69–70

FURTHER READING

Edwards A, Elwyn G 2001 Evidence-based patient choice: inevitable or impossible? Oxford University Press, Oxford
A good collection of essays on various approaches to the doctor–patient relationship, all within the general model of shared decision-making.

General Medical Council Codes of Conduct. Online. Available:http://www.gmc uk.org

Oakley J, Cocking D 2006 Virtue ethics and professional roles. Cambridge University Press, Cambridge
A broad account of several professions from a virtue ethics perspective.

Skene I 1990 You, your doctor and the law. Oxford University Press, Melbourne
A legal approach to the doctor patient relationship, focusing on doctors' responsibilities and patients' entitlements.

Stewart M, Brown J, Weston W, McWhinney I, McWilliam C, Freeman T 2003 Patient-centred medicine: transforming the clinical method, 2nd edn. Radcliffe Publishing, Oxford
A key text on patient-centred medicine.

Doctors, patients and professions

Part II

SPECIFIC
TOPICS

Consent

6

INTRODUCTION

Medical students often become aware of the issue of consent during their first surgical attachment. They see junior doctors asking patients to sign a 'consent form'. 'Consenting' the patient can become, for the junior doctor, yet another thing to do to the patient, like taking blood and obtaining a chest X-ray. From the legal point of view, consent is, effectively, a power of veto. A competent patient has the right to refuse any examination, investigation or treatment, but does not have the right to demand treatment. From the ethical point of view, the approach taken to consent is fundamental to the patient–doctor relationship (see Chapter 5), and a key test of the degree to which patient autonomy is respected.

THE CONCEPT OF INFORMED CONSENT

The philosophical basis of informed consent rests on the principle of patient autonomy (see Chapter 3). Lidz and colleagues (1984) have analysed valid consent (a more general concept than informed consent) using three principal components (Box 6.1) and two subsidiary components. The three principal components are incorporated into English law. The two subsidiary components, understanding and deciding, can be seen as elements of competence (see below). According to Lidz et al (1984, p. 23), for consent to be valid the doctor discloses information to a patient who is competent, the patient understands the information and voluntarily makes a decision.

Faden & Beauchamp (1986) have criticized this analysis as being too much centred on the provision of information. They argue that too central a focus on providing information is not in patients' interests. It is too easy to provide extensive information and then claim that the doctor has carried out her duty to the patient. Such an approach may be legally safe, but is not ethically right. They propose that informed consent should be thought of as 'autonomous authorization'. On this view, informed consent is a type of action. They wish to make a clear distinction between consent and assent. Assent may be mere submission to the doctor's authoritative order. The patient who assents does not call on his own authority. True informed consent requires that the patient does not merely assent but specifically authorizes the doctor to initiate the medical plan. Some patients may not wish to be given a great deal of information and may wish the doctor to make the decisions and choose the plan of management. But this situation is to be clearly differentiated from the

| **Box 6.1** | Three principal criteria for valid consent (see text) |

1. Informed
2. Competent
3. Voluntary (not coerced)

patient who passively assents to the doctor's decision. 'Autonomous authorization' for such patients involves two processes: the patient must first assume responsibility for decision-making, and then transfer that responsibility to the doctor.

OVERVIEW OF THE LAW ON CONSENT

There are two main areas of law concerned with consent: battery and negligence. Both are part of the civil, common law (see Chapter 4). In addition, there are some statutes of relevance, in particular the Mental Capacity Act 2005 (which is the major legislation governing those aged over 16 years who lack capacity; see Box 6.5 for an overview of the Act); the Children Act 1989, which governs some aspects of consent with regard to children (see Chapter 10); the Family Law Reform Act 1969 (see Chapter 10) which governs some aspects of consent with regard to children (minors) aged 16 and 17 years; and the Mental Health Act 1983 (see Chapter 11), which regulates some aspects of consent with regard to mentally disordered patients.

The law distinguishes between competent and incompetent patients. Competence refers to the ability to give or withhold consent, and is discussed below. The legal term for competence is capacity. We use the terms interchangeably in this book. There is a fundamental difference in the way the law deals with competent and incompetent patients (Fig. 6.1): competent adult patients may refuse any, even life-saving, treatment; the situation with regard to incompetent adults is more complex and needs more detailed consideration (see below). In brief, incompetent patients should be treated in their best interests. The legal concept of best interests, as we shall see, puts a great deal of weight on patients' previous views when competent, including any advance decisions that they have made, and including the views of any proxy decision-makers that they have appointed.

The three ethical components for valid consent (see Box 6.1) are also crucial in law. Doctors must, therefore, from a legal point of view, ensure that the patient is properly informed, has the legal capacity to give consent, and does so voluntarily (i.e. without coercion).

In English law, a person becomes adult on his or her 18th birthday. The Mental Capacity Act, however, applies to anyone aged 16 years and over. As we shall see in Chapter 10, this means that in relation to 16 and 17 year olds there is an overlap between the Act and common law. The law on consent to medical treatment with regard to those aged under 18 years ('minors') is rather more complex than with regard to adults (see Chapter 10).

In order to understand the law on consent, it is necessary to consider both battery and negligence.

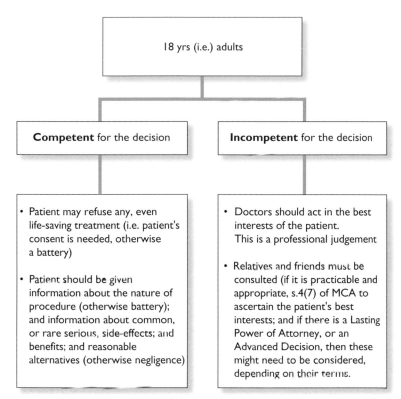

Fig. 6.1   Consent in English law.

Battery

In general, if one person touches another person without her consent, this constitutes a battery for which damages may be awarded (civil law) and for which, in extreme cases, a criminal prosecution might be brought. The key legal statement, with regard to the clinical setting, goes back to a judgment made in 1914 in the case of Schloendorff v Society of New York Hospital. The patient had given consent to an abdominal examination under anaesthetic but had specifically requested no operation. The surgeon removed a fibroid. Although this is a US case, the statement concerning battery has been absorbed into English common law. The judge in that case (J Cardozo) said: 'every human being of adult years and sound mind has a right to determine what shall be done with his own body; and a surgeon who performed an operation without the patient's consent commits an assault' (i.e. battery). In marked contrast to negligence (see below), there is no need to prove that the person touched has suffered harm as a result of the touching, in order for damages to be awarded.

The key legal reason why a doctor needs to have the consent of a patient before carrying out a procedure or treatment is that, without such consent, the patient could successfully sue the doctor for battery. In practice, however, more legal cases concerning the question of consent focus on negligence, because the issue is usually about the appropriate amount of information that should have been given to the patient.

Negligence

The legal concept of negligence is discussed in Chapter 4. We will discuss negligence here only in so far as it relates to consent. In order for patients to choose whether to accept a treatment (for example, an operation) or to undergo a diagnostic test, they need information. In particular they need information about the nature of the treatment, its benefits, risks and alternative possible treatments. A doctor may be negligent in not providing relevant information before the patient gives consent for the operation or procedure. In other words, a patient could successfully sue a doctor on the grounds that the doctor was negligent in not providing certain key information.

What information should be given for consent to be valid?

The nature of the procedure

The amount of information that a doctor needs to give to a patient in order for consent to be legally valid is an amalgamation of the law relating to battery and negligence.

From the point of view of *battery*, the key statement was given by J Bristow in Chatterton v Gerson [1981]. Bristow said: 'in my judgement once the patient is informed in broad terms of the nature of the procedure which is intended, and gives her consent, that consent is real, and the cause of the action on which to base a claim for failure to go into risks and implications is negligence, not trespass' (i.e. negligence not battery).

Let us take an example. A surgeon recommends a partial colectomy (removal of part of the colon) for severe diverticulitis. In order for the patient's consent to be valid, from the point of view of battery, the surgeon would need to inform the patient that the operation involved an abdominal incision, followed by removal of part of the colon, with subsequent rejoining of the two ends of the colon. If a colostomy were also being considered, then the patient ought to be told of that possibility. From the point of view of battery, it would not be necessary for the doctor to give any information about the risks, benefits or alternative treatments. However, from the point of view of negligence this would be important.

Risks and benefits

In general a doctor is not negligent 'if he has acted in accordance with the practice accepted as proper by a responsible body of medical men skilled in that particular art' (the Bolam test; see Chapter 4). There has, however, been legal concern that in much medical practice patients are not being given as much information about risks and benefits as should be given. In the case of Sidaway Board of Governors of the Bethlem Royal Hospital and Maudsley Hospital [1984], some of the Law Lords suggested that the courts could find that normal medical practice falls below acceptable standards.

Legal cases since Sidaway suggest that the courts will increasingly expect doctors to provide patients with the amount of information that a 'prudent' patient would want. This view is supported by the judgment in the case of Bolitho v Hackney Health Authority [1997] (see Chapter 4). In the case of Pearce v United Bristol Healthcare Trust [1998], one of the Law Lords stated that: 'if there is significant risk which would affect the judgement of a reasonable patient, then in the normal course it is the responsibility of the doctor to inform the patient of that significant risk, if the information is needed so that the patient can determine for him or herself as to what course he or she should adopt'. This suggests that in setting the standard of care the courts will look to the needs of the reasonable (i.e. prudent) patient (and to the GMC guidelines).

At what level of risk should doctors inform their patients?
The courts have been reluctant to give precise figures for risks that need to be disclosed, and recognize that doctors need to use their judgement in specific clinical situations. In the Sidaway case, Lord Bridge suggested that there would need to be a good reason not to inform a patient of a 10% risk of stroke following an operation. Since that case the standards of information provision expected of doctors have increased considerably. Doctors would now normally be expected to disclose much lower probabilities of serious side-effects. In an Australian case (Rogers v Whitaker [1992]), a doctor was found negligent for not warning of a risk of blindness following an eye operation where that risk was put at 1 in 14000.

What should the doctor do when the patient specifically asks for information about risks?
In the Sidaway case Lord Bridge said: 'Some patients make it clear that they wish to be well informed about risks. From the ethical point of view the issue is more about how best to inform, rather than whether to inform. If a patient asks for particular information they would be very unusual circumstances that would justify not being open and honest with the patient'. The guidelines from the General Medical Council (1998) state that doctors must respond honestly to any question from the patient and 'as far as possible, answer as fully as the patient wishes'.

The legal status of the 'consent form'

It is routine for patients to be asked to sign a consent form before undergoing surgery. Does this mean that it would be illegal to perform surgery on a competent patient without a signed form? The answer is no. From the legal point of view, the key thing is that the patient has given valid consent (see Box 6.1). That consent can be given verbally. The purpose of a written consent form for surgical procedures is twofold: first, it provides a mechanism to ensure that consent is obtained and to communicate that fact to other members of the healthcare team; second, from the legal point of view it provides *evidence* that the patient has given consent. The consent form has no other legal force; in particular, it is not a contract. One important implication of this is that a patient may withdraw consent after signing the consent form. A competent patient can withdraw consent at any time, in which case it would normally be illegal (battery) to proceed with the operation.

When can consent be implied?

Because touching without consent can constitute battery, a patient's consent is needed even when taking the pulse or examining the chest. And yet doctors rarely obtain specific consent for such routine parts of the medical examination. Does this mean that patients could successfully sue doctors much of the time? The answer is no, because the courts recognize the concept of 'implied consent'. If the doctor says, 'I would like to take your pulse' and the patient proffers her wrist and sits quietly while the doctor takes the pulse, then the patient's consent is taken to be implied by her behaviour. If, however, a competent patient were to say, 'There's no way you're going to take my pulse', it would constitute battery if the doctor went ahead and took the patient's pulse. The mere fact, however, that a person voluntarily comes to see a doctor, or is admitted to hospital, does not imply consent to any examination, investigation or treatment. A competent patient could come to the doctor and then refuse to be touched in any way.

Consent form disclaimers

In order to avoid being sued in battery the surgeon must describe 'the general nature of the operation'. This would normally include the fact that an incision will be made, the rough site of the incision, and what part or parts of the body will be removed. The surgeon may not know, until he is already carrying out the operation, exactly what needs to be done. What is the legal force of a consent form disclaimer to the effect that the surgeon will do whatever is necessary in the patient's best interests?

A doctor would normally be justified in proceeding without a patient's consent if a condition were discovered in an unconscious patient for which treatment was necessary (i.e. if it would in the circumstances be unreasonable to postpone treatment). In a Canadian case (Marshall v Curry [1933]) a grossly diseased testicle was discovered during a hernia operation. It was removed on the grounds both that removal was necessary for the hernia repair and because the gangrene was thought to be a threat to the patient's life. The court upheld the surgeon's action. In another Canadian case (Murray v McMurchy [1949]) a doctor was successfully sued in battery when he tied the patient's fallopian tubes during a caesarean section because he discovered fibroids in the uterine wall and was concerned about the hazards of a future pregnancy. These Canadian cases are likely to reflect English law. In the English case of Devi v West Midlands Regional Health Authority [1980], a woman of 29 years old who had four children and hoped for more was admitted to hospital for a minor operation on her womb. In the course of the operation her womb was found to be ruptured. She was sterilized, without her consent or knowledge, because it was feared that if she were to become pregnant again her womb would rupture. The patient won her claim.

We will now consider three hypothetical clinical situations. In none of these situations is the legal position certain because of the lack of relevant case law. We have given our view. Each doctor must make up her own mind as to what is right, based on legal and ethical judgement.

Case study: – the exploratory operation

Mr A has chronic abdominal pain. Investigations have not revealed a cause. A laparotomy (exploratory operation) is needed. It is explained to Mr A that the cause is not certain and permission is sought to carry out whatever is considered necessary at operation. Mr A wishes this to be done and so grants a *carte blanche* to the surgeon to remove whatever she thinks necessary. On laparotomy the surgeon discovers a bowel carcinoma. She removes the carcinoma and sufficient healthy bowel on either side to try to ensure that the entire tumour is removed.

As Mr A did not give explicit consent for the removal of the carcinoma and part of the bowel, could he successfully sue in battery on the grounds that the nature of the operation had not been sufficiently explained? The Department of Health has produced a standard consent form which includes the following statement for patients: 'I understand that any procedure in addition to those described on this form will only be carried out if it is necessary to save my life or to prevent serious harm to my health' (Department of Health 2002). In our view the surgeon should proceed with the operation. This is because the bowel carcinoma was thought to contribute to the presenting complaint, the patient has already given consent to appropriate treatment, including removal of what is thought necessary, and the surgery is necessary to prevent serious harm.

Case study: the additional finding

Mr A has intermittent abdominal pain. Investigations reveal gallstones, and the cause of the pain is thought to be due to this. Mr A gives consent for the operation involving removal of the gallbladder, and also for anything else to be done that is thought necessary. At operation, the surgeon finds that, although there are gallstones the cause of the pain is probably a carcinoma, which he discovers at the head of the pancreas. The surgeon removes not only the gallbladder but also the pancreatic carcinoma.

Because Mr A did not give explicit permission for the removal of part of his pancreas, could he successfully sue in battery on the grounds that he did not give this consent? In our view a surgeon in this situation should normally proceed with the operation because the carcinoma is thought to relate to the presenting complaint.

Case study: the incidental finding

Mrs B has acute abdominal pain. A diagnosis of appendicitis is made and Mrs B gives her consent for surgery, including removal of her appendix. At operation the surgeon discovers that, in addition to an acutely inflamed appendix, Mrs B also has an ovarian tumour. This tumour is not likely to have contributed to her acute abdominal pain. The surgeon considers that it is in Mrs B's best interests for the ovary containing the tumour to be removed. She therefore removes it. Could the surgeon be successfully sued for battery on the grounds that Mrs B did not give explicit permission for her ovary and ovarian tumour to be removed? Would it make any difference if Mrs B had explicitly given her consent for any procedure that the surgeon deemed, at surgery, to be in her best interests?

In this case the surgeon is on much shakier ground because the ovarian tumour is incidental to the presenting complaint. In our view, a patient might successfully sue in battery for removal of part of the body without consent, even if she gave consent for the surgeon to do 'whatever he judges to be in the patient's best interests', and even if what the surgeon did was in the patient's best interests! The surgeon would need to give good reasons why the removal of the ovarian tumour could not have been carried out at a later and separate operation, for which the patient's explicit consent could be sought. The key reason would have to be that delaying the operation would expose the patient to a significantly increased risk of death or serious harm. Such an argument might be used, for example, in the case of finding an aortic aneurysm, where the aneurysm could rupture at any time, and might also be used where the patient, perhaps because of chronic obstructive airway disease, is at high risk from a general anaesthetic (so that any further operation is dangerous). The normal risk of an operation, however, may not be sufficient to justify avoiding a further operation. What is legally advisable may therefore conflict both with what is in the patient's best interests and with what the patient would want. The surgeon could, of course, take the (legal) risk of doing the extra procedure on the grounds that the patient was very unlikely to want to sue.

Some key legal points in the law on consent are summarized in Box 6.2.

PATIENTS WHO LACK CAPACITY

In the legal and ethical analysis of treating people against their will, a great deal depends on whether the patient is competent (has legal capacity). The approach to competence endorsed by both law and most ethical analyses

---

Box 6.2 Some key legal principles relating to consent

- Competent adults have a legal right to refuse medical treatment, or demand withdrawal of treatment, even if this refusal results in death or permanent injury.
- Incompetent adults should be treated 'in their best interests' (Mental Capacity Act 2005).
- Under the Mental Capacity Act 2005, doctors (and other people) can make decisions on behalf of an adult who lacks capacity.
- A person is legally adult at age 18 years.
- Those aged 16–17 years can consent to treatment, but not necessarily refuse beneficial treatment (see Chapter 10).
- Those aged less than 16 years may, if competent, consent to treatment (see Chapter 10).
- A parent or guardian can give proxy consent on behalf of a minor (age less than 18 years).
- Parents and guardians are under a legal duty to act in the minor's best interests. If doctors and parents cannot agree the minor's best interests, a court may need to decide either who should judge best interests, or what those best interests are.
- The Mental Capacity Act defines an adult as a person of 16 years and over. There is thus an overlap between the Act and the common law in relation to young people aged 16 and 17 years (see Chapter 10).

(see Buchanan & Brock 1989) is what is known as the 'functional' approach. This focuses on the process by which the person comes to the particular decision. One implication of this approach is that competence refers to a person's capacity to make a particular decision or carry out a particular task at a particular time. A person may, at one time, be competent to make one decision (e.g. whether to take a particular medication) but not a different decision (e.g. whether she is capable of living alone), or vice versa.

Capacities needed for competence

Buchanan & Brock (1989) distinguished three central elements:

1. Understanding and communication
2. Reasoning and deliberation
3. The person must have a 'set of values or conception of the good'.

The first element is needed to ensure that the person can become informed and express a choice. This in turn requires cognitive (intellectual) abilities. The understanding requires not only an 'intellectual' understanding but also 'the ability to appreciate the nature and meaning of potential alternatives – what it would be like and "feel" like to be in possible future states …' (Buchanan & Brock 1989, p. 24). The second element requires sufficient short-term memory to retain the relevant information and allow the process of decision-making to take place. The third element, the set of values, must be 'at least minimally consistent, stable and affirmed as his or her own. This is needed in order to be able to evaluate particular outcomes as benefits or harms, goods or evils, and to assign different relative weight or importance to them' (p. 24).

Assessing capacity

There are many situations in which doctors need to assess a patient's capacity. Some involve the issue of whether the patient has capacity to consent to (or refuse) treatment. Others involve assessment outside the clinical context: for example, the doctor may be asked to assess a person's capacity to make a will.

The first two elements of Buchanan and Brock's analysis were effectively incorporated into English common law (Re C [1994]), and with slight amendment form the current four legal criteria for capacity specified in the Mental Capacity Act (see Box 6.3, which also summarizes other key legal principles relating to capacity).

The law in Scotland is different, mainly because of the Adults with Incapacity (Scotland) Act 2000 (see Box 6.6).

We suggest a three-step approach to assessing capacity that incorporates the ethical and legal considerations discussed above (summarized in Box 6.4).

Step 1: Identify the information relevant to the decision

Capacity is specific to a particular decision (see Box 6.3). The first step in assessing capacity is to clarify what information is critically relevant to making the decision. The critically relevant information includes the likely consequences

Box 6.3 Some key legal principles relating to capacity

The legal criteria for capacity (Mental Capacity Act 2005)

A person lacks capacity if 'he is unable to make a decision for himself in relation to the matter in question because of an impairment of, or a disturbance in, the functioning of the mind or brain'. (Section 2(1)).

A person is unable to make a decision (i.e. lacks capacity) if he or she is unable (Section 3(1)):

- to *understand* the information relevant to the decision,
- to *retain* that information,
- to *use or weigh* that information as part of the process of making the decision, or
- to *communicate* his decision (whether by talking, using sign language or any other means).

An imprudent decision is not, by itself, sufficient grounds for incapacity

A person should not be regarded as lacking capacity merely because she is making a decision that is unwise or against her best interests (see s.1(4) of Mental Capacity Act 2005). An unwise decision might alert a doctor to the need for assessment of capacity, but that assessment must be made by analysing the way the decision is made (see text), not from the decision itself.

Capacity is 'function specific'

A person is not 'globally' competent or incompetent. One can only talk of competence to do a particular thing. Thus a patient may be competent to make a will, but incompetent to consent, or refuse consent, to a particular operation (or vice versa). Indeed, a patient may be competent to consent to one type of treatment but not to another. A general statement to this effect was made in an Australian case as follows (Gibbons v Wright [1954]):

" the mental capacity required by the law in respect of any instrument is relative to the particular transaction which is being effected by means of the instrument, and may be described as the capacity to understand the nature of that transaction when it is explained.

The standard of proof is 'The balance of probabilities'

The usual standard for proof in civil cases is 'balance of probabilities', as opposed to 'beyond reasonable doubt'. Thus, in assessing capacity, courts will be concerned with whether the balance of probabilities favours capacity or lack of capacity (see s.2(4) of Mental Capacity Act 2005).

The presumption of capacity

An adult is presumed capable of doing something until the contrary is proved by acceptable evidence. The onus of proof therefore lies with showing that someone does not have capacity (see s.1(2) of Mental Capacity Act 2005).

The presumption of continuance

Once incapacity has been established, it is presumed to continue until the contrary is proved by acceptable evidence.

Capacity is, ultimately, a legal not a medical decision

" … it is for the court to decide [the question of capacity], although the court must have the evidence of experts in the medical profession who can indicate the meaning of symptoms and give some idea of the mental deterioration which takes place in cases of this kind' (Mr Justice Neville in Richmond v Richmond [1914]).

In practice, courts usually take considerable notice of doctors' assessments of capacity.

Enhancing capacity

Under the Mental Capacity Act 2005 doctors (and other carers) have a duty to ensure that information is given in the most appropriate way (such as using simple language and visual aids if helpful) and that steps are taken to try to enhance the patient's capacity (for example, by ensuring a quiet comfortable setting in which to talk with the patient).

Box 6.4   Assessment of competence: summary

Step 1: Identify the information relevant to the decision
For example:

* That a decision needs to be made
* The nature of the various reasonable decisions
* The pros and cons of each reasonable decision.

Step 2: Assess cognitive ability
With regard to the information identified in Step 1, assess whether the person has the cognitive ability to carry out the elements of the decision-making process:

* Understanding and believing the information
* Retaining the information
* Using and weighing the information and coming to a decision
* Communicating the decision.

Consider particularly the following conditions that can interfere with such ability:

* Acute confusional state (delirium)
* Dementia
* Learning disability
* Stroke
* Korsakoff's psychosis.

Step 3: Assess other factors that may interfere with decision-making
* Mental illness – delusions, hallucinations, affective disorder (depression, manic illness)
* Lack of maturity – when considering a minor's competence, consider both emotional and cognitive maturity.

of different decisions (e.g. different possible treatments, or treatment versus non-treatment), and understanding in broad terms what would be involved in carrying out a decision.

With regard to medical treatment, the Department of Health Code of Practice (1999) (to the Mental Health Act) identifies the following areas:

1. Understand what medical treatment is, and that somebody has said that he (the patient) needs it and why the treatment is being proposed.
2. Understand in broad terms the nature of the proposed treatment.
3. Understand the principal benefits and risks of the treatment.
4. Understand what will be the consequences of not receiving the proposed treatment.

Step 2: Assess cognitive ability

Understanding and believing the relevant information

Does the person have sufficient intellectual ability to understand the various aspects of the critically relevant information? The standard should not be set too high. Most healthy people without learning disability have the capacity to make decisions about their own health care and to understand the main points at issue.

A person may understand the information presented but not be capable of believing it because, for example, of a relevant delusion or other mental disorder. If this is the case then he or she might be assessed as lacking capacity. Patients should not, however, generally be judged as lacking capacity simply on the grounds that they do not believe the information from the doctor, because, for example, of skepticism about professionally based knowledge, or a strong belief in, for example, complementary therapies.

Retain the information

Can the person *retain* the information long enough to use it to come to a decision? Severe memory impairment, even in the absence of other intellectual deficits, may render someone incompetent for a specific task.

Use or weigh the information and make a choice

Has the person *sufficient intellectual ability* to weigh up the relevant information? Again, the standard for this should not be set too high. The main causes of cognitive impairment are: acute confusional state (delirium), dementia, learning disability, stroke, head injury, Korsakoff's psychosis and brain tumour.

Is the person able to communicate the decision?

Many patients, for example following stroke, may have difficulty communicating their views and decisions even though they have the capacity to make their own decisions. It is therefore important in assessing capacity to make every effort to ensure that difficulties in communication are overcome. This may involve a careful and patient approach to listening to the patient, or using writing if the problem is primarily one of speech difficulty. If, despite all reasonable attempts to enable the patient to communicate his decision, he is unable to do so then, according the Mental Capacity Act, he should be regarded as lacking capacity.

Step 3: Assess other factors that may interfere with competence

Cognitive impairment is only one factor that may interfere with the three elements of information processing. Other causes that need to be specifically addressed are as follows.

Mental illness

A *delusion* may interfere with *believing* the information; for example, a person suffering from a grandiose delusion may not believe that failure to treat is likely to have serious consequences, even though there is good evidence that it will. However, the fact that a person has delusional beliefs, for example as part of schizophrenia, does not necessarily render that person incompetent with regard to a particular decision. For the person to be incompetent, the delusion must interfere with the understanding, believing or decision-making process specific to the particular decision.

An *affective illness* (depression or mania) may interfere with the weighing-up of information and coming to a decision. For example, a person suffering from a depressive disorder may refuse beneficial treatment because she does not feel herself worthy of treatment.

It can be difficult to assess the effect of mental illness on competence to make a particular decision. When in doubt it may be helpful to ask: Is the decision likely to be different from what the person would decide if free from mental disorder?

Maturity

In the case of a *child*, is the choice likely to be due to lack of maturity, either cognitive or emotional? Is the child likely to come to a different decision when more mature? With children the assessment of competence may involve also an assessment of coercion. Indeed, the two concepts may overlap. An important question is: Is the child the subject of a relationship of a type that might have a marked impact on the ability to make a free choice? For example, children who are insecurely attached to their parents may be unable to muster sufficient autonomy to be free to make a decision. Instead, they may feel bound to comply with parental wishes. This can be particularly true of children who are being maltreated by one or other parent.

Enhancing capacity

A person's competence to make a decision depends not only on the person but also on the environment. The assessment of competence must not be treated like a school exam. If patient autonomy is to be properly respected, doctors should try to enable patients to have the competence to make decisions. This might be done in several ways:

- By treating any mental disorder that affects capacity and any physical disorder (such as a urinary tract disorder) that may be causing an acute confusional state.
- If capacity is likely to improve, to wait, if possible, until it does improve to allow the patient to be properly involved in decisions.
- To be aware of the possibility that medication may adversely affect capacity.

- If capacity fluctuates (e.g. it depends on the time of day), to assess capacity and discuss treatment if appropriate when the patient is at her best.
- If there is a need to assess capacity for different tasks or decisions, to assess these separately.
- To choose the environment that maximizes the patient's capacity, including minimizing distractions such as excessive noise.
- To consider whether the person might be helped if a relative or friend is with her.
- By allowing the person time to take in and process information.
- By making explanations simple and using aides mémoire, written information and diagrams, where these are likely to be helpful.

The Mental Capacity Act 2005 places on health professionals a duty to enhance capacity if possible and to enable decision-making. These include the duty not to treat a person as unable to make a decision unless all practicable steps to help him to do so have been taken without success (s.1(3)).

Making decisions for people who lack capacity

There are four theoretically possible approaches to making decisions about the health care of incompetent patients (Buchanan & Brock 1989):

1. Best interests
2. Proxy
3. Substituted judgement
4. Advance directives.

Best interests

One approach for a doctor faced with an incompetent patient is to ask which plan of management serves the patient's best interests. In Chapter 3 we outlined different approaches to the question of what is in a person's best interests. These different approaches will give different answers to the question of what is in a person's best interests in some clinical situations (see Case example of Alzheimer's disease on p. 36).

Proxy

An alternative approach is for a proxy to make decisions on behalf of an incompetent patient. This proxy essentially plays the role that the patient would play if competent. Such an approach of course leaves the proxy with the question: On what basis should the decision be made?

Substituted judgement

The criterion of substituted judgement asks the hypothetical question: Suppose the patient were (magically) able to become competent, what treatment would he choose? In order to try to answer this question the doctor could use a range of evidence: reports of what the patient has said about this kind of situation in the past; the kind of general values the patient held; and experience with other patients.

Advance directives

Definition
Advance directives are statements made by people at a time when they are competent, about how they would want to be treated in the future were they to become ill and at the same time incompetent to decide about or give consent for their treatment.

Purpose
A competent patient can help decide her own health care, and normally has the legal and ethical right to refuse any specific treatment. The purpose of advance directives is to extend such patient autonomy to include situations in which a person is no longer competent.

Types of advance directive
1. *Instruction directive* – a statement expressing a preference for, or a refusal of, specific treatments in certain specific future circumstances.
2. *General values/preferences statement* – a statement of a person's general values or preferences relevant to medical treatment.
3. *Proxy directive* – a directive authorizing another specific person to take the patient's part in making healthcare decisions, were she to become incompetent.
4. *Formal* – a formal directive is written and witnessed in the same way that a 'last will and testament' is created. This contrasts with an *informal* directive, which could arise, for example, from a conversation with a relative, doctor or nurse.
5. *Living will* – a term sometimes used synonymously with advance directive, and sometimes used in the more restricted sense of a formal instruction directive.
6. *Advance statement of health care* – synonymous with advance directive.
7. *Advance decision* – the term used in the Mental Capacity Act 2005 for what is essentially a formal instruction directive.

Some reasons in favour of respect for advance directives
1. They respect, and extend, patient autonomy.
2. US evidence suggests that many patients become less anxious about the possibility of unwanted treatments, and doctors who have had experience with advance directives have usually found them helpful.
3. In the USA, at any rate, they are expected to lower healthcare costs because it is thought many people would want less aggressive treatment than they would otherwise get.

Some reasons against advance directives
1. Anecdotal experience suggests that many patients want in prospect less aggressive treatment than they want when seriously ill. This sheds doubt on whether people can imagine future situations sufficiently vividly for their present views to be a good guide to their future wishes.

2. The statements made in the directive will need to be interpreted when applied to the specific situation. The patient's actual condition may be different from that implied by any of the statements in the advance directive.
3. The person might have changed her mind since making the decision (and while still competent) without altering the directive.

The legal approach to adults who lack capacity

As we have seen, a procedure can be undertaken on a competent patient only with that patient's informed consent.

With regard to incompetent adults, current law uses elements from all four of the approaches outlined above. For people aged 16 years and over, the main relevant statute is the Mental Capacity Act 2005 (MCA; Box 6.5). The central legal position in both common law and in the MCA is that incompetent adults should be treated in whatever way serves their best interests. If there is no *Lasting Power of Attorney* (see below), and no *advance decision* (see below) that the patient has made, then doctors have the duty to assess what is in a patient's best interests (see Chapter 3). Under the MCA doctors have a legal duty to consult a range of people when determining the best interests of a person who lacks capacity (see Box 6.5 and p. 91).

Section five (s.5) of the MCA enables those caring for an incompetent adult (e.g. doctors or other health professionals) to make decisions in the absence of consent. In effect s.5 allows such actions to be taken as if the person concerned

---

Box 6.5 Overview of the Mental Capacity Act 2005

1. The Act came into force in 2007.
2. It applies to people aged 16 years and over.
3. The Act applies primarily to those who lack capacity. It states, however, that 'a person is not to be treated as unable to make a decision unless all practicable steps to help him to do so have been taken without success'. The Act also states that 'A person is not to be treated as unable to make a decision merely because he makes an unwise decision'.
4. The Act covers the following areas:
   - It provides the legal criteria for *lack of capacity* (see Box 6.3).
   - It provides the legal definition of *best interests* (see Chapter 3, p. 38).
   - It states that doctors have a *duty to consult friends and relatives* of a patient in order to help determine the patient's best interests, if this is practicable and appropriate. The doctor must also consult a person named in any Lasting Power of Attorney, or Deputy appointed by the court (see p. 86).
   - It provides for a person, when competent, to appoint a *Lasting Power of Attorney* (see p. 86).
   - It provides for a person when competent to create an *advance decision to refuse treatment* (see p. 86).
   - It gives some *legal protection* to doctors and other carers in their determination of a patient's best interests.
   - It created the Court of Protection to make decisions if necessary relating to the MCA

had capacity and had given consent, and provides carers and decision-makers with protection from any liability for their actions, so long as they can show that the act was in the best interests of the person lacking capacity. There is no need for professionals to obtain any formal powers or authority to act. The actions in question are those carried out 'in connection with the care or treatment' of the person lacking capacity. The category is thus wide enough to include the range of medical management, including, for example, diagnosis as well as treatment.

There are circumstances when the doctor, or other carers, believe that what is in the best interests of the patient (who lacks capacity) involves the use of threats or force in order to impose (an aspect of the) treatment that the patient is resisting, or in order to restrict the patient's liberty of movement. Such use of threats or force is called *restraint*. For such restraint to be lawful two conditions must be satisfied (s.6 of the MCA): first, the doctor reasonably believes it to be necessary in order to prevent harm to the patient, and second the use of restraint must be proportionate to its value.

In determining best interests the MCA can be seen as trying, as far as is possible, to extend to patients who lack capacity the same respect for autonomy that is intrinsic to the law with regard to adult patients who have capacity. In assessing best interests the MCA gives a great deal of weight to what the person would have wanted (i.e. to substituted judgement) and to any statements made by the person, when competent, about how they wish to be treated (i.e. to advance directives, or advance decisions as they are called in the Act). It is, of course, frequently the case that the patient never considered and never spoke about what she would have wanted in the circumstances that have arisen. It is therefore often not possible for doctors, or for relatives and friends, to judge best interests on the basis of what the person would have wanted. In such cases some judgement has to be made about the patient's best interests, not on the basis of judging what the person might have wanted, but on the basis of objective, external judgements about what is in the person's best interests. Such judgement might, for example, be based on the 'mental state theory' of best interests (see Chapter 3) and be a judgement about the patient's likely quality of life given different management options. Even if the patient had made a clear advance decision that covered the situation, on both mental state theories and objective list theories (although not on the view taken by the MCA; see below) the best interests of the patient may not be served by following this advance decision (see Case example on Alzheimer's disease, p. 36).

If no valid advance decision exists then the doctor, with the help of friends and relatives, should try and make a *substituted judgement*. If there is insufficient evidence on which to base such a substituted judgement, the doctor should judge best interests on the basis of what seems reasonable, perhaps using the approach of *mental state theories*, that is, trying to judge which management approach would maximize the patient's quality of life.

The Act recognizes the difficulties in judging the best interests of an incompetent patient and provides protection (s.4(9)) to a person (e.g. a doctor) who acts or makes a decision in the reasonable belief that he is doing so in the best interests of the person who lacks capacity. A doctor must be able to point to objective reasons to demonstrate why he believed he was acting in the person's best interests, and, even if it is subsequently shown that a doctor was mistaken in his opinion of best interests, he will still receive the protection of the Act providing that it was a reasonable decision.

The law in Scotland is different in important respects from that in England and Wales with regard to incompetent patients aged 16 years and over (Box 6.6) and with regard to children (see Chapter 10). The Mental Health (Care and Treatment) Act 2003 governs some aspects of consent in Scotland (see Chapter 11). Note too that the Department of Health is revising its guidance on consent generally (see http://www.dh.gov.uk/en/Policyandguidance/Healthandsocialcaretopics/Consent/index.htm).

Lasting Power of Attorney (LPA)

Section 9 of the MCA introduces the provision for a *Lasting Power of Attorney*. Under such a power a person (the 'donor') when competent may confer authority (to the 'donee(s)') so that the donee can make decisions (if the donor becomes incompetent) about any specified matters of personal welfare and any specified matters of property. The donor must be at least 18 years old (as must the donee) and the process of conferring this authority must be properly registered. More than one donee may be appointed and in such a case the donor can specify whether they can act (or make decisions) only together or separately. The ability to nominate a *proxy* decision-maker for matters of personal welfare, which can include decisions about medical management, has been possible in English law only since the MCA came into force.

If the Lasting Power of Attorney authorizes the donee to make decisions about the donor's personal welfare, this can extend to the giving or refusing of consent to the carrying out or continuation of treatment by a person providing health care (e.g. by a doctor). This power, however, would authorize the donee only in the giving or refusing of consent to life-sustaining treatment if this had been specifically stated when the power was given.

The powers that may be covered under 'matters of personal welfare' include: deciding where the donor is to live (and so may be relevant to decisions such as whether a person with dementia should live in a nursing home); prohibiting a named person from having contact with the donor; medical care and giving direction that a doctor should pass medical care to another doctor.

The Court of Protection can also appoint a Deputy to make healthcare decisions on behalf of a patient, although a deputy cannot be appointed if there is a LPA.

In Scotland there is also provision for proxy consent for incompetent adults (see Box 6.6).

Advance decisions

Sections 24–26 of the MCA set out the provisions that enable competent adults aged 18 years and over to make advance decisions to refuse treatment. The Act defines an advance decision as 'a decision to refuse specified future medical treatment (and the continuation of treatment) which is made when the patient had capacity and was 18 or over' (s.24). An advance decision must specify the treatment that is to be refused and will apply only at a time when the patient lacks capacity. The effect of a valid advance decision is to enable the person to

Box 6.6 The Adults with Incapacity (Scotland) Act 2000 (http://www.opsi.gov.uk/legislation/scotland/acts2000/20000004.htm)

This Act provides comprehensive legislation concerning the welfare of adults who are incapable ('by reason of mental disorder or inability to communicate') of managing their own affairs or of giving consent, e.g. for medical treatment. It covers the management of property and financial affairs, and medical treatment and research. There is no similar legislation in England and Wales.

Definition of adult
A person who has attained the age of 16 years (s1(6)).

Least restrictive intervention
The Act states as a general principle that: 'such intervention shall be the least restrictive option in relation to the freedom of the adult, consistent with the purpose of the intervention' (s1(3)).

Definition of incapacity

" ... 'incapable' means incapable of:
(a) acting; or
(b) making decisions; or
(c) communicating decisions; or
(d) understanding decisions; or
(e) retaining the memory of decisions,

" ... by reason of mental disorder or of inability to communicate because of physical disability; but a person shall not fall within this definition by reason only of a lack or deficiency in a faculty of communication if that lack or deficiency can be made good by human or mechanical aid (whether of an interpretative nature or otherwise); and 'incapacity' shall be construed accordingly.

This definition of incapacity is, strictly speaking, relevant only to this Act: it is not necessarily the definition applicable in common law, although judges might use it as a guide in such instances.

Medical treatment where there is no guardian of the patient
If a doctor believes a patient to be incapable of giving consent to treatment then he or she may certify this:

" The 'medical practitioner primarily responsible for the medical treatment of the adult shall have, during the period specified in the certificate, authority to do what is reasonable in the circumstances, in relation to the medical treatment, to safeguard or promote the physical or mental health of the adult (s47(2)).

In order to decide what it is reasonable to do, the Act specifies the general approach that is to be taken (an approach that is relevant to all aspects of welfare covered by the Act, and not only to medical interventions). This could be seen as, in effect, outlining an approach to determining a patient's 'best interests' (although this approach is clearly legally valid only in situations covered by this Act):

66 In determining if an intervention is to be made and, if so, what intervention is to be made, account shall be taken of:

(a) the present and past wishes and feelings of the adult so far as they can be ascertained by any means of communication, whether human or by mechanical aid (whether of an interpretative nature or otherwise) appropriate to the adult;

(b) the views of the nearest relative and the primary carer of the adult, in so far as it is reasonable and practicable to do so; the views of-

(i) any guardian, continuing attorney or welfare attorney of the adult who has powers relating to the proposed intervention; and

(ii) any person whom the sheriff has directed to be consulted,

(c) in so far as it is reasonable and practicable to do so; and

(d) the views of any other person appearing to the person responsible for authorizing or effecting the intervention to have an interest in the welfare of the adult or in the proposed intervention, where these views have been made known to the person responsible, in so far as it is reasonable and practicable to do so. (s1(4))

Medical treatment where there is a guardian

If there is a guardian, welfare attorney or other authorized person the doctor ('medical practitioner primarily responsible for the medical treatment') should obtain the consent of that person to any proposed medical treatment. If there is disagreement between the doctor and the guardian as to the medical treatment:

the medical practitioner shall request the Mental Welfare Commission to nominate a medical practitioner … to give an opinion as to the medical 66 treatment proposed … Where the nominated medical practitioner certifies that, in his opinion, having regard to all the circumstances and having consulted the guardian … the proposed medical treatment should be given, the medical practitioner primarily responsible for the medical treatment of the adult may give the treatment … Where the nominated medical practitioner certifies that, in his opinion … the proposed medical treatment … should not be given, the medical practitioner primarily responsible for the medical treatment of the adult, … may apply to the Court of Session for a determination as to whether the proposed treatment should be given or not. (s.50)

A doctor may have to act rapidly, without having time to use the above procedures, in order to preserve life or prevent serious deterioration in the patient's medical condition.

Medical research

This Act also addresses the issue of medical research involving adults without capacity. See Chapter 14 for further details.

refuse the treatment when she no longer has capacity. Note that advance decisions do not empower patients to demand a particular treatment but only to refuse treatment. This is consistent with the position with regard to patients with capacity who can refuse any treatment but cannot necessarily demand a particular treatment.

Except in the case of life-sustaining treatment, advance decisions can be oral or written, and they have the same legal status as contemporaneous competent decisions to refuse treatment.

If the advance decision covers life-sustaining treatment, specific formalities must be followed. Life-sustaining treatment is treatment that in the view of the person providing health care is necessary to sustain life (s.4(10)). According to the Code of Practice this would include artificial nutrition and hydration but not basic or essential care (such as warmth, shelter and hygiene measures to maintain body cleanliness and the offer of oral food and water).

The formalities required for an advance decision refusing life-sustaining treatment are that:

1. the advance decision must be in writing
2. it must be signed by the maker (or by another person in the maker's presence and by his direction)
3. the signature must be witnessed by a witness who must also sign the document (in the maker's presence)
4. the document must be verified by a specific statement made by the maker expressly stating that the advance decision is to apply to the specified treatment 'even if life is at risk'
5. the specific statement must also be signed by the maker (or by someone else at his direction), in the presence of a witness who must also sign the statement.

An advance decision may be invalid in certain circumstances (s.25). These are that the patient:

1. has withdrawn the decision while he had capacity to do so
2. has overridden the decision by creating a Lasting Power of Attorney that covers the decision in question (see p. 86) and that was made after the advance decision
3. has done something inconsistent with the advance decision.

An advance decision may be invalid (i.e. not applicable to the treatment in question) if the circumstances are different from those set out in the advance decision, or if there are reasonable grounds for believing that circumstances have now arisen that were not anticipated by the person when making the advance decision and that would have affected the advance decision had she anticipated them (s.25(4)). There are further issues that are not explicitly stated in the Act but that must, in our view, be relevant to the question of the validity of the advance decision. These are:

• Is the advance decision (whether written or reported by a friend or relative) genuinely that of the patient?
• Did the patient have capacity to make the decision at the time it was made?
• Was the patient in possession of the relevant facts at the time of making the decision?

Under the MCA, when a doctor is satisfied that a valid and applicable advance decision to refuse treatment exists, anyone who provides treatment contrary to the advance decision may be liable to a claim for damages. Just as in relation to treatment generally, however, doctors are protected from liability in two sets of circumstances. First, a doctor will not incur liability for providing treatment unless 'satisfied' that a valid and applicable advance decision to refuse treatment exists (s.26(2)). Second, doctors will not be liable for the consequences of withholding or withdrawing treatment if they 'reasonably believe' that a valid and applicable advance decision exists refusing such treatment (s.26(3)). Interestingly, there are thus different standards of certainty in these two situations ('satisfaction' in one case and 'reasonable belief' in the other). It has been suggested that the higher standard, namely satisfaction, is appropriate in so far as a valid and applicable advance decision is as effective as a competent patient's refusal. To disregard such a refusal would therefore be a battery and potentially a criminal offence too. As regards the arguably lower standard of 'reasonable belief', it seems that failure to treat (in the absence of reasonable belief) that a valid and applicable advance decision exists is likely to constitute negligence (Bartlett 2005). The Code of Practice contains guidance for when concerns about the existence, validity or applicability might arise.

It is likely that many advance decisions will be relevant to the circumstances that actually arise but that their application will not be straightforward. Doctors will need to exercise considerable judgement in interpreting advance decisions that are ambiguous in their application to the situation that arises. In many circumstances advance decisions will be one, but only one, piece of evidence in coming to a decision about the patient's best interests. If by 'best interests' what is meant is 'what the patient would have wanted', this masks an important ambiguity. Does it mean what the patient would have said she wanted at the time of writing the advance directive had the exact circumstances that in fact occurred been described? Or does it mean what the patient would want if (magically) she regained capacity? These two may differ, either because people fail properly to imagine the future situation adequately, or because the experience, for example of being close to death, alters people's values (see discussion of strengths and weaknesses of advance directives above).

The position in law, at least since the MCA, appears to be that if a valid advance decision exists that covers the circumstances that have arisen, then it must be followed. The Code of Practice to the MCA states (clause 9.52): 'If healthcare professionals are satisfied that an advance decision to refuse treatment exists, is valid and applicable, they must follow it and not provide the treatment refused in the advance decision'. The difficulty for doctors will be to judge whether an advance directive is valid. As we have seen, the Act says (s.25(4)) that the advance decision does not apply if there are 'reasonable grounds for believing that circumstances exist which [the patient] did not anticipate at the time of the advance decision and which would have affected his decision had he anticipated them' then.

Suppose that a person writes an advance decision to the effect that, were he to suffer from Alzheimer's disease, he should not be treated for pneumonia but should instead be allowed to die. Suppose further that this person suffers from Alzheimer's disease but appears to enjoy life. He gets pneumonia.

Should we treat him? The advance decision says *no*, but we may not know whether, when the advance decision was written, the person had anticipated that life with Alzheimer's disease would (for that person) be enjoyable. In such circumstances doctors will need to make judgements in the light of the Act's position that, if the person when they made the advance decision had correctly imagined the current circumstances (e.g. that they would be happy when suffering from dementia) then the decision must be respected, and the Act's guidance on how best interests are to be determined.

As regards Scotland, the position is less clear mainly because the Adults with Incapacity (Scotland) Act 2000 does not deal directly with the issue of advance decisions to refuse treatment. The Act does, however, state that account shall be taken of the present and past wishes of the adult when interventionist activity is being taken (s.1(4)). This provision presumably allows for a valid advance decision to refuse treatment to be determinative (see further Box 6.6).

The role of the family

When patients are not capable of making decisions for themselves, clinicians usually involve families or close friends. There are five different types of information that a doctor may wish to gather from patients' relatives:

1. Explicit instructions that the patient had given to the family.
2. A general view of the patient's values.
3. Information about the patient's quality of life and likely quality of life. Relatives are often in a better position than doctors to judge these issues.
4. The relatives' opinion of what is best for the patient.
5. The relatives' opinion as to what is best for themselves. If a particular management decision will go strongly against the interests of the relatives, it is unlikely in the long run to be in the best interests of the patient. Furthermore, it is important to many people that they should not become a burden to their families (Nelson & Nelson 1995).

The MCA imposes a legal duty on doctors to consult a range of people when determining the best interests of a person who lacks capacity. Section 4(7) states that the decision-makers (e.g. doctors and other health professionals) must take into account, if it is practicable and appropriate to consult them, the views of:

- anyone named by the person as someone to be consulted on the matter in question or on matters of that kind
- anyone engaged in caring for the person or interested in his or her welfare
- any donee of a Lasting Power of Attorney
- any deputy appointed by the court
- as to what would be in the person's best interests, and, in particular, as to the matters mentioned in subsection 6 (i.e. the person's past and present wishes and feelings, beliefs and values).

CHILDREN AND CONSENT

The complex area of consent to medical treatment in those under 18 years old (minors) is discussed in Chapter 10.

REFERENCES

Bartlett P 2005 Blackstone's guide to the Mental Capacity Act. Oxford University Press, Oxford

Bolitho v City and Hackney HA [1997] 4 All ER771 HL

Buchanan A E, Brock D W 1989 Deciding for others – the ethics of surrogate decision making. Cambridge University Press, Cambridge

Chatterton v Gerson [1981] QB 432

Department of Health 1983 Mental Health Act 1983: Code of Practice, 3rd edn. HMSO, London

Department of Health 2002 Patient agreement to investigation or treatment. Consent form 1. Online. Available:http://www.doh.gov.uk

Devi v West Midlands Regional Health Authority [1980] CLY 687

Faden R R, Beauchamp T L 1986 A history and theory of informed consent. Oxford University Press, Oxford

General Medical Council 1998 Seeking patients' consent: the ethical considerations. Online. Available:http://www.

gmc-uk.org/guidance/current/library/consent.asp 12 Jun 2007

Gibbons v Wright [1954] 91 CLR 423, at p 428

Lidz C W, Meise A, Zerubavel E, Carter M, Sestak R M, Roth L H 1984 Informed consent – a study of decision making in psychiatry. Guilford Press, New York

Marshall v Curry [1933] 3 DLR 260

Murray v McMurchy [1949] 2 DLR 442

Nelson H E, Nelson J L 1995 The patient in the family – an ethics of medicine and families. Routledge, New York

Pearce v United Bristol Healthcare Trust [1998] 48 BMLR 118

Re C (Adult Refusal of Treatment) [1994] 1 All ER 819 (FD)

Richmond v Richmond [1914] III LT 273

Rogers v Whitaker [1992] 4 Med LR 79

Schloendorff v Society of New York Hospital [1914] 105NE 92

Sidaway v Board of Governors of the Bethlem Royal Hospital and the Maudsley Hospital. [1984] 1 All ER 1018, CA; [1985] 1 All ER 643, HL

FURTHER READING

Legal aspects of consent

See list of further reading to Chapter 4. Many of the core textbooks on medical ethics discuss consent in some detail (see Further reading: medical ethics in Chapter 2).

Buchanan A E, Brock D W 1990 Deciding for others: the ethics of surrogate decision making. Cambridge University Press, Cambridge

A thorough philosophical account of consent and, in particular, on making decisions on behalf of incompetent people.

Dworkin G 1988 The theory and practice of autonomy. Cambridge University Press, Cambridge

The chapter on consent, representation and proxy consent provides an excellent account of the relation between autonomy and informed consent.

Faden R, Beauchamp T 1986 A history and theory of informed consent. Oxford University Press, Oxford

This provides a legal and philosophical history of the emerging concept of informed consent to medical treatment.

Manson N, O'Neill O 2007 Rethinking informed consent in bioethics. Cambridge University Press, Cambridge

A critical look at the way in which informed consent in medicine has developed over the last decades.

Other Useful Books

Beyleveld D, Brownsword R 2007 Consent in the law. Hart, Oxford

British Medical Association 2001 Consent, rights and choices in health care for children and young people. BMA, London

British Medical Association 2001 Consent tool kit. BMA, London

Department of Health 2001 Consent: What you have a right to know: a guide for relatives and carers. DoH, London

Donnelly M 2002 Consent: bridging the gap between doctor and patient. Cork University Press, Cork

Farndon P, Douglas F 2006 Consent and confidentiality in genetic practice: guidance on genetic testing and sharing genetic information/ a report of the Joint Committee on Medical. Genetics Royal College of Physicians, London

Gilberthorpe J 1999 Consent to treatment. Medical Defence Union, London

Useful Papers

Clarke S, Oakley J 2004 Informed consent and surgeons' performance. Journal of Medicine and Philosophy F 29(1):11–35

Fraser J 2005 Ethics of HIV testing in general practice without informed consent: a case series. Journal of Medical Ethics 31(12):698–699

Harris J, Holm S 2003 Should we presume moral turpitude in our children? – Small children and consent to medical research. Theoretical Medicine and Bioethics 24(2):121–129

Kottow M 2004 The battering of informed consent. Journal of Medical Ethics 30(6):565–569

Lynoe N, Hoeyer K 2005 Quantitative aspects of informed consent: considering the dose response curve when estimating quantity of information. Journal of Medical Ethics 31(12):736–738

Newson A 2006 Should parental refusals of newborn screening be respected?. Cambridge Quarterly of Healthcare Ethics 15(2):152–160

Parker M 2004 Consent to HIV testing and consequentialism in health care ethics. Health Care Ethics Committee Forum 16(1):45–52

Skene L, Smallwood R 2002 Informed consent: lessons from Australia. British Medical Journal 324:39–41

White S M 2005 Consent for anaesthesia. Journal of Medical Ethics 30(3):286–290

Williams K 2000 Comprehending disclosure: must patients understand the risks they run? Medical Law International 4:97–109

Worthington R 2002 Clinical issues on consent: some philosophical concerns. Journal of Medical Ethics 28 377–380

6

Consent

7 Confidentiality

Medical students often find that their friends and acquaintances turn to them for support at difficult times. There is, it seems, a strong public perception that doctors, and medical students, can be trusted to keep confidences. Confidentiality is one of the cornerstones of trust that enables patients to be open with doctors about their symptoms and problems, and to undergo physical examination. From the moment that medical students start their clinical training they have access to confidential information. They will be expected to have the same standards of confidentiality as qualified doctors.

THE ENFORCEMENT OF PATIENT CONFIDENTIALITY

If a patient considers that a doctor has wrongly breached confidentiality, he can pursue his grievance in several ways: by complaining to the doctor (or, in the case of a junior doctor, to the doctor's consultant); by taking the complaint to the doctor's employer, or to the General Medical Council (GMC); or by taking the case to court.

THE ETHICAL BASIS FOR MEDICAL CONFIDENTIALITY

Definition

Much of the information a patient gives a doctor, and which a doctor gains about a patient in her professional duties, is confidential. By this it is meant that the doctor should not divulge that information to another person without the agreement (possibly implied) of the patient. Beauchamp & Childress (2001, pp. 305–306) explain confidentiality as being present 'when one person discloses information to another … and the person to whom the information is disclosed pledges not to divulge that information to a third party without the confider's permission'.

Case example

A doctor comes home after a tiring day in the clinic. He tells his wife that he saw a specific patient in the clinic, naming that patient. He goes on to tell his wife that the reason why this patient came to see him was that she had a sore throat and cold.

How serious a breach of confidentiality is this? Would it have been a more serious breach if the patient had seen the doctor because she was: pregnant; worried that she was HIV positive; or suffering from a depressive disorder?

Is the severity of the breach of confidentiality affected by what the doctor's wife does with this information? In particular, is it affected by whether: she tells no-one else (keeps it completely secret), or she tells several of her friends that this particular patient came to see her husband, and tells her friends the reason for the visit?

Four grounds for the importance of confidentiality

Respect for patient autonomy

An important principle in medical ethics is respect for patient autonomy (see Chapters 1 and 3). This principle emphasizes the patient's right to have control over his own life. It implies that a person has the right, by and large, to decide who should have access to personal information about himself. It is this principle that, in this view, underpins the importance of medical confidentiality. If this approach is applied to the above case, the key issues are: first, whether the patient gave permission to the doctor to share her confidences with his wife; and second, whether the patient minds that the doctor's wife (and her friends) knows this information. If the patient did not give permission to the doctor for him to tell his wife, there has been a breach of confidentiality.

On one view the doctor has committed a serious breach of confidentiality, whatever condition the patient suffers from and whatever his wife does with the information. On another interpretation, the seriousness of the breach depends on what view the patient would take of the breach. If the patient would not mind whether the doctor's wife knew that she had a sore throat, then the breach could be seen as minor. Because the doctor does not know what view the patient might take, in practice he should not tell his wife anyway. On this interpretation, however, the breach is likely to be much more serious if the patient were worried about her HIV status, and if the wife told her friends.

Can there be a serious breach of confidentiality if the patient never knows about the breach? On the view of confidentiality that considers that respect for patient autonomy is of key importance, the answer is yes. Suppose that the patient has a strong desire that her doctor's wife not know about her worries that she is HIV positive: her autonomy has not been respected if the doctor tells his wife, whether or not the patient knows this.

Implied promise

Some views of the doctor–patient relationship (see Chapter 5) see it as having elements of an implied contract. Such a contract may include an implied promise that doctors keep information about their patients confidential. Patients generally expect doctors to treat information confidentially, and professional guidelines emphasize the importance of high standards of confidentiality. Indeed, confidentiality is one of the central and most universal of doctors' codes of ethics. Thus patients may reasonably believe that when they come to their doctor there is an understanding that what they say will be kept confidential. If the doctor subsequently breaches confidentiality the patient may feel that the doctor has broken an implied promise.

Confidentiality

This view of confidentiality is different from that of patient autonomy. It does not ultimately depend on what the patient would want or believes. It depends on a concept of the doctor–patient relationship that is independent of what the patient believes. There are, however, two problems with this view: first, there has been no explicit promise, so the issue of an implied promise is to some extent a fiction; and, second, it raises the whole issue of why it is important to keep promises. The reason for the importance of keeping promises is likely to be grounded in one of the other theories that also underpin confidentiality.

Virtue ethics

Unlike patient autonomy, virtue ethics (see Chapter 2) focuses on the position of the doctor rather than that of the patient. This approach concentrates on the question of what makes a virtuous person, rather than what it is right to do in particular circumstances. One of the characteristics of a virtuous doctor, it might be argued, is that she is trustworthy and respects her patients' confidences. On this view, what the doctor in the case above does in talking to his wife is to act in a way contrary to that of the virtuous doctor. The degree of seriousness of the breach of confidentiality depends on the analysis of the reasons for espousing virtue ethics. However, it is the breach of confidentiality that is the critical lapse of virtue and so, on this view, the seriousness is not much affected by the specific differences envisaged in the various scenarios.

Consequentialism

On this view it is the consequences of the breach of confidentiality that determine the seriousness of the breach, and, indeed, that underlie whether breaching confidentiality is wrong in the first place. There are several different types of consequence that could be relevant here, and the analysis of the situation depends in part on how these are viewed.

The particular patient might discover the breach in confidentiality, with several possible consequences: she is angry or upset; she loses trust in that particular doctor; her loss of trust results in her receiving poorer health care because of a reluctance to see the doctor; she loses trust in doctors in general – and this might lead to her receiving poorer health care.

There may be an effect on others. The specific patient may, for example, make a complaint that becomes known more widely leading to other people losing trust in that specific doctor. This might lead to poorer health care for a larger number of people. This wider group of people may also lose trust in doctors more generally, with a deleterious effect on health care. If the profession does not set a very high standard of confidentiality then patients may have insufficient trust in doctors, with resulting poor health. The issue is not just about ill-health: there are other consequences of untreated illness. For example, if people with uncontrolled epilepsy drive, they may kill other road users. There is a public interest in ensuring that such people receive good health care in order to maximize control of the epilepsy.

In English law confidentiality is seen as important because of its consequences, and the relevant consequences are that it is in the public interest for people to trust their doctors so that they receive treatment for disease – both because it is a general public interest for people to receive good health care, and because of consequences of illness on others.

PROFESSIONAL GUIDELINES

Although not legally binding, the GMC guidelines (Boxes 7.1 & 7.2) are particularly important for four reasons:

1. A patient with a serious grievance is more likely to complain to the GMC than to sue.
2. The courts take a great deal of notice of the GMC guidelines (see below).
3. The guidelines represent the medical profession's self-imposed standards and amount to a public statement of what standard patients can expect from their doctor.
4. They are clear and well thought out.

WHAT COUNTS AS IDENTIFYING A PATIENT?

Case example: Globerg's syndrome

Professor P is giving a talk at a conference about a rare, but recently described, syndrome known as Globerg's syndrome. Professor P has collected the largest series of patients suffering from this syndrome in the world. There is debate as to the relative roles of psychological and physical causes of this syndrome. Professor P describes seven patients with the syndrome. He refers to the patients by initials: Mrs PQ, Mr SR, etc., and briefly describes the personality of these people and their medical histories. He concludes that there is no clear psychological or personality aspect that emerges. The only striking point is that all seven had taken a holiday in the Mediterranean within 3 months of the first symptoms.

Suppose that one of the subjects in Professor P's series sued Professor P on the grounds of breach of confidentiality. Suppose that this subject argued that the information about his personality and medical history – and even his holiday destination – was given to Professor P within a confidential medical consultation. Professor P had no right to inform the conference audience of these particulars. How would the law deal with such a complaint?

The first question is whether the patient gave consent to the particular disclosure of information. If the patient did give valid consent then there has not been a breach of confidentiality. The second question is whether the patient can be identified from the information provided by Professor P. The issue is not whether the patient has been named (although if she has been named it will almost certainly be a breach of confidentiality), nor whether the initials used are or are not the correct ones, but whether the patient can be identified. If, for example, the patient is suffering from rare symptoms or is one of a small community, particular care must be taken to ensure that the patient cannot be identified. If a patient is in fact identified, then in law the doctor will have breached his obligation of confidence despite the fact that he took reasonable steps to anonymize the disclosure.

Confidentiality

Box 7.1 Confidentiality and the GMC: general points (abbreviated From GMC guidelines at http://www.gmc-uk.org)

Principles of confidentiality

Patients have a right to expect that information about them will be held in confidence by their doctors. Confidentiality is central to trust between doctors and patients.

Without assurances about confidentiality, patients may be reluctant to give doctors the information they need in order to provide good care. If you are asked to provide information about patients you should:

1. seek the patient's consent to disclosure of information wherever possible, whether or not you judge that the patient can be identified from the disclosure
2. anonymize data, where unidentifiable data will serve the purpose
3. keep disclosures to the minimum necessary.

Information about patients is requested for a wide variety of purposes, including education, research, monitoring and epidemiology, public health surveillance, clinical audit, administration and planning. You have a duty to protect patients' privacy and respect their autonomy. When asked to provide information you should follow the guidance given above.

You must always be prepared to justify your decisions in accordance with this guidance.

Disclosure within teams

Where patients have consented to treatment, express consent is not usually needed before relevant personal information is shared to enable the treatment to be provided.

You should make sure that patients are aware that personal information about them will be shared within the healthcare team, unless they object, and of the reasons for this.

You must respect the wishes of any patient who objects to particular information being shared with others providing care, except where this would put others at risk of death or serious harm.

You must make sure that anyone to whom you disclose personal information understands that it is given to them in confidence, which they must respect.

Circumstances may arise where a patient cannot be informed about the sharing of information, for example because of a medical emergency. In these cases you should pass relevant information promptly to those providing the patient's care.

Disclosures that will have personal consequences for patients (e.g. to employers)

You must obtain express consent where patients may be personally affected by the disclosure, for example when disclosing personal information to a patient's employer. When seeking express consent you must make sure that patients are given enough information on which to base their decision, the reasons for the disclosure, and the likely consequences of the disclosure. You should also explain how much information will be disclosed, and to whom it will be given. If the patient withholds consent, or consent cannot be obtained, disclosures may be made only where they can be justified in the public interest, usually where it is essential to protect the patient, or someone else, from risk of death or serious harm.

Disclosures that are unlikely to have personal consequences for patients

Disclosure of information about patients for purposes such as epidemiology, public health safety or the administration of health services, or for use in education or training, clinical or medical audit, or research is unlikely to have personal consequences for the patient. In these circumstances you should still obtain patients' express consent to the use of identifiable data, or arrange for members of the healthcare team to anonymize records.

Where information is needed for the above purposes, and you are satisfied that it is not practicable either to obtain express consent to disclosure, or for a member of the healthcare team to anonymize records, data may be disclosed without express consent only where it is essential for the purpose. Such disclosures must be kept to the minimum necessary. In all such cases you must be satisfied that patients have been told, or have had access to written material informing them:

1. that their records may be disclosed to persons outside the team that provided their care
2. of the purpose and extent of the disclosure, for example to produce anonymized data for use in education, administration, research or audit
3. that the person given access to records will be subject to a duty of confidentiality
4. that they have a right to object to such a process and that their objection will be respected, except where the disclosure is essential to protect the patient, or someone else, from risk of death or serious harm.

Publication of case histories and photographs

You must obtain express consent from patients before publishing personal information about them as individuals in media to which the public has access, for example in journals or textbooks, whether or not you believe the patient can be identified. Express consent must therefore be sought to the publication of, for example, case histories about, or photographs of, patients.

Disclosure after a patient's death

You have an obligation to keep personal information confidential after a patient dies. Information may need to be disclosed to assist a coroner, procurator fiscal or other similar officer in connection with an inquest or fatal accident inquiry; as part of national confidential enquiries; or on death certificates.

In connection with judicial or other statutory proceedings

You must disclose information to satisfy a specific statutory requirement, such as notification of a known or suspected communicable disease, and if ordered to do so by a judge or presiding officer of a court. You should object if attempts are made to compel you to disclose what appear to you to be irrelevant matters.

You should not disclose personal information to a third party such as a solicitor, police officer or officer of a court without the patient's express consent, except in unusual circumstances, such as to prevent serious harm to another person.

Confidentiality

Box 7.2 Confidentiality and the GMC: the interests of others (abbreviated from GMC guidelines at http://www.gmc-uk.org)

The public interest

In cases where you have considered all the available means of obtaining consent and are satisfied that it is not practicable to do so, or that patients are not competent to give consent, or, exceptionally, in cases where patients withhold consent, personal information may be disclosed in the public interest where the benefits to an individual or to society of the disclosure outweigh the public's and the patient's interest in keeping the information confidential.

In all such cases you must weigh the possible harm (both to the patient and to the overall trust between doctors and patients) against the benefits that are likely to arise from the release of information.

Risk of harm to patient or others

Disclosure of personal information without consent may be justified where failure to do so may expose the patient or others to risk of death or serious harm. Where third parties are exposed to a risk so serious that it outweighs the patient's privacy interest, you should seek consent to disclosure where practicable. If it is not practicable, you should disclose information promptly to an appropriate person or authority. You should generally inform the patient before disclosing the information.

Such circumstances may arise, for example:

- where a colleague, who is also a patient, is placing patients at risk as a result of illness or other medical condition. If you are in doubt about whether disclosure is justified you should consult an experienced colleague, or seek advice from a professional organization. The safety of patients must come first at all times
- where a patient continues to drive, against medical advice, when unfit to do so. In such circumstances you should disclose relevant information to the medical adviser of the Driver and Vehicle Licensing Agency (DVLA) without delay
- where a disclosure may assist in the prevention or detection of a serious crime. Serious crimes, in this context, will put someone at risk of death or serious harm, and will usually be crimes against the person, such as abuse of children.

Driving against medical advice

The DVLA (see above) needs to know when driving licence holders have a condition that may affect their safety as a driver either now or in the future. Where patients have such conditions you should make sure that they understand that the condition may impair their ability to drive, and explain that they have a legal duty to inform the DVLA about the condition. If patients continue to drive when they are not fit to do so, you should make every reasonable effort to persuade them to stop. If you do not manage to persuade patients to stop driving, or you are given or find evidence that a patient is continuing to drive contrary to advice, you should disclose relevant medical information immediately, in confidence, to the medical adviser at the DVLA. Before giving information to the DVLA you should try to inform the patient of your decision to do so. Once the DVLA has been informed, you should also write to the patient to confirm that a disclosure has been made.

If a patient is incapable of understanding your advice, for example because of dementia, you should inform the DVLA immediately.

Crime

Prompt disclosure to an appropriate person or authority may be necessary for the prevention or detection of a serious crime.

According to the 2003 NHS Confidentiality Code of Practice, staff are permitted to disclose personal information:

> ❝ to prevent and support the detection, investigation and punishment of serious crime and/or prevent abuse or serious harm to others where they judge on a case by case basis, that the public good that would be achieved by disclosure outweighs both the obligation of confidentiality to individual patients and the broader public interest in the provision of a confidential service.

The Code acknowledges that although the concept of 'serious crime' is unclear it does include rape, murder, manslaughter, treason, kidnapping and child abuse. As to the risk of harm, the Code states that this would include disclosures to prevent child abuse, neglect, assault and traffic accidents, and the spread of infectious diseases.

HIV and AIDS (guidelines from General Medical Council 1995)

The GMC believes that, where HIV infection or AIDS has been diagnosed, any difficulties that arise concerning confidentiality will usually be overcome if doctors are prepared to discuss openly and honestly with patients the implications of their condition and the need to secure the safety of others.

If, having considered the matter carefully in the light of such counselling, the patient still refuses to allow the general practitioner to be informed, then their request for privacy should be respected. The only exception to that general principle arises where the doctor judges that the failure to disclose would put the health of any of the healthcare team at serious risk. The GMC believes that, in such a situation, it would not be improper to disclose such information as that person needs to know.

Disclosure to patient's spouse or sexual partner

The GMC has reached the view that there are grounds for such a disclosure only where there is a serious and identifiable risk to a specific individual who, if not so informed, would be exposed to infection. Therefore, when a person is found to be infected in this way, the doctor must discuss with the patient the question of informing a spouse or other sexual partner. The GMC believes that most such patients will agree to disclosure in these circumstances, but where such consent is withheld the doctor may consider it a duty to seek to ensure that any sexual partner is informed, in order to safeguard such persons from infection.

THE LEGAL APPROACH TO CONFIDENTIALITY: THE BALANCING OF PUBLIC INTERESTS

Box 7.3 summarizes the key legal aspects of confidentiality. There is, however, important statute law that covers specific situations, summarized in Box 7.4.

The balancing of public interests

The legal basis for confidentiality is not as clear as one might expect (Herring 2006). It is probably best to see a doctor's legal obligation as a public, not a

Box 7.3 Key legal aspects of confidentiality

There is a general legal obligation for doctors to keep confidential what patients tell them. This obligation is not absolute:

- There are situations when the law obliges doctors to breach confidentiality.
- There are situations when the law allows doctors to breach confidentiality.

In both of these situations it is important that the doctor breaches confidentiality only to the relevant person(s) or authority(ies).

The general obligation for doctors to maintain confidentiality is a public not a private interest (see main text). In other words, from the legal perspective what is important is the public interest for patients to be able to trust their doctors to maintain confidentiality. Therefore, the issue of when it is lawful, and when not lawful, for a doctor to breach confidentiality is often a question of balancing public interests (not of balancing a private versus a public interest).

The General Medical Council (GMC) provides professional guidelines on the issue of confidentiality. Although these do not have the force of law, they are taken seriously by the courts. No breach of confidentiality has occurred if:

- a patient gives consent, or
- the patient cannot be identified.

Sharing information about patients with other members of the healthcare team, for the purpose of providing the best treatment, is not generally viewed by the law as a breach of confidentiality.

A doctor must take reasonable precautions to prevent confidential information from falling into the wrong hands (i.e. confidential medical information must be kept reasonably secure).

The NHS Confidentiality Code of Practice for NHS staff (Department of Health 2003) is a lengthy and detailed document that describes what a confidential service looks like, provides a description of the main legal requirements, recommends a generic decision support tool for sharing/disclosing information, and lists examples of particular situations for sharing information.

Four steps to how lawyers look at clinical confidentiality (with acknowledgement and thanks to Charles Foster, barrister) are the following:

1. Was the information given to the clinician 'in circumstances of confidentiality'? Almost all disclosures to doctors occur in the context of a relationship in which confidentiality is expected, but if the information is already in the public domain then any confidentiality that it might originally have had will have evaporated.
2. Is the information of a private or intimate nature? Most information given to a doctor in a clinical setting will be, but perhaps some (such as the patient travelled on the number 37 bus) may not. It is, however, wise for doctors to assume that all information given to them is confidential.
3. Has the doctor disclosed the information without the consent of the patient? An unauthorized disclosure need not be deliberate: it can be inadvertent, as when a doctor is overheard in a lift, or leaves patient notes on a bus.
4. Does the public interest in non-disclosure outweigh the public interest in disclosure? See main text for a discussion of this aspect of confidentiality.

If the answer to all four questions is *yes* then, from the legal point of view, there has been a culpable breach of confidentiality.

Box 7.4   Statutes relevant to medical confidentiality

NB: Most legal aspects of confidentiality are governed by common law. The following statues govern the law in restricted circumstances.

Public Health (Control of Diseases) Act 1984 (Notifiable Diseases)
A doctor must notify the relevant local authority officer (usually a public health consultant) if he or she suspects a patient of having a notifiable disease or food poisoning. The following information must be provided (by completing a specific certificate): patient's name, age, sex, address, suspected disease, approximate date of onset and date of admission to hospital (if appropriate). An up-to-date list of notifiable diseases can be obtained from NHS Direct at http://www.nhsdirect.nhs.uk.

Abortion Act 1967
A doctor carrying out a termination of pregnancy must notify the relevant Chief Medical Officer, including giving the name and address of the woman concerned.

Notification of births and deaths – Births and Deaths Registration Act 1953
Parents have a legal duty to register the details (child's name, sex, date and place of birth, parents' names, places of birth, address and father's occupation) of a birth with the local registrar within 42 days. The doctor or midwife normally has a duty to inform the district medical officer of the birth within 6 hours.

Stillbirths (a baby born dead after the 24th week of pregnancy) must also be registered. Doctors attending patients during their last illness must sign a death certificate, giving cause of death (to their best knowledge). The certificate must be sent to the registrar. The registrar must inform the coroner of deaths that occur without attendance of a doctor at the last illness, or during an operation, or while the effects of an anaesthetic persist.

Road Traffic Act 1988
All citizens, including doctors, must provide the police, on request, with information (name, address) that might identify a driver alleged to have committed a traffic offence (see Box 7.6). This would not normally justify providing clinical information without the patient's consent, or a court order.

Human Fertilization and Embryology Act 1990, modified by the Human Fertilization and Embryology (Disclosure of Information) Act 1992
This Act regulates assisted reproduction and research on human embryos outside the human body (see Chapter 9, p. 149). Relevant to confidentiality are the following:

- The Human Fertilization and Embryology Authority keeps a register recording the names of all those for whom infertility treatments under the Act were provided, and of all those born, or probably born, as a result of such treatments. The doctors providing such treatments must therefore provide the names of the relevant patients to the register.
- Individuals aged over 18 years are entitled to find out whether they are on the register, and whether the register shows that their parents may not be their genetic parents, and whether they are related to a person they propose to marry.
- The confidentiality of gamete donors is strictly protected.
- The patient's consent is normally needed before information, e.g. that the patient has undergone treatment for infertility, is passed to someone else – even to the patient's own general practitioner (GP).

NHS Venereal Diseases Regulations 1974

This requires health authorities to take all necessary steps to ensure that information capable of identifying patients with sexually transmitted diseases should not be disclosed except for the purpose of treating the disease and preventing its spread. Such disclosure, furthermore, can be made only to a doctor, or to someone working on a doctor's instruction in connection with treatment or prevention. This allows contact tracing. However, it does not allow those working in a genitourinary clinic to inform an insurance company of a patient's sexually transmitted disease – even with the patient's consent. Case notes from genitourinary clinics are kept separate from other hospital records. GPs are not routinely informed of the patient's attendance at such clinics, although the patient may request that the GP be informed.

The Children Act 1989

See p. 154.

Terrorism Act 2000

The Act imposes a duty on health professionals to report their suspicions that a person has been involved in terrorist activities. This duty of disclosure applies even if the health professional has not specifically been asked for information.

The Human Rights Act 1998

Article 8 of the Convention on Human Rights states that: 'Everyone has the right to respect for his private ... life' (see main text for impact on medical confidentiality).

private, interest. It is for this reason that the obligation of confidentiality is not absolute. Because the duty of confidentiality is thus qualified, there are circumstances in which doctors can justifiably breach confidentiality. Some of these arise from legislation (see below). The most problematic justification is, however, the public interest criterion: that a breach is justified if the public interest in breaching confidentiality outweighs the public interest in maintaining confidentiality. It is problematic because there is little guidance from the courts as to the meaning of public interest.

A key case that established four important principles was that of W v Egdell [1990]. The first principle is that in order for the disclosure of confidential information to be justified there must be a serious risk of danger to the public (including to an individual). In other words the 'public interest' in maintaining medical confidentiality is strong. It seems likely that a doctor who breached medical confidentiality in order to help the police with regard to a crime against property could be found liable. Second, the GMC's guidelines on confidentiality, although not law, are taken very seriously by the courts. Third, disclosure should be limited to those with a legitimate interest in knowing the information. Fourth, only the minimum information necessary to protect the public should be disclosed.

The impact of the Human Rights Act 1998 (HRA) on confidentiality

Prior to the HRA, medical confidentiality was seen as a *public* interest. The HRA, and the case of Campbell v MGN [2004] (see below), established, more clearly than before, that in English law people have a *private* right to confidentiality. However, because this is not absolute, and as the public interest in medical confidentiality is considered to be strong, the HRA has had relatively little impact on medical confidentiality. Its impact has been greater in other settings, such as confidentiality and the media, where the private right to confidentiality has given greater protection to individual privacy than previously.

The leading case on the impact of the Human Rights Act 1998 on confidentiality is Campbell v MGN [2004]. Although no medical practitioner was involved in disclosing medical information (the case was about the publication of details of a famous model's drug therapy), several important points were made by the judges. These are worth noting as they would undoubtedly influence a court's approach should a case alleging breach of medical confidentiality arise.

First, the case marked a shift in language, away from the idea of balancing public interests to a balance of Article rights. The relevant Articles are 8 (right to respect for private life) and 10 (right to freedom of expression). This means that, although the balancing exercise is basically the same as balancing public interests, it must be more 'carefully focused and penetrating'. Second, by emphasizing the values underpinning respect for private life, namely privacy and personal autonomy, the need for a confidential relationship becomes less important. In other words, the right to privacy attaches to private information, irrespective of the circumstances in which that information was disclosed.

Situations when doctors are legally obliged to maintain confidentiality

Most breaches of medical confidentiality that would be considered by the GMC as misconduct are inadvertent and a result of carelessness. Breaching confidentiality in order to amuse one's dinner guests, for example, is likely to be taken extremely seriously, both by the courts and by the GMC.

Case example: in the supermarket

Dr B is a general practitioner in a small country town. Three days ago she saw Miss Elaine X in her surgery. Miss X is a 20-year-old student who had been feeling unusually tired for over a month. Dr B had sent off a number of blood tests. Dr B is shopping in the local small supermarket when she bumps into Miss X's mother. 'Oh, doctor, have you had the blood test results back on Elaine?'. What should Dr B reply? It is potentially a breach of confidentiality for Dr B even to confirm to Mrs X that her adult daughter has been to see her, let alone to tell Mrs X the test results, unless of course Miss X has given her consent. Dr B would be wise to use a bland phrase for all such occasions, such as: 'I'm afraid I cannot discuss any of my patients outside the surgery'. It is unsafe to assume that Miss X does not mind her mother knowing she has visited the doctor.

Situations when specific statutes impose a legal duty to disclose confidential information

There are a number of situations when the law imposes a duty on doctors to disclose specific information to a specific person, or people. This is mainly through specific statutes (see Box 7.4).

Situations when doctors may have discretion

Because the law sees confidentiality as a matter of public interest, there is a wide range of situations where it is unclear whether the public interest is best served by the doctor maintaining confidentiality or by breaching it. It is likely that, in many instances, the courts would allow doctors to exercise discretion: in other words, the courts would not find against doctors whether they breached or maintained confidentiality, as long as the doctor had acted thoughtfully and could provide a coherent explanation for his action. The GMC provides useful guidance (see Boxes 7.1 & 7.2). Box 7.5 summarizes legal considerations concerning when doctors should or should not breach confidentiality.

Case example: the police phone the casualty officer

Box 7.6 summarizes some key issues for a casualty officer if phoned by the police enquiring about a patient in the course of investigating a possible crime.

CONFIDENTIALITY AND THE HEALTHCARE TEAM

See Box 7.1 for a summary of the GMC's guidance.

CONFIDENTIALITY AND MEDICAL STUDENTS

The position of medical students raises two issues: first, the question of students' access to confidential information, and second, their legal responsibilities with regard to maintaining confidentiality. If they are to be properly educated, students need to have access to confidential information about patients. Although in practice clinical students are often part of the healthcare team, the prime reason for their access to confidential information is for the purpose of students' own education. The GMC states: 'Patients' consent to disclosure of information for teaching and audit must be obtained unless the data have been effectively anonymized'.

There is little doubt from the legal point of view that patients have the right to refuse to see medical students, and to refuse to allow medical students access to their notes. It might be argued that patients should not normally exercise such a right; that a patient cannot expect, on the one hand, to be looked after by well trained doctors and, on the other hand, not be prepared to enable medical students to receive training.

Medical students, just like doctors, have a duty to keep confidential information about patients that they learn in the course of their clinical studies. It seems unlikely that courts would sanction breaches of confidentiality in students that they would not allow in doctors. Furthermore, students would be expected, when they introduce themselves, to make it clear to patients that they are students and not doctors.

Occasionally a patient may tell a student something and ask the student not to tell anyone else – not even the doctors and nurses. The student will have to use some judgement in such circumstances. It is probably safer for the student to share the information with the relevant consultant, rather than withhold information that may be important, either for the sake of the patient or in the

---

Box 7.5 Summary of when doctors should or should not breach confidentiality

When doctors should not breach confidentiality (unless with consent of patient)

- 'Casual breaches', e.g. for amusement, or carelessly.
- Simply to satisfy another person's curiosity.
- To prevent minor crime, or to help conviction in the case of minor crime. Most crime against property would probably count as minor crimes in this context.
- To prevent minor harm to someone else.
- In the case of doctors working in a genitourinary clinic, no information that might identify a patient examined or treated for any sexually transmitted disease should be provided to a third party, except in a few specific situations (see Box 7.6).
- A doctor should not write a report, or fill in a form, disclosing confidential information (e.g. for an insurance company) without the patient's consent (preferably written).

NB: It would be unwise for a doctor to lie in order to protect patient confidentiality, for example to write on an insurance form that the patient has not had an HIV test when in fact she had. If the patient subsequently made an insurance claim and the lie was discovered, not only might the insurance company refuse to pay but the patient might successfully sue the doctor because the doctor's actions had led to her not being insured.

When doctors must breach confidentiality (to specific authorities only)

- Notifiable diseases
- Termination of pregnancy
- Births
- Deaths
- To police, on request. name and address of driver of vehicle who is alleged to be guilty of offence under Road Traffic Act 1988
- Search warrant signed by circuit judge
- Under court orders.

When doctors have discretion (see main text)

- Sharing information with other members of the healthcare team in the interests of the patient
- Patient continuing to drive who is not medically fit to do so (NB: The GMC advises doctors to inform DVLA medical officer)
- When a third party is at significant risk of harm (e.g. spouse of HIV-positive person)
- The detection or prevention of serious crime (but see Box 7.2).

---

public interest. It is unwise for students to promise to keep information confidential from the consultant in advance of knowing what that information is.

CONFIDENTIALITY AND PUBLICATION

Similar issues arise with regard to publication both of written material and pictures. Most journals now require explicit consent from patients if their case history or image is to be used in publication. The editor of the *British Medical Journal* wrote: 'Authors and editors must thus ensure that patients have given

Box 7.6   When the police phone the casualty officer: six steps that the casualty office should take

1. Write down the caller's name, rank and police station.
2. Ask the caller for information as to why the request is being made and the nature of the suspected crime under investigation.
3. Say that he will phone back, and put the phone down.
4. If there is a patient who fits the description, the casualty officer needs to do a number of things:
   - It would be sensible to discuss the situation with a senior doctor.
   - If the police were investigating a road traffic accident then the hospital would have to provide the name and address (but not clinical details) of any person for whom there were reasonable grounds to suppose that they might have been the driver involved (see Box 7.4).
   - If the crime was not serious (e.g. a crime against property not involving physical damage to anyone), then if the casualty officer were to inform the police she could be in breach of GMC guidelines.
   - If the crime did involve significant injury then the casualty officer and her seniors would probably be legally safe to inform the police.
   - Consider whether to ask the patient for permission to inform the police. However, this should be done only if the doctors are happy not to inform the police if the patient refuses consent.
5. Check the phone number of the caller's police station through some independent source (e.g. the phone book). The reason for this is to ensure that the phone call was genuinely from the police, and not from someone impersonating the police, such as an unscrupulous reporter or someone wishing to harm the patient.
6. Having decided, after discussion with seniors, on what information to provide, the police can be phoned back.

The casualty officer should not tell a lie. If the decision has been taken not to tell the police, the casualty officer should not falsely say, 'There is no one fitting your description' but, 'I'm afraid we cannot provide confidential information in these circumstances'. Such a reply is, of course, likely to make the police suspicious that there is someone fitting the description, but there seems to be no way round this.

their consent to publication whenever there is a possibility that the patient may be identified' (Smith 1995, p. 1241).

In practice, the journal editors consider that patients may be identified from most case histories even where some of the details have been changed.

The GMC guidelines on visual and audio recording of patients require that patients give permission even when they could not be identified. (General Medical Council 1997, Hood et al 1998). Such a position gives patients rights akin to ownership, rather than confidentiality over an image of themselves.

CONFIDENTIALITY AND THE INCOMPETENT PATIENT

The incompetent patient cannot, by definition, give consent for information to be passed on to someone else. The general legal criterion, in the case of incompetent patients, is for doctors to act in the patient's best interests (as defined by the

Mental Capacity Act; see Chapters 3 and 6). Sharing information about diagnosis, treatment and prognosis with close relatives or key carers would normally be seen as in a patient's best interests. However, an incompetent patient has the same legal protection from casual breaches of confidentiality as a competent patient, and the same protection from being harmed through a breach of confidentiality.

CONFIDENTIALITY AND CHILDREN

The key legal issue is whether the child is competent to give or withhold permission for information to be shared (see Chapter 10). A child aged 16 years and above is assumed competent unless there are specific grounds (such as learning disability) for doubting this. The doctor owes the obligation of confidentiality to the child and not to the parents. Thus the doctor must generally seek the child's permission, either explicitly or inferred from the child's conduct, in order to discuss the case with the parents. This is also the case for a child aged less than 16 years who is 'Gillick competent'. However, even with a competent child the situation is not the same as with a competent adult. This is because a doctor has an obligation to act in a child's best interests. What this means in practice is that if a child refuses disclosure to her parents, but the doctor believes that the child's best interests in fact require that the matter be discussed with the parents, then it is generally thought that that disclosure would be lawful. The doctor must be prepared to justify such disclosure as being necessary to avoid a demonstrable risk of harm to the child.

When a child patient is not competent, the doctor would normally be acting lawfully in discussing her medical treatment with the parents, and, indeed, parental consent for treatment would normally be necessary (see Chapter 10).

The legal position in Scotland is different. The Age of Legal Capacity (Scotland) Act 1991 gives various legal rights to children under 16 years old, including the right to confidentiality if the child has the competence to understand the relevant issues.

PATIENTS AND THEIR MEDICAL NOTES

A series of Acts gives patients the legal right to see their medical notes (health records), medical reports, personal data held on computer and their personal file held by social services. Boxes 7.7 and 7.8 summarize the legal position.

Court proceedings, medical records and the doctor

Doctors may be asked to show the medical records of a patient to, for example, a solicitor because they are relevant evidence in court proceedings. The general principle is that records (or copies of the records) may be released only with the permission of the patient, or in response to a court order (in which case the order must be complied with). The procedure is slightly different in different settings.

The police have no right to inspect a person's medical records – although a doctor may consider it right to breach a patient's confidentiality to the police in some circumstances. A circuit judge (but not a magistrate), however, can order the medical records to be released to the police.

Box 7.7 Statutes relevant to patients' access to records

Data Protection Act 1998
See Box 7.8.

Access to Medical Reports Act 1988
Gives patients the restricted right of access to any medical report relating to them that has been supplied by a doctor (medical practitioner) for employment or insurance purposes.

Access to Health Records Act 1990
This has been replaced by the Data Protection Act 1998, except in relation to the records of deceased persons. The executor or administrator of a deceased person's estate may apply under the Access to Health Records Act 1990 for access to health records; the Data Protection Act 1998 does not cover this situation.

Box 7.8 Data Protection Act 1998

This Act sets out eight principles that apply to both computer records and records held in manual form (e.g. patients' medical notes). These principles are designed to ensure that personal data shall be accurate, relevant, held only for specific defined purposes for which the user has been registered, not kept for longer than is necessary, and not disclosed to any unauthorized persons.

A key term is 'data subjects'. These are the people to whom the data apply, e.g. patients or participants in research. The Act gives statutory right for data subjects to have access to personal information held on them, subject to certain exceptions (see below). The Act enables data subjects:

1. to be informed as to whether personal data are processed
2. to be given a description of the data held, the purposes for which they are processed, and knowledge of the persons to whom the data may be disclosed
3. to be given a copy of the information constituting the data
4. to be given information on the source of the information.

NB: The Act defines the 'processing' of data as 'obtaining, recording, or carrying out any operation including retrieval or consultation, or use of information, and disclosure'.

The data subject also has the right of rectification, i.e. the right to have inaccuracies in the data corrected. Data subjects may seek compensation for any harm suffered as a result of the inaccuracy.

For a patient to gain access to his personal health record a request must be made in writing. A response must be given by the appropriate person or institution within 40 days of the request, or the applicant must be informed that there are grounds for withholding the information. Information can be withheld in certain circumstances, for example:

• when access 'would be likely to cause serious harm to the physical or mental health or condition of the data subject or any other person'

- where the request for access is made by another person on behalf of the data subject, such as a parent or child, and if the data subject had provided the information in the expectation that it would not be disclosed
- where 'Giving access would reveal the identity of another person, unless that person has given consent to the disclosure or it is reasonable to comply with the access request without that consent. This does not apply if the third party is a health professional who has been involved in the care of the patient unless serious harm to that health professional's physical or mental health or condition is likely to be caused by giving access.'

Box 7.9 Guidelines to doctors when writing in patients' medical notes (healthcare records) (based on recommendations of the Medical Defence Union)

The primary function of medical records is the communication of health information between professionals, and recording information to help the doctor in the future care of the patient. Records should be:

- legible
- date and time recorded
- signed, and name also written clearly.

Use only approved, unambiguous abbreviations. Records should relate primarily to diagnosis and management. Offensive remarks and jokes do not go down well in court.
  Errors should be:

- corrected by crossing through with a single line
- signed and dated.

A patient cannot dictate what goes into the notes. Never alter or add to notes, especially after notification of a complaint or claim, in the hope that it will be assumed they were written contemporaneously.

If a coroner asks to see the medical records of a dead patient, this should be complied with. On the other hand, if a life assurance company requests the medical records of a dead patient, this should be complied with only with the consent of a personal representation of the dead person's estate.

Box 7.9 gives guidelines for doctors in writing medical notes.

Children's medical records

A child of 16 years or more, and a 'Gillick competent' child aged less than 16 years (see Chapter 10) can give consent for the release of her medical records to a third party. Otherwise, consent must be given by a person with 'parental responsibility' (see Chapter 10). In Scotland, the Age of Legal Capacity (Scotland) Act 1991 gives statutory rights to 'mature' children under 16 years of age to give consent to the release of medical records.

REFERENCES

Beauchamp T L, Childress J F 2001 Principles of biomedical ethics, 5th edn. Oxford University Press, Oxford

Campbell v MGN [2004] UKHL 22

Department of Health 2003 Confidentiality: NHS Code of Practice. Department of Health, London. Online. Available:http://www.dh.gov.uk

General Medical Council 1995 HIV and AIDS: the ethical considerations. GMC, London. Online. Available:http://www.gmc-uk.org/guidance/archive/hiv_and_aids_oct_1995.pdf4 Jul 2007

General Medical Council 1997 Making and using visual and audio recordings of patients. GMC, London

General Medical Council 2000 Confidentiality: protecting and providing information. GMC, London. Online. Available:http://www.gmc-uk.org/guidance/current/library/confidentiality.asp12 Jun 2007

Herring J 2006 Medical health law and ethics. Oxford University Press, Oxford

Hood C A, Hope T, Dove P 1998 Videos, photographs, and patient consent. British Medical Journal 316:1009–1011

Smith R 1995 Publishing information about patients. British Medical Journal 311:1240–1241

W v Egdell [1990] 1 All ER 835

FURTHER READING

Most medical law textbooks (see Further Reading to Chapter 4) and general books on medical ethics (see Further Reading to chapter 2) address confidentiality.

McHale J 1993 Medical confidentiality and legal privilege. Routledge, London

This legal textbook focuses on medical confidentiality and addresses ethical as well as legal issues.

Genetics

8

A code combines the allure of a secret with the challenge of a puzzle. Breaking the 'genetic code' suggests more than mere understanding of mechanisms of protein production, biological development and heredity. It is as though, in a secular world, we have discovered the fundamental language of nature. No wonder that the claims for genetics are grand, and that they attract such widespread ethical concerns. However, few of the ethical issues discussed in the context of modern medical genetics are unique to that context, although genetic tests and therapies may make common some ethical problems that have, until now, been rare. We will consider some of the ethical issues relevant to modern medical genetics under five headings: genetic information, genetic testing, reproductive choice, gene therapy and cloning.

GENETIC INFORMATION

Non-directive counselling

Genetic counselling has been defined as 'the process by which patients or relatives at risk of a disorder that may be hereditary are advised of the consequences of the disorder, the probability of developing and transmitting it and of the way in which this may be prevented or ameliorated' (Harper 1988). The idea of 'non-directive counselling' was one of the first explicit models of the doctor–patient relationship that influenced practice and challenged the paternalistic model (see Chapter 5). In the context of reproductive choice, the purpose of non-directive counselling is to uphold the personal nature of reproductive choice and to ensure that counsellors avoid passing judgement on the worthiness of the life of a person affected with a genetic condition (Murray 1996). It is a clear and definitive response to the coercive practices of eugenics in the early 20th century and it distances clinical genetics from those eugenic practices. The case of Bob (Box 8.1) challenges the view that non-directive counselling is always the right approach. Box 8.2 summarizes some arguments for and against such counselling.

GENETIC INFORMATION AND THE LAW

As genetic information becomes increasingly important and available, questions about confidentiality may become more complex. In the absence of any specific legislation or case law concerning genetic confidentiality it has

Box 8.1 The case of Bob – a challenge to non-directive counselling

Bob's mother died from bowel cancer at the age of 32 years. She was found to have familial adenomatous polyposis. This genetic disorder involves the development of many polyps in the bowel and leads in time to almost certain bowel cancer. Colonoscopy can detect cancerous lesions early, and treatment is effective. Prophylactic colectomy is also an option. A genetic counsellor explains these facts. Bob understands them. The counsellor also explains that there is a 50% chance that Bob has inherited the gene. Bob states that he does not wish to have either a genetic test or a colonoscopy. The counsellor ensures that Bob has understood the key facts. Two years later Bob develops cancer and dies.

Box 8.2 Arguments for and against non-directive counselling

For
- It reduces the risk of coercion.
- The patient is best placed to make decisions about genetic testing.
- The patient's values, not the counsellor's, are paramount.
- It promotes active autonomous decision-making.

Against
- It is not possible, even in theory, because any way of presenting the information has some effect on decision-making and is therefore biasing.
- Patients may want and need advice and direction (see Chapters 3 & 5).
- It denies patients the opportunity for moral dialogue about their choices.
- It allows patients to make wrong decisions without discussion.
- It leaves no place for persuasion.
- It is inconsistent with other areas of medical practice where advice is given.

been suggested that the law could take several approaches. Herring (2006, pp. 177–181), for example, suggests the following options:

1. *The traditional confidentiality approach.* According to this approach only where there is a high risk of significant harm to another would a breach of confidentiality be justifiable. Factors to be taken into account in reaching a decision would therefore include the risk of the relative suffering from the illness, the severity of the illness, the availability of a cure or treatment, and so on.
2. *A human rights approach.* Under a rights-based approach the central question would be the extent to which the exception contained in Article 8(2) of the Human Rights Act would justify breaching confidentiality. Very strong reasons would be required to justify disclosure given that the genetic information might be regarded as even more private than other medical information, because it is related to arguably the most intimate part of a person.
3. *A property approach.* Such an approach reflects a widely held belief by the public that a person's genetic information belongs not just to them but

also to their relatives. This means that a daughter could claim (under the Data Protection Act 1998) that information about her mother is information held about her.

The absence of case law in this area means that currently it is not possible to say which approach will be taken. In the absence of such case law perhaps the safest approach is the traditional one using the core General Medical Council (GMC) standard that a breach of confidentiality is justified only 'where failure to do so may expose the patient or others to risk of death or serious harm'. Better still, if possible, is to gain the patient's consent to inform relevant relatives of genetic information that may be important to them.

GENETIC TESTING

Genetic tests are medical tests. What makes them unusual (although not unique) is that the results may provide significant medical information not only for the person who has the test, but also for her genetically related relatives. For this reason genetic tests often raise issues of confidentiality that are unusual with other medical tests. Current GMC guidelines, and case law, do not treat medical confidentiality as absolute (see Chapter 7). Box 8.3 describes two hypothetical, but realistic, clinical scenarios that raise questions of whether or not the confidentiality of the patient undergoing the test should be breached.

Competent adults

The British Medical Association (1998, p. 72) states that the following factors should be considered before disclosing genetic information to relatives without the consent of the patient:

- The severity of the disorder
- The level of predictability of the condition
- What action relatives could take to protect themselves or make more informed reproductive decisions
- The level of harm and benefit of giving or withholding the information
- The reason given for refusing to share the information.

Case 1 (see Box 8.3), involving the question of whether to disclose non-paternity, presents a situation where clinicians vary considerably in their practice. Anecdotal evidence suggests that most favour telling a 'white lie' to the husband and letting the woman know the implications of the test. Lucassen & Parker (2001) argue against this practice, on the grounds both that it does not sufficiently respect the man's interest in knowing the facts, and that it is contrary to the principle that doctors should not lie to patients except in most unusual circumstances. Case 2 (see Box 8.3) describes a situation where the patient has probably broken the terms of her contract with the fertility clinic and may have committed a crime. Professional guidelines do not suggest that doctors should breach confidentiality simply on the grounds that a patient has broken the law (see Chapter 7); however, in this case a child may be conceived with a serious genetic problem.

Box 8.3 Two clinical scenarios that raise questions of whether the confidentiality of the patient undergoing the test should be breached

Case 1: Non-paternity

John and Sarah attend the genetics clinic after the diagnosis of an autosomal recessive condition in their newborn baby. The disorder is severe and debilitating, and there is a high chance that the child will die in the first year. The gene for this disorder has just been mapped, and there is a possibility that prenatal diagnosis would be possible in a future pregnancy. John and Sarah give their consent for a blood sample to be taken for DNA extraction, for themselves and from their affected child. Molecular analysis of these samples shows that John is not the biological father of the child.

At the first consultation, when the condition was explained to them, they were told that there was a 25% chance that any future baby of theirs would be affected. The carrier frequency for this condition is about 1 in 1000, and thus the chance that John is also a carrier (as he is not the biological father) is negligible.

Should the geneticist disclose the finding of non-paternity to the parents when they come back to the clinic as part of their ongoing counselling? Although they did not seek information about paternity, it is of direct relevance to their understanding of the probability of an affected child in future pregnancies (Lucassen & Parker 2001).

Case 2: Eggs donated to a fertility clinic

A woman whose mother has Huntington's disease tests positive for the condition, although as yet she has no symptoms. During the post-test counselling the woman reveals that she donated eggs to a private fertility clinic 6 months ago. She refuses permission for the counsellor to contact the clinic because she is afraid she will get into trouble.

Case 3: Duchenne muscular dystrophy (based on Parker & Lucassen 2004)

A 4-year-old boy has been diagnosed with Duchenne muscular dystrophy (DMD), a severe, progressive muscle-wasting disease associated with a life expectancy of 20–30 years. DMD is an X-linked recessive genetic condition. The boy's mother, Helen, is shown to be a carrier for the mutation; this means that any sons she has will have a 50% chance of inheriting the condition.

Helen's sister, Penelope, is 10 weeks' pregnant. She knows that her nephew has speech and development delay but does not know the diagnosis. Her family doctor referred her to the clinical genetics unit. Penelope told the geneticist that she would want to terminate her pregnancy were her fetus to have a serious genetic condition. From the information given to the doctor by Penelope it would not be usual practice to test her to see whether she is a carrier for DMD, or to test her fetus. Furthermore, for technical reasons, it would probably not be possible to test reliably without using information from her nephew and sister about the precise mutation responsible for her nephew's DMD.

At her next meeting with the clinical geneticist, Helen says that she knows that her sister is pregnant and that she understands that the pregnancy could be affected. She also says that she has not discussed this with her sister, both because they are not close and because she suspects that if her sister's fetus were tested and found to be affected Penelope would terminate the pregnancy. Helen feels very strongly that this would be wrong. Helen tells the geneticist that she wants her test results and information about her son to remain confidential.

Should the geneticists who are advising both sisters respect Helen's wishes, and her confidentiality, with the result that Penelope would remain ignorant of the genetic risk to her fetus? Or should the geneticists use the information they have as a result of testing Helen and her son to test Penelope or her fetus and provide Penelope with the information she would want in order to make her reproductive choices?

Case 3 raises the question of what should be the principles that govern genetic confidentiality within families. On the 'personal account model' (Parker & Lucassen 2004). which is the traditional approach discussed in Chapter 7, the question is whether the harm to Penelope and her fetus is sufficiently severe to justify the breach of Helen's confidentiality. This is not a simple question to answer. How important is reproductive choice? To Penelope it is very important, but it is not clear that failure to provide her with the information about her nephew, or to test her using information gained from testing him, amounts to 'risk of death or serious harm'. And how is one to evaluate the risks to Penelope's fetus, or potential future child? On one view the greatest harm would be termination of pregnancy. On such a view breaching confidentiality is more likely to cause harm than prevent it. On another view – the view that the fetus is not a person but that the future potential child is – it might be argued that failure to breach confidentiality could lead to the harm of having the serious condition of Duchenne muscular dystrophy (DMD) – a harm that could have been prevented. On yet another view, as the choice is between a child existing with DMD, or not existing (if the fetus is aborted), then even though DMD is a serious condition it is better than not existing at all (see discussion of the non-identity issue, p. 145).

Parker & Lucassen (2004) propose an alternative model: the 'joint account model'. This is similar to the 'property approach' outlined by Herring in a legal context (see above). According to this model 'genetic information is shared by more than one person, much like information about a joint bank account' (Parker & Lucassen 2004). Thus, the ethical position is 'not about the appropriate limits to confidentiality but is analogous to me asking my bank manager not to reveal information about a joint account to my fellow account holders'.

The first model sees genetic information as essentially personal, the second as belonging to families. According to the first model the presumption is that genetic information remains confidential to the individual unless there are very good reasons why someone else should have access to that information. According to the second model the presumption is that genetic information is to be shared with family members who have an interest in the information unless there are very good reasons for excluding them from knowing.

Incompetent adults

The same principles apply to genetic testing as to other medical testing in incompetent adults (see Chapter 6). On rare occasions it may be desirable to perform genetic testing on incompetent adults solely for the benefit of members of the family. The British Medical Association (BMA 1998, p. 79) states that this may be ethically justified, taking account of the following factors:

1. The potential harm to the individual of the test
2. The degree of harm or benefit to others
3. Any previous expressed wishes of the incompetent individual
4. Whether the information can be obtained by other means, e.g. testing other relatives
5. Whether there are grounds for believing that most competent adults would wish to help others in this way.

The BMA notes that such testing of incompetent people, even if ethically justified, may constitute battery in law (unless it is carried out according to the principles of the Mental Capacity Act 2005; see p. 76). If time permits, it would be desirable to obtain court authorization for such testing. The testing previously obtained specimens, or of specimens obtained for therapeutic purposes, may not be battery and may be lawful as long as any relevant provisions in the Human Tissue Act 2004 are followed (see Chapter 12).

Genetic testing and children

Should predictive testing be carried out on children, or should such tests be offered only once the person is adult and can decide for herself? The UK Clinical Genetics Society (1994), the American Society for Human Genetics (1995) and the Human Genetics Society of Australasia (2005) have all published guidelines that strongly advise against genetic testing in children for a disease in which surveillance, or pre-emptive or definitive medical treatment, is not available in childhood. Box 8.4 gives arguments for and against predictive testing in children.

REPRODUCTIVE CHOICE

Genetics allied to modern reproductive technologies can, potentially, provide would-be parents with enormous reproductive choice. What should be the limits on such choice? We will consider three issues: prenatal selection in general, sex selection in particular and the issue of whether reproductive choice can amount to discrimination against the disabled.

Prenatal genetic testing

Prenatal genetic tests aim to detect genetic abnormalities, such as cystic fibrosis, in an embryo or fetus with a view to termination of pregnancy or, in the case of preimplantation diagnosis, to be used to guide selection of an embryo for implantation. In Box 8.5 we consider five ethical issues raised by the possibility of prenatal genetic testing.

The legal regulation of prenatal genetic diagnosis

There have been several legal cases involving the issue of 'saviour siblings'. This situation occurs when a child exists with a serious condition that could be treated through a 'transplant' from a close relative with compatible tissue. The

> **Box 8.4** Arguments for and against predictive genetic testing in children (based on Savulescu 2001a, b)
>
> **For**
> 1. Information about one's predisposition to disease can *be beneficial in a non-medical sense* to allow more informed decision-making about educational and career choices.
> 2. *Self-knowledge* can promote more autonomous decision-making about one's life.
> 3. Testing can *resolve uncertainty* in parents and children, thereby reducing anxiety.
> 4. Testing can show *respect for parental autonomy* if the parents wish the child to have the test, and thus avoids *professional paternalism*.
> 5. Participation of a child in decisions about testing can promote the *development of autonomy*.
> 6. Early testing may result in *better psychosocial adjustment* than later testing, when lifestyle and life plans have been more firmly established.
>
> **Against**
> 1. Predictive testing *fails to respect the child's later autonomy* to decide whether to have testing or not, and violates the future adult's *'right not to know'*.
> 2. Testing breaches the child's *confidentiality*, as the parents will know the result.
> 3. Testing may *cause harm* to the child by causing disturbed family dynamics, as parents may treat that child differently; and parents, or the child, may become depressed and anxious. The child might experience discrimination and stigmatization, and develop low self-esteem.
> 4. Parents may develop a sense of *guilt*.

relevant 'transplant' is either umbilical cord blood stem cells or bone marrow from the donor. If no close family member exists with compatible tissue, the child's parents may wish to conceive a child and use preimplantation genetic testing and embryo selection to ensure that the implanted embryo will develop into a child who could act as donor to their existing sick child. In a recent case, Quintavalle v HFEA [2005], the House of Lords considered the legality of the Human Fertilisation and Embryology Authority's (HFEA's) licence allowing a clinic to use Human Leukocyte Antigen (HLA) typing to test embryos. This information was needed to establish whether stem cells could provide a cure for an existing child suffering from a potentially fatal blood disorder. The House of Lords unanimously agreed that a treatment licence could be granted (i.e. one designed to produce a child who would be a compatible tissue donor). In so doing the court endorsed guidance from the HFEA (2004) stating that preimplantation genetic diagnosis and HLA typing licences, albeit as a last resort, could be granted provided certain factors were taken into account. These included the condition of the existing child, the prognosis and whether there were any alternative sources of tissue for treatment.

Sex selection

What limits, if any, should be placed on reproductive choice? This question is particularly pertinent as more and more genetic tests become available for minor abnormalities and for characteristics that are not disease states at all, such as

Box 8.5   Five ethical issues raised by the possibility of prenatal genetic testing

The ethics of termination of pregnancy
Because, in most cases, the only intervention available to prevent a child being born with a genetic disorder is termination of the pregnancy, the ethical issues associated with this are central (see Chapter 9). Preimplantation genetic testing, followed by embryo selection, does not require termination of a pregnancy, although it does usually involve discarding embryos and the use of IVF.

Which conditions should be tested for?
Termination of pregnancy, or embryo selection, following genetic testing is normally limited to 'significant disability' associated with either chromosomal abnormalities, such as Down's syndrome, or single gene disorders, such as cystic fibrosis or Duchenne muscular dystrophy. How significant should the disability be in order to justify either termination of pregnancy or embryo selection? Does the answer depend on which of these two methods is used, and, in the case of termination of pregnancy, does it depend on the fetal age? Are chromosomal abnormalities such as those associated with Turner's or Klinefelter's syndrome sufficiently serious to justify selection? Is it for the parents to decide, and, if so, should there be any restrictions on the grounds used for their decision? Should parents be allowed to select any embryo on the basis of its sex (see text), and should they be able to choose an embryo whose genetic profile suggests that the child is likely to have what they see as desirable characteristics (e.g. high intelligence) or to avoid what they see as undesirable characteristics (e.g. aggressive behaviour, colour blindness)?

Cost-effectiveness
Should prenatal genetic testing be evaluated for its cost-effectiveness, and, if so, what should the outcome measures be? Some argue that clinical genetics is about providing education and choice, and so it is difficult to evaluate its cost-effectiveness. Others argue that the reduction in the proportion of people born with disability is an important outcome, and the savings from not having to treat disability can be included in the evaluation of its cost-effectiveness (Beaudet 1990).

Public health and coercion
Is public health, or the public interest, a legitimate goal of clinical genetics? Should the state encourage, or even enforce, genetic testing in some circumstances for the purpose of reducing the number of people born with some disease or disability? Consider testing for the carrier state of thalassaemia in Cyprus, where the Church must authorize marriage. Prior to such authorization couples must have thalassaemia carrier testing. There is no obligation to have prenatal diagnosis on the basis of the result. However, the vast majority of those tested choose to have prenatal diagnosis, and today virtually no babies with thalassaemia are born in Cyprus. Currently, around 50% of the supply of blood for transfusion is used to treat people with thalassaemia, and this accounts for about 20% of the 'drug budget'. If screening for thalassaemia had not been introduced, there would have been more than twice as many people in Cyprus with thalassaemia today.

There is an element of coercion in the carrier testing programme in Cyprus, as people who want to marry must have such testing. However, the programme increases informed decision-making about reproduction and thus increases autonomy.

The carrier testing programme is also in the public interest. Some would argue that coercion may be justified in the public interest if:

- there is a significant health problem
- the intervention will be an effective way of promoting the public interest
- there is no effective, or less coercive, alternative.

Prenatal testing for conditions that begin in adulthood

Prenatal testing is currently offered for some adult-onset conditions such as Huntington's disease. However, it is not routinely offered for familial breast or bowel cancer, nor for predisposition to adult-onset dementias such as Alzheimer's disease. Should a pregnant woman be allowed to choose to have her fetus tested for genetic predisposition to adult-onset conditions with a view to termination of pregnancy if the test is positive?

Arguments against testing include the following:

1. If the fetus is found to have the adult-onset condition and the couple decide not to proceed with termination, then they will know that the child born will have a predisposition to a serious adult-onset condition. This breaches the confidentiality of that person and may remove the option of that individual not to know his or her genetic status.
2. Several decades of good life is enough.
3. In the case of hereditary breast cancer, it is not certain that cancer will develop.
4. In the case of inherited bowel cancer, there are effective surveillance measures (colonoscopy).

Arguments in favour of testing include the following:

1. Termination of pregnancy is available in practice – at least early in pregnancy – for any condition. Indeed, the vast majority of terminations are for normal fetuses, so it is discriminatory to refuse termination for these conditions.
2. Couples may decide not to have any children if they cannot have testing.
3. It may cause significant psychological distress to a couple to be uncertain whether they have a child with an adult-onset condition.
4. It is better, other things being equal, that children are born without a predisposition to adult-onset disease than that children are born with such a predisposition.

physical and intellectual abilities or psychological characteristics. One key example is sex selection. Should couples be allowed to select the sex of their child, if they so wish. The Ethics Committee of the American Society of Reproductive Medicine (1999) concluded that to use preimplantation genetic diagnosis and sex selection for non-medical reasons is normally inappropriate and 'should be discouraged'. Some of the Committee's arguments are summarized in Box 8.6.

Arguments in favour of sex selection include the following:

1. We should respect couples' 'procreative autonomy'.
2. It is sometimes argued that sex selection would add to discrimination against women because selection would lead to relatively more male babies. However, this does not seem true. Some 90% of couples in the West who come forward for sex selection do so in order to balance sex within the family, and in both the USA and the UK just over half of such couples choose

> **Box 8.6** Some of the arguments considered by the American Society of Reproductive Medicine (1999) against sex selection
>
> 1. Gender should not be a reason to value one person over another.
> 2. Sex selection may 'contribute to a society's gender stereotyping and overall gender discrimination'.
> 3. It is 'unreasonable for individuals who do not otherwise need IVF to undertake its burdens and expense solely to select the gender of their offspring'.
> 4. It may represent a misallocation of limited medical resources.

a girl (Batzofin 1987, Lui & Rose 1995). In any case, it might be argued that discrimination against women should be tackled through changing the social and legal arrangements that result in such discrimination, rather than through controlling reproduction (Savulescu 2001b).

3. A woman should be left to make her own autonomous decision about the risks and benefits of various methods of sex selection.
4. Sex selection is not a misallocation of medical resources if it is fully funded privately.
5. The physical risks of harm are low.
6. There are no clear and overriding psychological risks to the child (e.g. owing to the child's not meeting the expectations of his or her parents). Most parents have some expectations and come to accept and love the child they have.
7. The desire to select sex itself does not necessarily reflect a dysfunctional parental psychology, nor does it necessarily result in harm to other siblings.
8. It is sometimes argued that, in selecting the sex of their child, parents are using their child to fulfil their own desires, and that this fails to respect the child as a person. However, this argument is in danger of proving too much. Parents have many desires related to their children: perhaps to have a companion, to hold a marriage together, to be a friend to the first child, and so on. It is unlikely that any parent ever desires a child simply as an end in itself (whatever that might mean). Provided that parents love their child as an end in itself, it is not clear that sex selection has any harmful effects on the child.
9. Without sex selection, without a unique sperm and egg uniting, that particular child would not have existed. Even if the child is disadvantaged psychologically, this is wrong *from the child's perspective* only if its life is so bad that it is not worth living (see Chapter 9 for further discussion of this issue).

Discrimination against the disabled

Prenatal diagnosis followed by termination of pregnancy, or embryo selection, has been the object of considerable criticism on the general grounds that it discriminates against the disabled (for further discussion of disability see also Chapter 15). Newell (1994) has claimed that prenatal diagnosis is 'a technology of oppression and control' which 'devalues' the lives of those with disabilities. We will consider three arguments in support of this view based on the analysis of Buchanan and colleagues (2000).

The expressivist objection

According to this objection the new genetics expresses a negative judgement about people with impairments, and such judgements constitute an injustice and a violation of the right of people with impairments to be regarded as people of equal worth. This is captured in the slogan that prenatal testing implies 'better dead than disabled'. There are two responses to this. The first is that it conflates judgements about people with impairments and judgements about impairment. We can have a negative attitude towards deafness without having a negative attitude towards Beethoven, for example. Indeed, we use education, diet and medicine to bring about what we judge to be better lives for our children. The whole of medical testing and treatment is based on the assumption that some lives are better than others. Why else would a particular test or therapy be developed? People with impairments can lead full and worthwhile lives, and are clearly entitled to equal concern and respect, but that does not imply that we cannot value impairments negatively.

The second response is to argue that the expressivist objection assumes that embryos or fetuses are persons with a right to life, and that selection through prenatal testing is like eliminating impairments by killing children or adults. This is a controversial assumption (see Chapter 9). If termination of pregnancy is tolerated, it can be argued that parents should have the choice of whether to have a normal child in the future rather than this disabled child now. Indeed, more than 95% of terminations are for social reasons and not on the basis of impairment. Imagine that a woman decides not to have a child because she is unemployed and has insufficient financial resources: we should not conclude that this implies that it is better to be dead than poor.

Loss of support argument

According to this argument, a reduction in the number of people with impairments will result in a loss of public support for those with impairment. There is little empirical evidence to support this claim. Indeed, increased resources were given to those with thalassaemia in Greece following the introduction of carrier testing. Moreover, this argument focuses on those who exist with impairments, and excludes the interests of those in whom an impairment might be prevented or treated. The use of folate in pregnancy reduces the incidence of spina bifida. Should we not continue to promote the use of folate in pregnancy even if this results in less support to existing people with spina bifida? In some cases the individual himself has an interest in not having an impairment, e.g. in not being paralysed by spina bifida. In other cases parents and other siblings have an interest in the family not having a child with an impairment. These legitimate interests are ignored by the loss of support argument.

The unique culture argument

According to some deaf people we should not use cochlear implants and other interventions to treat deafness because deafness is not an impairment, it is another culture. Signing, it is claimed, is a unique form of communication. This argument could be extended to other impairments and to genetic testing for them. One response to this view is to argue that, even if signing is like another form of communication, it is not an exclusive or a superior form. Just as being fluent in one language does not preclude a person from being fluent in another, so too, being able to hear does not preclude one from being able to sign. It is better to be able to communicate in two ways rather than one. Moreover, even if deafness were a unique culture, in our society being deaf is limiting. The strongest reason for rejecting the unique culture argument is that if deafness is not valued as worse than having normal hearing, then there would be nothing objectionable about parents rendering their children deaf. This is a conclusion that few people would accept.

GENE THERAPY

Gene therapy is in its infancy. There are two broad types: somatic and germline therapy. Somatic gene therapy uses genetic methods to treat disease in an individual. Like most treatments it directly affects only the target individual. Somatic gene therapy aimed at curing disease is no different in principle from any other disease treatment. Being new, it has considerable potential risks, but that is a feature of most new treatments. The interesting ethical issues for somatic gene therapy arise because of the potential (not yet realized) of enhancing human characteristics. Box 8.7. examines some arguments for and against such use.

Germline therapy is different in that the therapeutic intervention affects not only the target patient but also, potentially, that person's descendants, through genetic changes in the germline. We will not consider this type of therapy here. Further reading about germline therapy is given at the end of the chapter.

CLONING

A cloned cell has a genome that is a near-identical copy of the genome of its parent or 'progenitor' cell. There are two methods of genome cloning: fission and fusion (Box 8.8) (Savulescu 2005). Cloning can be divided into *therapeutic cloning* and *reproductive cloning*. Therapeutic cloning involves using cloning processes to produce embryonic stem cells, tissues or whole organs for research and transplantation. Reproductive cloning is the use of cloning to grow a living person who shares the DNA of the progenitor.

Therapeutic cloning

The possibility of therapeutic cloning centres on the concept of stem cells. Stem cells have the ability to develop into different mature cell types. *Totipotent* stem cells are cells with the potential to form a complete animal if placed in a uterus. They are early embryos. *Pluripotent* stem cells are immature stem cells with the potential to develop into any of the mature cell types in the adult (liver, lung, skin, blood, etc.), but cannot by themselves form a complete animal if placed in a uterus.

Therapeutic cloning research has been set back by the revelations that Korean cloning scientist, Woo Suk Hwang, faked cloning a human embryo and faked deriving embryonic stem cell lines (Saunders & Savulescu 2007). However, cloning research remains one of the hottest and most important revolutions in medical research. Scientists in the UK have applied to use rabbit eggs to mix with human DNA to produce, through cloning, embryonic stem cell lines (ES) of cells that are pluripotent (Savulescu 2007).

Box 8.7 Arguments for and against genetic enhancement

Imagine that there is a newly developed somatic cell therapy kit targeted at the brain cells of children that increases IQ by 20 points. A couple wish to buy this kit to help their daughter's school progress and increase her chance of being able to attend university. The daughter's current IQ is 98. Are there overriding ethical objections to this use of gene therapy? Or is it little different, from an ethical point of view, from the use of specialist teachers in helping children's intellectual development?

Objections to genetic enhancement and responses to these objections

1. Genetic enhancement is an unnatural way of enhancing people's abilities. It is 'playing God'.
Response: Genetic enhancement is no more unnatural than vaccination, the treatment of cancer or cosmetic surgery. If it is natural for some people to have these traits, why not others? Moreover, it is the improvement of well-being or human flourishing that is important, not what is or is not 'natural'.

2. Enhancing ourselves through genetic manipulation is a form of hubris (excessive pride). It is underpinned by an arrogance about what is of value.
Response: This objection would apply equally to environmental manipulations, such as education.

3. The enhancement of a narrow range of socially valued traits will result in a loss of genetic diversity, which is bad in itself and leaves the population more vulnerable to environmental insult.
Response: It is likely that genetic enhancement will be practised by only a minority of people, and so will have little impact on diversity worldwide. Furthermore, it is not clear that such variation is still necessary for survival, or for human flourishing. We are able to control our environment to an enormous extent, and genetic diversity might be introduced by deliberate genetic intervention should this prove necessary in the future.

4. Enhancement will result in intolerance of differences: as more and more people share similar qualities, they will be less tolerant of those who do not have those qualities.
Response: It is not clear that enhancement will reduce differences – it may increase them. Even if it does reduce differences, this may lead to difference becoming more highly valued. Moreover, tolerance of a quality is not necessarily dependent on there being large numbers of people with that quality. Tolerance is an attitude, under voluntary control, not determined by the biology of people around us.

5. Genetic enhancement limits freedom of choice both for the individual involved and, in the case of germline therapy, for future generations.
Response: Many choices made by parents affect the future choices available for their children (e.g. the choice of school). It is in any case a question of different choices, not of fewer choices. The child who does not have a genetic enhancement will be denied the life choices associated with that enhancement. In many cases, enhancement will increase options open to children and increase freedom. Similarly, we make all kinds of decisions within a society that alter the choices that will be open to future generations. There is nothing unique about genetic enhancement.

6. Enhancement would result in some people obtaining unfair advantage. In practice, those who are rich would be more able to purchase such enhancements than those who are poor. This would entrench privilege and increase injustice.
Response: Enhancements could be used to promote justice by making them freely available and enabling everyone to start life without genetic disadvantage. Enhancements may correct for the effects of the genetic lottery.

7. Enhancement is 'cheating', like the use of performance-enhancing drugs in sport.
Response: The natural distribution of talent is unfair. It would be unfair not to correct for natural injustice. Cheating occurs only when there are rules or laws preventing enhancement. Drinking coffee is not cheating.

8. Enhancement may engender a culture where perfection is expected and people have a constant fear of failure and rejection.
Response: The same danger is inherent in environmental manipulations (such as special schools or elite sporting institutes). Steps need to be taken to reduce this danger, but it would be wrong to go to the extreme of preventing people from improving skills and abilities, whether this is through special education, good diet or genetic enhancement.

Some arguments in favour of genetic enhancement, and responses to these arguments

1. There should be a presumption in favour of liberty for people to pursue what they believe is good for themselves and their children.
Response: Liberty can be restricted in the public interest.

2. We already allow, and indeed often encourage, people to enhance both their own abilities and attributes and those of their children through environmental manipulation. It would be inconsistent to prevent such enhancement through genetic means.
Response: Environmental manipulations are not as irreversible and do not produce such dramatic changes. Genetic manipulations have the potential to produce irreversible dramatic changes, and could even raise the question of whether they amount to changing the identity of the person.

3. Distributive justice may require enhancement – to correct for the natural injustices.
Response: Social change is a preferable way of correcting for injustice than is changing people.

4. Genetic methods may be a more cost-effective way of bringing about desirable changes than environmental manipulations, and may therefore be a more efficient use of resources.
Response: Efficiency is not the only value: tolerance, and equal consideration of individuals as they exist, are also important.

> **Box 8.8** Two methods of cloning
>
> **Cloning by fission**
>
> *Blastocyst division*
> Twinning is induced in a blastocyst by the application of heat or mechanical stress.
> The blastocyst splits in two, and the two halves continue to grow into complete
> embryos. At most, two identical embryos can be created using this method.
>
> *Blastomere separation*
> The coating of an early embryo (blastocyst) is removed and the cells (blastomeres)
> are placed in a solution that separates them. Each of these blastomeres is
> undifferentiated and can grow into an embryo. This technique can produce eight
> embryos at most, but can be repeated for each new embryo to produce larger
> number of cloned embryos.
>
> **Cloning by fusion**
> Fusion is achieved through the process of somatic cell nuclear transfer (SCNT).
> The nucleus is removed from a somatic cell and implanted into the cytoplasm of a
> denucleated egg. The egg reprogrammes the somatic cell's DNA so that a complete
> embryo can be grown out of this cell. Using this technique, a theoretically endless
> number of clones can be created from the same individual. SCNT is the only method
> currently available that might be used to clone existing or pre-existing people.

One likely application of therapeutic cloning is in the treatment of leukaemia, and more broadly in various types of tissue and organ transplantation.
Therapeutic cloning is important for four reasons. First, there is a shortage
of tissue for transplantation. Second, there are problems with the compatibility of tissue transplanted from another individual, requiring immunosup-
pressive therapy with serious side-effects. Cloned tissue from the individual
needing the transplant would be compatible. Third, the role of transplantation might be expanded to include common diseases such as heart attack and
stroke. Fourth, cloning may prove to be a cost-efficient means of preventing
disability and morbidity, and of promoting distributive justice.

Using this kind of technology, one day we may be able to take a skin cell
from a patient with leukaemia, clone it, derive embryonic stem cells, produce
blood stem cells, and transfer the blood cells back as a transplant after chemotherapy. Because the cells would come from the patient, there would be
no need for drugs (which can be lethal) to prevent rejection. And we could
produce tissue to repair damaged organs such as the heart and brain with
no capacity for regeneration, providing radical new treatments for stroke and
heart attack, Parkinson's disease and many other diseases. This is regenera-
tive medicine. It is the holy grail of medicine.

Cloning might also be used to study in a radically new way any disease in
a culture dish. Cloning a single skin cell from a patient with a disease, using
a human or non-human (e.g. rabbit) egg, could be used to produce inexhaust-
ible amounts of cells and tissue with that disease. Experiments could be carried out on the tissue to understand why disease occurs. It could be used to
understand the genetic contribution to disease and to test vast arrays of new
drugs that could not be tested in human people. Cloning might also reduce the

need for animal experimentation because human cells and tissues, not people or animals, could be used to test new drugs. This represents a new avenue of experimentation – developing cellular models of human disease.

The main ethical issue raised by the production of embryonic stem cells and therapeutic cloning is that of producing and destroying embryos for the purposes of research, or tissue for transplantation. If the embryo is considered to have a moral status similar to, say, that of a child, then embryo research would normally be wrong. On this view, in-vitro fertilization (IVF) and almost any termination of pregnancy would also be wrong (see Chapter 9). Those who support such embryo research argue that if some of the embryos produced during IVF would be otherwise discarded (as normally they would) then what could be wrong with using those embryos for research and then destroying them? This counter-argument is less persuasive if the embryos are created solely for the research and would not otherwise exist. Views about the moral status of the embryo (see Chapter 9) are then more crucial. It remains the case, however, that in a society that accepts that embryos (and fetuses) may be destroyed (such as in discarding embryos created during IVF, as a result of the use of intrauterine devices, and by termination of pregnancy) there would need to be a special justification for banning embryo research. Furthermore, for every live birth up to five embryos miscarry. In attempting to have a child by natural conception, we implicitly accept that this loss is a price worth paying to produce a new life (Harris 2000). If the loss of embryos is an acceptable price to pay to produce a new life, is it not also an acceptable price to pay to save an existing life?

There are four further objections to therapeutic cloning. First, fusion cloning normally requires removing eggs from women and this is associated with discomfort and some risk of harm. It is not clear, however, that such discomfort and harms are greater than are accepted in medical research (see Chapter 14) in other settings. Second, because the technologies around cloning are expensive, the benefits of cloning may be enjoyed only by the rich, and this is unjust. This objection may be countered through arguing that some benefits may involve the development of therapeutic techniques and drugs, using cellular models of common human diseases such as cancer and diabetes, that will benefit poor as well as rich. A second counter is that in due course the technology will become cheaper and will potentially benefit rich and poor alike. A third counter is that such inequity is common across the range of human benefits. The response to such inequity is not to ban the development of useful technology but to address directly the sources of poverty. A third objection to therapeutic cloning involving embryonic stem cells is that the benefits of such research can be developed equally using adult stem cell research, and such research does not face the moral problems that arise from producing and destroying embryos. There are some types of research, however, that cannot be carried out using adult stem cells. Adult stem cells are not immortal and cannot be used to develop cellular models of disease in the way that embryonic stem cells can. The fourth objection is that the transplantation of tissue created from cloning for therapeutic purposes might introduce new infections (analogous, for example, to the introduction of bovine spongiform encephalitis), because tissue is often grown on a medium made from non-human animal products, or the cloning might involve non-human animal eggs.

The use of non-human animal eggs to develop cellular models of human disease can overcome some of these objections. These models would require few or no human eggs in order to produce vast amounts of tissue for the study of disease (because this tissue, once produced, is potentially immortal). The research might result in the development of drugs for common conditions that afflict people all round the world, including in poor countries. And there would be no risk of infection from drugs developed this way: the risk of infection applies only when cloned tissue is used for transplantation.

The use of non-human eggs, however, raises another possible moral objection: that we should not create human clones using animal eggs or new human–non-human hybrids or chimeras because they are unnatural and cross some kind of ethical line. In fact scientists have been inserting human genes into animals to create animal models of human disease for over 20 years. More recently, scientists have introduced human embryonic cells into animals to study development and disease. For more than a decade we have had the power to create human–non-human chimeras by fusing embryos. Indeed, we have already created new animals such as the 'geep', brought into being by fusing a goat and sheep embryo. Novel life forms have been created and could be created. Given that, in the case of therapeutic cloning research, the research will be closely regulated and the embryos destroyed, the creation of human–non-human hybrids through cloning does not raise new ethical issues. The 'chimeras' that may be created in cloning research might best be seen, not as some esoteric and worrying form of new species, but as biological material or tissue for studying disease.

A final objection to therapeutic cloning is that, although not wrong in itself, it will lead down a slippery slope (see Chapter 1) to reproductive cloning. One response to this objection is to argue that there is a clear distinction between the two types of cloning, that is, there is a clear barrier that will prevent slipping down the slippery slope. The UK has already banned reproductive cloning, and any scientist in the UK who clones a human person would face criminal charges. To ban therapeutic cloning because of objections to reproductive cloning, on this view, is to throw the baby out with the bath water. A second response is to question whether reproductive cloning is necessarily unethical.

Reproductive cloning

Reproductive cloning is the production of a (near-identical) genetic copy of an existing or previously existing person. Live animals have been cloned using both fission methods (in the cattle industry) and somatic cell nuclear transfer (SCNT; see Box 8.8), in cases such as the one that produced Dolly the sheep. So far there have been no confirmed cases of the deliberate cloning of a human embryo that has developed into a live baby.

The Human Reproductive Cloning Act 2001 aims to prevent human reproductive cloning by making it a criminal offence to place a human embryo in the womb of a woman unless the embryo has been created by fertilization. Reproductive cloning is illegal in many other countries (e.g. Australia) and several international declarations prohibit it.

Box 8.9 summarizes some arguments for and against reproductive cloning.

Box 8.9   Some arguments for and against reproductive cloning

For

1. Liberty – we should be free to reproduce however we choose.
Response: The harm to a clone and society in general justifies constraint on this freedom.

2. For medical reasons – clones could be created as a compatible source of protein, cells, tissue or organs. This is already taking place without cloning through the creation of 'saviour siblings' (see p. 118). Cloning would ensure the best possible match.
Response: Such a use, as with 'saviour siblings', is wrong because it uses people as an *instrument* for the benefit of others (see 'instrumentalization' below).

3. Freedom of scientific enquiry – the knowledge gained by human cloning will be invaluable in gaining scientific knowledge.
Response: The potential for harm to the clone and society constrains the pursuit of knowledge.

4. To achieve a sense of immortality – while we may die, our clone may live on. This would give us a greater sense of connectedness with the future.
Response: Clones are different people. Any sense of connectedness with the future would be based on false assumptions about personal identity.

5. Eugenic selection – cloning could be used to reproduce especially gifted individuals, such as Einstein.
Response: Clones will be different people from the 'original'. Eugenic selection is based on a crude genetic determinism which suggests that people are merely the product of their genes.

6. Treatment of infertility.
Response: Cloning is necessary for the treatment of infertility only in the case of mitochondrial disease. Such diseases are rare. Moreover, there are other ways for people to have a baby using donor gametes.

7. Replacement of a dead relative.
Response: The relative will not be replaced (even if this were desirable), as the clone will be a different person.

8. Negative attitudes to cloning represent a new form of discrimination: *clonism*. To label the creation of a clone as an affront to human dignity (see below) is like saying that creating a black person is an affront to human dignity. People deserve equal concern and respect regardless of the origin of their genome. Clones are not 'genetic bastards': they are people who deserve equal respect and concern with everyone else.
Response: This analogy is unconvincing. No one is saying that a person who is a clone should in any way be discriminated against. But from that it does not follow that it was not wrong to have used cloning in the first place. In believing that it is wrong to clone humans, one is not 'expressing' a negative view towards individuals created by cloning (see also 'expressivist argument', p. 123).

9. Most arguments against cloning assume that the clone is the same person as the 'original', but, just as identical twins are not the same person, neither are clones.

Much opposition to cloning is also based on a crude genetic determinism that underplays the importance of environment (and, perhaps, freedom of the will) in determining the kind of person we are.

Response: Many arguments against cloning do not make these assumptions. Cloning will reduce originality as clones will be more similar to one another than non-clones.

Against

1. Cloning is an affront to human dignity – this claim has been made by the European Parliament, UNESCO and the World Health Organization. The *Additional Protocol to the Convention for the Protection of Human Rights and Dignity of the Human Being with regard to the Application of Biology and Medicine, on the Prohibition of Cloning Human Beings (1998)*, for example (http://conventions.coe.int/treaty/en/treaties/html/168. htm) states in its preamble that: 'the instrumentalisation of human beings through the deliberate creation of genetically identical human beings is contrary to human dignity and thus constitutes a misuse of biology and medicine' and goes on to say in Article 1: 'Any intervention seeking to create a human being genetically identical to another human being, whether living or dead, is prohibited'.

Response: What is human dignity and how is cloning an affront to it? Approximately 1 in 300 live births are identical twins (and therefore clones) and this does not seem to represent any threat to human dignity. Are identical twins an affront to human dignity?

2. Cloning is liable to abuse – dictators and other evil people will clone multiple copies of themselves, or use cloning technology to produce large armies of clones.

Response: This argument assumes genetic determinism. A different time and circumstances will ensure that the clone is not a replica. Moreover, It would be an inefficient means for a dictator to impose his will. We have much more to fear from dictators than cloning – such as their use of weapons.

3. Cloning allows eugenic selection – this criticism has been put forward by the European Parliament.

Response: Many other current techniques could be used for eugenic purposes, such as preimplantation diagnosis, prenatal testing, abortion and sterilization. Should these also be prohibited? The eugenics practised by the Nazis was an atrocity both because it was motivated by racism and because it was imposed by the state on individuals without their agreement. The choice by parents to have a child without a serious genetically determined disease is quite different from what the Nazis did.

4. Instrumentalization – cloning uses people as a means.

Response: People have children for a variety of motives. What is important is how a child is treated and loved, not the reasons her parents had for conceiving her. See discussion of sex selection (p. 119).

5. Clones will live in the shadow of the 'original' person.

Response: Many people live in the shadow of their parents, or others, without excessive untoward effect. In any case, cloning does not significantly increase risks from high expectations. A clone may well *benefit* from fore-knowledge of his genetic inheritance – his talents, limitations and disease propensities.

6. Cloning would reduce genetic variation.

Response: Identical twins occur at a rate of 3.5 per 1000. This does not affect genetic diversity. It is likely that only a small proportion of any population would be clones, and so cloning would have little impact on genetic diversity.

7. Right to genetic individuality – the European Parliament claimed, in the context of cloning, that the individual has a right to his or her own genetic identity.

Response: It is clear that twins are autonomous individuals. Identical twins do not seem deficient in any way, as is manifested by the absence of objection to drugs that increase the rate of twinning, and by the fact that little research into preventing twinning is carried out.

8. Safety – cloning increases the risk of serious genetic malformation, cancer or shortened lifespan.

Response: This is currently a valid objection because the science of cloning is in its infancy. Further research on cloning and improved techniques are likely to reduce the risks so that they are comparable with those of normal reproduction. If cloning and other forms of artificial reproduction were to be safer and more efficient than natural reproduction, we would have a reason to employ these artificial rather than natural methods.

REFERENCES

American Society for Human Genetics/ Advisory Council on Medical Genetics 1995 Points to consider: ethical, legal and psychological implications of genetic testing in children and adolescents. American Journal of Human Genetics 57:1233–1241

Batzofin J H 1987 XY sperm separation for sex selection. Urologic Clinics of North America 14:609–618

Beaudet A L 1990 Carrier screening for cystic fibrosis. American Journal of Human Genetics 47:603–605

British Medical Association 1998 Human genetics: choice and responsibility. BMA, London

Buchanan A, Brock D W, Daniels N, Winkler D 2000 From chance to choice: genetics and justice. Cambridge University Press, Cambridge

Clinical Genetics Society (UK) Working Party 1994 The genetic testing of children. Journal of Medical Genetics 31:785–797

Ethics Committee of the American Society of Reproductive Medicine 1999 Sex selection and preimplantation genetic diagnosis. Fertility and Sterility 72:595–598

Harper P S 1988 Practical genetic counselling. Butterworths, London

Harris J 2000 The ethical use of human embryonic stem cells in research and therapy. Paper presented to the National Taiwan University Hospital, 27 June 2000

Herring J 2006 Medical health law and ethics. Oxford University Press, Oxford

Human Fertilisation and Embryology Authority 2004 New guidance on pre-implantation tissue typing. CH(04)05. Online. Available: http://www.hfea.gov.uk/en/599.html 18 Jun 2007

Human Genetics Society of Australasia 2005 Predictive genetic testing of children and adolescents. Online. Available: http://hgsa.com.au/images/UserFiles/Attachments/Predictivetesting(General) APRIL2005.pdf 24 Jun 2007

Lucassen A, Parker M 2001 Revealing false paternity: some ethical considerations. Lancet 357:1033

Lui P, Rose G A 1995 Social aspects of over 800 couples coming forward for gender selection of their children. Human Reproduction 10:968–971

Murray T 1996 The worth of a child. University of California Press, Berkeley

Newell C 1994 A critique of the construction of prenatal diagnosis and disability. In: McKie J (ed.) Ethical issues in prenatal diagnosis and termination of pregnancy. Centre for Human Bioethics, Monash University, Melbourne, pp. 89–96

Parker M, Lucassen A 2004 Genetic information: a joint account?. British Medical Journal 329:165–167

Quintavalle v HFEA [2003] EWCA Civ 667

Saunders R, Savulescu J 2007 Research ethics and Hwanggate: what can we learn from the Korean cloning fraud? Journal of Medical Ethics (in press)

Savulescu J 2001a Predictive genetic testing in children. Medical Journal of Australia 175:379–381

Savulescu J 2001b In defense of selection for nondisease genes. American Journal of Bioethics 1:16–19

Savulescu J 2005 The ethics of cloning. Medicine 33:18–20

Savulescu J 2007 The case for creating human–nonhuman cell lines. Bioethics Forum Online. Available: http://www. bioethicsforum.org/research-cloning-hybrid-embryos.asp 18 Jun 2007

FURTHER READING

General

Agar N 2003 Liberal eugenics. Blackwell, Oxford

British Medical Association 1998 Human genetics: choice and responsibility. Oxford University Press, Oxford
The British Medical Association's position on ethics and genetics.

Buchanan A, Brock D W, Daniels N, Wikler D 2000 From chance to choice: genetics and justice. Cambridge University Press, Cambridge
One of the best books on ethics and the new genetics which covers the literature thoroughly. Highly recommended.

Chadwick R F (ed.) 1990 Ethics, reproduction, and genetic control. Routledge, London

Harris J 1998 Clones, genes and immortality. Oxford University Press, Oxford
An updated version of Harris's influential 'Wonderwoman and superman' (Oxford University Press, Oxford, 1992).

Mehlman M J, Botkin R 1998 Access to the genome: the challenge to equality. Georgetown University Press, Washington, DC

Human Cloning

British Medical Association 2007 BMA position on human 'cloning'. Online. Available: http://www.bma.org.uk/ ap.nsf/Content/Humancloningposition 18 Jun 2007

Devolder K, Savulescu J 2006 The moral imperative to conduct embryonic stem cell and cloning research. Cambridge Quarterly of Health Care Ethics 15(1):7–21

European Commission 1997 Opinion of the group of advisers on the ethical implications of biotechnology to the European Commission: ethical aspects of cloning techniques. European Commission, Luxemburg

Ezzell C 2003 Ma's eyes, not her ways. Clones can vary in behavioral – and physical – traits. Scientific American 288(4):30

Fukuyama F 2002 Our posthuman future. Consequences of the biotechnology revolution. Farrar, Straus & Giroux, New York

Harris J 1997 'Goodbye Dolly?' The ethics of human cloning. Journal of Medical Ethics 23:353–360

House of Lords Select Committee 2002 Stem cell research - report. Stationery Office, London. Online. Available: http://www.parliament.the-stationery-office.co.uk/pa/ld200102/ldselect/ldstem/83/8301.htm 18 Jun 2007

Humber J, Almeder R (eds) 1998 Human cloning: biomedical ethical reviews. Humana Press, Totowa, NJ

Kass L R 2002 Human cloning and human dignity: an ethical inquiry. The President's Council on Bioethics, Washington, DC. Online. Available: http://www.bioethics.gov/reports/ cloningreport/fullreport.html 18 Jun 2007

Kass L R, Wilson J Q 1998 The ethics of human cloning. American Enterprise Institute, Washington, DC

Klotzko A J (ed.) 2001 The cloning source-book. Oxford University Press, Oxford

Klotzko A J 2002 A clone of your own. Oxford University Press, Oxford

Lott J P, Savulescu J 2007 Towards a global human embryonic stem cell bank. American Journal of Bioethics (in press)

McGee G (ed.) 2000 The human cloning debate, 2nd edn. Berkeley Hills Books, Berkeley

Nussbaum M C, Sunstein C R (eds.) 1998 Clones and clones: facts and fantasies about human cloning. W W Norton, New York

A collection of important essays on cloning from a variety of perspectives.

Pence G E (ed.) 1998 Flesh of my flesh: the ethics of cloning humans (a reader). Rowman & Littlefield, New York

Pence G E 1998 Who's afraid of human cloning? Rowman & Littlefield, Oxford

Ruse M, Sheppard A (eds) 2001 Cloning: responsible science or technomadness? Prometheus Books, New York

Savulescu J 2006 Solving the stem cell and cloning puzzle. Bioethics Forum. Online. Available: http://www.bioethicsforum. org/australian-debate-on-stem-cells-and-cloning.asp 21 Sept 2006

Savulescu J, Persson I 2003 Reproduction and embryo research: bringing embryos into existence for different purposes, or not at all. Festschrift edition of the Journal of Medical Ethics in honour of Raanan Gillon. Journal of Medical Ethics 29:265–266

Silver L M 1998 Remaking Eden: cloning and beyond in a brave new world. Weidenfeld & Nicolson, London

Stock G 2003 Redesigning humans: our inevitable genetic future. Houghton Mifflin, Boston

Tooley M 1998 The moral status of the cloning of humans. In: Humber J M, Almeder R F (eds) Human cloning. Humana Press, Totowa, NJ, pp. 65–101

A philosophical rebuttal of many of the objections to cloning.

Warnock M 2002 Making babies: is there a right to have children? Oxford University Press, Oxford

Eugenics

Caplan A L, McGee G, Magnus D 1999 What is immoral about eugenics? British Medical Journal 319:1284–1285

Kevles D J 1995 In the name of eugenics: genetics and the uses of human heredity. Harvard University Press, Cambridge, MA

A landmark history of eugenics.

Wikler D 1999 Can we learn from eugenics? Journal of Medical Ethics 25:183–194

A good overview and analysis of eugenics.

Disability rights and genetics

Parens E, Asch A (eds) 2000 Prenatal testing and disability rights Georgetown University Press, Washington, DC

Genetic enhancement

Holtug N 1999 Does justice require genetic enhancements? Journal of Medical Ethics 25:137–143

Juengst E T 1997 Can enhancement be distinguished from prevention in genetic medicine? Journal of Medicine and Philosophy 1997; 22:91–98

McGee G 1997 The perfect baby: a pragmatic approach to genetics. Rowman & Littlefield, Lanham, MD

Parens E (ed.) 1998 Enhancing human traits: ethical and social implications. Georgetown University Press, Washington, DC

An excellent collection of essays on genetic enhancement.

Gene therapy

Anderson W F 1985 Human gene therapy: scientific and ethical considerations. Journal of Medicine and Philosophy 10:275–291

Chadwick R 1998 Gene therapy. In: Kuhse H, Singer P (eds) A companion to bioethics. Blackwell, Oxford, pp. 189–197

Coutts M C 1994 Human gene therapy (bibliography). Kennedy Institute of Ethics Journal 4:63–83

Extended reading on gene therapy.

Harris J 1993 Is gene therapy a form of eugenics?. Bioethics 7:178–187

Holtug N 1997 Altering humans – the case for and against human gene therapy. Cambridge Quarterly of Healthcare Ethics 6:157–174

Walters L, Palmer G 1996 The ethics of human gene therapy. Oxford University Press, New York

Genetic research

Annas G J, Elias S (eds) 1992 Gene mapping: using law and ethics as guides. Oxford University Press, New York

Erwin E, Gendin S, Kleiman L (eds) 1994 Ethical issues in scientific research: an anthology. Garland, New York

Marteau T, Richards M (eds) 1996 The troubled helix: social and psychological implications of the new human genetics. Cambridge University Press, Cambridge

Genetic testing

Chadwick R F 1999 The ethics of genetic screening. Kluwer Academic, Dordrecht

Chadwick R F, Shickle D (eds) 1997 The right to know and the right not to know. Ashgate, Aldershot

Clarke A (ed.) 1998 The genetic testing of children. Bios Scientific, Oxford

Davis D S 1997 Genetic dilemmas and the child's right to an open future. Hastings Center Report 27:7–15

Robertson R, Savulescu J 2001 Is there a case in favour of predictive testing of children? Bioethics 15:26–49

Counselling

Biesecker B B 1998 Future directions in genetic counselling: practical and ethics considerations. Kennedy Institute of Ethics Journal 8:145–160

Chadwick R, ten Have H, Husted J, et al 1998 Genetic screening and ethics: European perspectives. Journal of Medicine and Philosophy 23:255–273

Rhodes R 1998 Genetic links, family ties, and social bonds: rights and responsibilities in the face of genetic knowledge. Journal of Medicine and Philosophy 23:10–30

Human genome project

Murphy T F, Lappe M A (eds) 1994 Justice and the human genome project. University of California Press, Berkeley

Murray T, Rothstein M, Murray R (eds) 1996 The human genome project and the future of health care. Indiana University Press, Bloomington, IN

Further papers on ethics and genetics

Baylis F, Robert J S 2004 The inevitability of genetic enhancement technologies. Bioethics 18(1):1–26

Burley J, Harris J 2004 A companion to genethics. Blackwell, Oxford

Caulfield T, Knowles L, Meslin E M 2004 Law and policy in the era of reproductive genetics. Journal of Medical Ethics 30(4):414–417

Corrigan O P 2005 Pharmacogenetics, ethical issues: review of the Nuffield Council on Bioethics Report. Journal of Medical Ethics 31(3):144–148

Evans M, Bergum V, Bamforth S et al 2004 Relational ethics and genetic counselling. Nursing Ethics 11(5):459–471

Hansson S O 2004 The ethics of biobanks. Cambridge Quarterly of Healthcare Ethics 13(4):319–326

Lewens T 2005 What is genethics? Journal of Medical Ethics 30(3):326–328

Manson N C 2004 Presenting behavioural genetics: spin, ideology and our narrative interests. Journal of Medical Ethics 30(6):601–604

Newson A 2004 The nature and significance of behavioural genetic information. Theoretical Medicine and Bioethics 25(2):89–111

Parens E 2004 Genetic differences and human identities: on why talking about behavioural genetics in important and difficult. Hastings Center Report 34(1):S1–S36

Parens E 2005 Authenticity and ambivalence: toward understanding the enhancement debate. Hastings Center Report 35(3):34–41

Wilson J 2005 To know or not to know? Genetic ignorance, autonomy and paternalism. Bioethics 19(5–6):493–504

9 Reproductive medicine

Most adults are left to reproduce, whether by choice or not, without interference from the state. The main role of medicine in the process of reproduction is to help ensure that mother and baby are healthy. Medical technology, however, can increase reproductive choice for three main reasons:

1. It provides the possibility of terminating the pregnancy (abortion), and this is carried out most safely in a clinical setting.
2. It provides the means of assisting conception, using an increasing array of techniques.
3. It makes available a range of investigations that help predict the likely health status, and much more, of the fetus or potential child.

To what extent should the state, or health professionals, control reproductive choice? In this chapter we discuss abortion, maternal–fetal relationships and assisted reproduction. Before turning to the issue of abortion we will outline four approaches to the issue of reproductive choice.

FOUR APPROACHES TO THE ISSUE OF REPRODUCTIVE CHOICE

Procreative autonomy – the interests of parents

This approach emphasizes the value, or perhaps the right, of adults to make their own reproductive choices. According to this approach, state or professional interference should be kept to a minimum and exercised only in rather extreme situations. This position has been taken by a number of liberal philosophers (e.g. Dworkin 1993, Harris 1997, 1998, Robertson 1994, Strong 1997).

The interests of the future child

This perspective emphasizes the interests of the future child and is particularly relevant to assisted reproduction. Because we can prevent access to assisted reproduction, we should, on this view, do so where we (the health professionals or the state) believe that preventing access is in the interests of the potential or future child.

The interests of the state

Reproductive choices affect the composition of the future population. The state therefore has an interest in what choices are made. Such interests may be relevant where the future child will require significant resources in its care, or where allowing couples choice (for example to select the sex of their children; see Chapter 8) could have undesirable consequences for the population as a whole.

Preserving life

Central to the issue of abortion is the morality of killing a fetus. Even if considerable weight is given to procreative autonomy, many would take the view that reproductive choice should not be enabled through killing an already existing fetus.

ABORTION

We will use the term 'abortion' in the normal (but not the medical) sense to mean the intentional termination of pregnancy with the resulting death of the embryo or fetus. At the heart of much of the debate around abortion, embryo experimentation and in-vitro fertilization is the question of the moral status of the embryo and fetus. Is it wrong to kill human embryos and fetuses, and, if it is, is that wrong significant enough to outweigh other goods?

Many different positions are taken on this issue. What all agree is that there are very few justifications, if any, for killing a child or adult. Such killing is a serious wrong. The child (normally) develops from the fertilized egg. At what stage in the development of the human organism from egg to child does it become a significant wrong to kill the organism? Some answer this question by identifying a point in the developmental process when such killing passes from being morally unimportant (or almost so) to being morally extremely serious – on a par with the killing of a child. Others deny that there is a point at which there is a sudden large change in moral status. Instead, through the developmental period, the wrong of killing increases so that there has to be increasing justification for allowing an abortion. Whichever of these two positions is taken, grounds have to be given for why it is that the moral status is different at different times in development.

Four views on what is important in determining the moral status of the embryo

Identity as a human organism

According to this view there are essentially no good grounds for according a different moral status to the human being at different stages in its development. If it is wrong to kill the child then it would have been just as wrong to kill that child at any stage in its existence. The fundamental reason, on this view, is that the embryo is the same entity – it has the same identity – as the child into which it develops. Most supporters of this position put the moment at when the embryo attains full moral status as conception, although some have argued that an individual cannot be said to exist until the potential for twinning is lost (e.g. Warnock Committee Report 1984). This is on the grounds that, until this point, the embryo could become two different people. It is thought that twinning ceases to be a possibility at about 14 days after conception. The term 'pre-embryo' is sometimes used for the entity before 14 days to assert that it is a different entity from that after 14 days.

The potential to be a person

This argument goes as follows: it is wrong to kill a child; if you kill an embryo or fetus, at any stage, you are carrying out an act that will have the effect that the potential future child will not exist. You are in effect killing a potential child. This argument differs from the argument about human identity in that it does not accord fetuses and embryos moral status for what they are, but because of what they have the potential to become.

Identity as a person

The view that an embryo, from the point of conception, has the same moral status as a child is sometimes called the right-to-life, or the pro-life position. The main alternative is the view that the moral status of an embryo depends on its properties, and not on its identity or potential. This view is often expressed as follows: it is very wrong to kill a *person* (in most situations), but a human embryo is not a person. A person is a human being that has certain characteristics. An embryo or fetus is a moral entity at the point when it becomes a person. The important moral issue is: what determines the stage during development when a human organism becomes a person?

Many different answers have been given to this question. Most proponents of this approach hold that being a person must involve some degree of consciousness. We, as persons, are conscious minds as well as physical bodies. Conscious life, it is thought, or at least the perception of pain, starts at about 24 weeks' gestation (Anand & Hickey 1987). On most forms of this view, therefore, fetuses of less than 24 weeks do not have moral status.

However, consciousness in the sense of feeling pain seems a rather minimal condition for being a person. Even quite primitive animals feel pain, and yet we do not accord them anything like the status of human persons in terms of the morality of killing. What is it that distinguishes a human being from a non-human animal, such that the one has a strong right to life and the other does not? Features such as the number of chromosomes seem irrelevant. Some philosophers have focused on *self-consciousness* as the hallmark of being a person (Singer 1993, Tooley 1983). These philosophers argue that what is wrong with killing a self-conscious being is the frustration of those desires that the being has for its own future: its future-directed plans and goals. Other candidates for the mental capacities that are important to being a person include rationality (the ability to reason) and the ability to form relationships. Some religious traditions confer moral status at the point when the soul enters the body (ensoulment). Various times, from conception to birth, have been proposed as the moment of ensoulment. The problem with this position is providing objective criteria for identifying that moment.

The value given to the human organism by others is crucial (conferred moral status)

Some have argued that moral status need not be based only on intrinsic properties of the entity, but that it can be conferred by others (Strong 1997). Benn (1984) and Feinberg (1984) have argued that conferring moral status at birth can be justified in terms of the consequences for others and in terms of fostering concern, warmth and sympathy for others. Feinberg argues that it is because infants are so similar to persons that we should confer status on them in a symbolic way. Englehardt (1973) argues that at birth the infant takes on an important social role, and that this justifies conferring moral status.

On all these closely related views, a strong prohibition on killing infants is justified both because those close to the infant care strongly for it, and because without such strong prohibition there is a danger that we will relax the strong prohibition on killing older babies and children. It is for these reasons that killing a human infant, or a child with severe learning difficulties, is morally more serious than killing an animal (such as an adult ape), even if the non-human animal possesses more of the morally important features of a person.

Problems with these four views

Each of the four views outlined above faces problems, which is why the issue of abortion remains so difficult. The first position confers moral status on what is just one cell or a few cells. It implies that killing that cell (or that early embryo) is, from a moral point of view, the same as killing a 10-year-old child. Such a position faces particular difficulties when the reasons a woman has for wanting an abortion are very powerful – for example, that she has become pregnant as a result of rape. This view also implies that taking postcoital contraception (such as the 'morning-after pill') or using an intrauterine contraceptive device amounts, morally, to murdering an adult.

The second position faces the same difficulties as the first, and other problems as well. The argument is likely to prove too much. A single sperm about to be injected into an egg constitutes a potential person, but it seems absurd to object to the disposal of either the egg or the sperm on the grounds that they constitute a potential person (Singer 1985). Furthermore, each couple could give birth to many potential people. Contraception and sexual abstinence both prevent some of these potential persons from coming into existence. Are they therefore morally wrong (Singer & Kuhse 1987)? Cloning raises further problems for this position, as all somatic human cells are potential people. It seems absurd to suggest that destroying somatic cells would be (a serious) wrong.

If the first two positions appear to give too much moral protection to very early embryos, the third may give too little protection to infants and people with severe learning difficulties. It also faces problems in justifying the particular feature, or group of features, that is taken to characterize a person.

The fourth position helps justify some of our intuitions about the moral importance of infants. However, to many it seems to justify these intuitions for the wrong reasons. It seems to suggest that we should not kill an infant on grounds such as that the infant's parents (and a few others) would be terribly upset. For many this is not the fundamental reason why we should not kill newborn children.

One view that is intuitively attractive to many people is that the moral status of the fetus develops as the fetus itself develops. On this view it may be wrong to kill even an early fetus, but the degree of wrong would be very much less than killing a late fetus. Furthermore, the grounds that would justify killing a fetus need to become stronger and stronger as the fetus develops. Parental convenience may be sufficient to justify the abortion of an early fetus, but it would need something much more significant to justify the abortion

Reproductive medicine

of an older fetus. Such a position is not easily compatible with either of the first two positions. However, the third and fourth positions can be adapted to allow the idea that the concept of a person, whether based on internal criteria or conferred by others, or a mixture of both, can admit of degrees, and that therefore the wrong in killing a fetus can change through development.

The morality of abortion

When is it wrong for a woman to have an abortion? When should the state prevent a woman from having an abortion? Although these questions are related, they are not the same. We may consider that it is morally wrong to lie to our friends, in many circumstances, without believing that it should be made illegal.

The answer to the first of the above questions is often taken to be: once the embryo or fetus acquires moral status. However, for many people this is only part of the picture, because the reasons why the woman wants the abortion are also crucial (Box 9.1). Those who believe that the grounds that justify abortion must be increasingly powerful as the fetus develops must take the view that the moral status of the embryo increases (either in stepwise or in continuous fashion) during development.

The rights and interests of women

Despite the wide range of quite different views on abortion considered above, they all share one assumption. This is that, if the fetus had the same moral status as, say, a normal adult, then it would be (almost always) wrong for a woman to have an abortion, and (almost always) right for the state to prevent

---

Box 9.1 Some circumstances and reasons for an abortion that might affect its ethical status

1. The pregnancy is the result of rape.
2. The woman is only 16 years old.
3. Having a child would interfere with the woman's career.
4. The expected time of birth coincides with a planned holiday.
5. The woman would be a single mother and very poor.
6. The couple already have three children. This pregnancy was the result of carelessness, by the couple, over contraception.
7. As for 6, but the pregnancy resulted from a failure of contraception that cannot be blamed on the couple.
8. The woman is depressed and feels unable to cope with motherhood.
9. Prenatal testing has revealed that the child will be severely physically handicapped and is likely to die in childhood.
10. Prenatal testing has revealed that the child will have severe learning disabilities.

the woman from having an abortion. Thomson (1971) denies this assumption and gives the following analogy:

The case of the connected violinist

Imagine that you wake up one day with your circulatory system connected to another person. It transpires that you are connected to a famous violinist. This man has a fatal kidney condition. However, if he remains connected to your circulatory system, he will eventually be cured. You are the only person who can save his life. His fans have kidnapped you and connected you up. 'But', they say, 'good news. It is only for 9 months and then he will be fully recovered and you can be disconnected.'

Thomson argues that it would be highly laudable if you were to choose to remain connected to the violinist and thus save his life, but you are not morally required to remain connected, even though the violinist has a right to life. The key point of this analogy is to suggest that, even if we grant the fetus full moral status as a human person, it does not necessarily follow that abortion is morally repugnant, and, in particular, a woman does not have a moral obligation to continue with a pregnancy and has the right to control what is done to her body. Thus the abortion debate should not depend exclusively on the issue of the moral status of the embryo.

Many feminists argue that a woman has a right to choose abortion on more general principles. Benschof (1985) claims that a right to abortion is grounded in a right to 'privacy, autonomy and bodily integrity'. Petchesky (1985) argues that decisions about abortion should place more emphasis on the social situations that place women in the situation of seeking an abortion (see Box 9.1), and should give central emphasis to their own moral judgements. Warren (1991) argues that making abortion illegal fails to respect women's right to liberty, self-determination and freedom from bodily harm, because carrying a pregnancy is arduous and risky (see also Holmes & Purdy 1992, Purdy 1996, Warren 1988).

Abortion law

There are two key statutes relevant to abortion: the Offences Against the Person Act and the Abortion Act.

The Offences Against the Person Act 1861

The Offences Against the Person Act 1861 remains the definitive law in England. It gives statutory grounds to the effect that abortion is a crime except where subsequent legislation provides protection against criminal prosecution.

The Abortion Act 1967, amended 1990

The Abortion Act was designed to tackle two main issues. The first was increasing concern at the number of 'back-street abortions', despite their being illegal. These were often medically quite unsafe, and an increasing number of women were being admitted to hospital with complications resulting from such abortions. The second was the lack of clarity over the question of when a doctor could carry out an abortion for the sake of the mother's health. Doctors, acting in good faith in the interests of their parents, faced the possibility of criminal charges.

The Act gives a doctor ('medical practitioner') who carries out an abortion within the terms of the Act immunity from prosecution. It does not decriminalize abortion in general. Nor does it provide protection for anyone other than the doctor (and for nurses as well, following the House of Lords ruling in Royal College of Nursing of UK v DHSS [1981]). Box 9.2 gives some of the important sections of the amended Act. Five points need emphasis:

1. Prior to 24 weeks a doctor may carry out an abortion, with the woman's consent, on very wide grounds (Section 1(1a)). By far the majority of abortions in England are carried out under this section.
2. After 24 weeks abortion is lawful only either to prevent risk of considerable harm to the mother, or for the sake of the fetus/child (see Box 9.2 for exact wording). In practice, most abortions after 24 weeks are done on grounds of fetal impairment (i.e. under Section 1(1d)).
3. Except in an emergency two doctors are required to be of the opinion that abortion is justified on one of the grounds stated in the Act.
4. It is generally assumed that when the Act states that 'pregnancy has not exceeded its 24th week' it means 24 weeks since the first day of the woman's last period. But this is not clear.
5. It is not clear what the approach should be to deciding whether an abortion is legal under Section 1(1d). The Royal College of Obstetricians and Gynaecologists (1996) has given guidance on this. The courts have not so far had to decide on the interpretation of Section 1(1d). Box 9.3 summarizes some points concerning legal aspects of abortion, and of fetal damage.

Box 9.2 The Abortion Act 1967 as amended in 1990

Section 1

Medical termination of pregnancy

(1) Subject to the provisions of this section, a person shall not be guilty of an offence under the law relating to abortion when a pregnancy is terminated by a registered medical practitioner if two registered medical practitioners are of the opinion, formed in good faith:

(a) that the pregnancy has not exceeded its 24th week and that the continuance of the pregnancy would involve risk, greater than if the pregnancy were terminated, of injury to the physical or mental health of the pregnant woman or any existing children of her family; or

(b) that the termination is necessary to prevent grave permanent injury to the physical or mental health of the pregnant woman; or

(c) that the continuance of the pregnancy would involve risk to the life of the pregnant woman, greater than if the pregnancy were terminated; or

(d) that there is a substantial risk that if the child were born it would suffer from such physical or mental abnormalities as to be seriously handicapped.

(2) In determining whether the continuance of a pregnancy would involve such risk of injury to health as mentioned in para (a) or (b) of sub-section (1) of this section, account may be taken of the pregnant woman's actual or reasonably foreseeable environment.

Box 9.3 Some key points in the law on abortion and fetal damage

1. Doctors may refuse to carry out an abortion on grounds of conscientious objection (Section 4 of the Abortion Act). The burden of proof lies with the doctor to show that he or she did have a conscientious objection. Conscientious objection is not a defence, however, if the abortion 'is necessary to save the life or to prevent grave permanent injury to the physical or mental health of a pregnant woman'.
2. The Abortion Act does not give a woman the right to demand an abortion. However, a doctor might be found negligent either for not advising a woman (in appropriate circumstances) of the possibility of an abortion, or for not carrying out an abortion, where appropriate, under Sections 1 (1b, 1c) (unless due to conscientious objection; see above).
3. The fetus has no right to life. Thus, its status in law is dramatically affected by birth. A fetus cannot be the subject of child protection under the Children Act (see Chapter 10).
4. A fetus probably has no legal right to be aborted. In other words, damages could not be claimed on the grounds that had doctors acted differently (e.g. advised abortion) the child would not have been born, and that it would have been better for the child not to have been born.
5. A woman has a legal right to refuse an abortion.
6. The father of a fetus has no legal right to prevent a woman from having an abortion – and no right to be consulted about it. Under Article 8 of The Human Rights Act (see Chapter 4) it may be possible for a father to claim some rights with regard to abortion. Such a claim, made in 1980 to the European Commission, was, however, rejected.

Intrauterine contraceptive devices (IUCDs) and 'morning-after' pills

The combined effect of R (John Smeaton on Behalf of SPUC) v The Secretary of State for Health et al [2002] and the Prescription Only Medicines (Human Use) Amendment Order 2000 is that:

1. it is legal for a pharmacist to dispense emergency contraception without a doctor's prescription; and
2. interceptive methods of contraception, such as the intrauterine device and the morning-after pill, which are designed to prevent implantation, are classified as contraceptive techniques. As such they are not governed by the Abortion Act 1967.

The living abortus

In carrying out a late abortion (under the Abortion Act) a doctor would be wise to ensure that the fetus is killed while it is still inside the uterus. If the fetus is alive outside the uterus it may acquire the legal protection of any newborn baby. Killing it may be murder.

MATERNAL–FETAL RELATIONS

Legal considerations

Enforcing caesarian section for the sake of the fetus

Over the last decade a number of cases have been heard in the courts concerning the legality of enforcing a caesarean section on an unwilling woman. Most cases have been heard in great haste and without legal representation for the pregnant woman. The Royal College of Obstetricians and Gynaecologists produced guidelines (2006, p. 11) that state:

" In caring for the pregnant woman, an obstetrician must respect the woman's autonomy and her legal right to refuse any recommended course of action … The use of judicial authority to implement treatment regimens in order to protect the fetus violates the pregnant woman's autonomy and should be avoided unless stringent criteria are met.

The Court of Appeal Judges (in Re MB (An Adult: Medical Treatment) [1997]) stated:

" A competent woman, who has the capacity to decide, may, for religious reasons, other reasons, for rational or irrational reasons or for no reason at all, choose not to have medical intervention, even though the consequence may be the death or serious handicap of the child she bears, or her own death. In that event the courts do not have the jurisdiction to declare medical intervention lawful and the question of her own best interests, objectively considered, does not arise…

The courts have interpreted common law as giving a competent woman the right to refuse treatment even where the life of the fetus is at grave risk. However, they fall over backwards to find the woman incompetent in order, perhaps, to justify saving the fetus, and perhaps on the view that the woman will be glad afterwards that that was the decision taken.

The principles established in Re MB have been confirmed most recently in Bolton Hospitals NHS Trust v O [2003]. The case involved a pregnant woman (with post-traumatic stress) who was held to be temporarily incompetent owing to panic induced by flashbacks. As a consequence a caesarean section could be carried out without her consent, i.e. it was in her best interests. It is likely that a similar outcome would now result if best interests were determined according to the Mental Capacity Act 2005.

Restraining a pregnant woman's lifestyle for the sake of the fetus

Under the Congenital Disabilities (Civil Liability) Act 1976 a damaged child, who would not have been born damaged were it not for the negligence of the defendant (for example a doctor), can make a claim and recover damages. This Act specifically excludes the case where the damage is a result of actions by the mother (except in the case of negligent driving).

Ethical considerations

A key distinction is considering Fetal interests and their relationship to material interests, is that between identity-preserving and identity-altering interventions

(Box 9.4). Most cases of maternal–fetal conflict relate to identity-preserving interventions involving potentially avoidable damage to the fetus. Consider the issue of whether pregnant women should be constrained from engaging in lifestyles, or making choices, that will lead to significant harm to the future child.

Arguments against constraining a pregnant woman's behaviour for the sake of the fetus (or future child)

1. *Autonomy* – such constraints infringe the woman's autonomy. This argument could be supplemented using a similar argument to that of Thomson (see above, the case of the connected violinist) in the context of abortion.
2. *Privacy* – the woman has a right not to have her body invaded or even touched without consent. Many constraints on her behaviour would involve such battery.
3. *Fetal status* – in English law the fetus has no status as a person until birth. The rights of a person (the woman) should not be subjugated to the rights, if any, of an entity that is not a person.
4. *Public policy* – the likely consequences of allowing fetal interests to affect the legal provisions for restraining people's behaviour are undesirable. A liberal society rightly draws back from the spectre of either imprisoning or impoverishing pregnant women for behaviour that would be tolerated in men, or in women who are not pregnant.
5. Even if there are good arguments that it is morally wrong for a pregnant woman to behave in ways that might harm the fetus or future child, it does not follow that such behaviour should be the subject of legal restraint.

Box 9.4 Identity-preserving and identity-altering interventions

In thinking about the ethical issues raised by decisions or interventions in reproductive medicine it is important to distinguish between an *identity-preserving* and an *identity-altering* intervention or decision.

An example of an *identity-preserving intervention* is when a pregnant woman drinks large amounts of alcohol. If the child is subsequently born with some brain damage as a result, it has been harmed by the mother's alcohol intake.

An example of an *identity-altering decision* is when a woman decides to delay reproduction from, for example, age 30 years to age 40 years. A different child will be born as a result of her decision. Suppose that she has a child (child A) at age 40 years that is born with Down's syndrome. The likelihood is that, had she conceived a child at age 30 years, it would not have suffered from Down's syndrome. Has child A been harmed as a result of her decision to delay reproduction? The decision has altered the identity of the child who is born. Had she conceived at age 30 years she would have given birth to a different child. Because child A would not have come into existence at all, had the woman not decided to delay reproduction, it is not clear that child A has been harmed by having Down's syndrome as a result of her decision. On one view of harm, the decision could have harmed child A only if it would have been better for A not to have existed at all than to exist with Down's syndrome.

An argument in favour of constraining a pregnant woman's behaviour for the sake of the fetus (or future child)

A classic example of justified state restraint is the banning of the sedative thalidomide. This sedative had no significant adverse effects on mothers. However, if taken during fetal gestation, it interfered with limb development. Rather than informing women of these possible effects and allowing them to choose whether to take this sedative, the state rightly banned it in the interests of future people.

In so far as a pregnant woman's behaviour causes harm to the child who will exist, the state may be justified in constraining such behaviour. Such constraint would be on the basis of the principle of preventing harm to others.

ASSISTED REPRODUCTION

Assisted reproduction has come of age. Louise Brown, the first 'test-tube' baby, will be 30 years old in 2008. Since Louise Brown's conception, which was made possible through in-vitro fertilization (IVF), several even more sophisticated techniques have been developed (Lockwood 2003). Some believe that IVF and related techniques are always wrong. Four arguments in support of this view are summarized in Box 9.5.

Box 9.5 Four reasons for considering IVF, and some other types of fertility treatment, as ethically wrong

1. Killing embryos is wrong

Some types of fertility treatment involve the production of embryos that are subsequently not used in treatment and are destroyed. The force of this argument depends on the moral status accorded to embryos (see text).

2. IVF is unnatural

The argument about unnaturalness is used in many situations involving modern technology. There are three major problems with the argument in general. The first is to determine what is natural and what unnatural. The second is that so much of medicine (and indeed so much of modern life) is unnatural. Few would argue that intravenous antibiotics should not be given to someone with septicaemia. The third is to provide reasons why something that is unnatural is therefore morally wrong.

3. IVF is harmful to marriage

Reproductive technologies separate the procreative aspects of marriage from the conjugal aspects. Some argue that this is harmful to the institution of marriage. The problem with this is to clarify in what way this is harmful to the marriage.

4. IVF harms women

Some argue that the new reproductive technologies harm women. These arguments centre on claims that men control these technologies and hence control female reproduction. Furthermore, such technologies help to perpetuate a view that women cannot be completely fulfilled unless they have children. This in turn is part of a value system that leads to women's opportunities and ability to compete with men being reduced because of being tied to child production and child care.

Many women take the opposite view and see the reproductive technologies as enhancing their freedom and choice by enabling them to have children if they so wish.

Box 9.6 gives some examples of categories of people who might seek medical help in having a child. Should any of these be refused help even if they are willing to pay for the total costs of treatment?

In deciding whether, or when, it is right to veto a request for help, or in deciding priorities for treatment, there are three main interests that are potentially important: those of the (potential) child, those of the couple, and those of society more generally.

The interests of the (potential) child

Most discussions, and the law, place the interests of the child that may result from the assisted reproduction as of paramount importance. However, it is not as clear as might at first be thought, what these interests are. There are generally three approaches to this question.

The analogy with adoption
The first approach sees the issue as broadly analogous to that of adoption. The central question is: which couple, out of all the available couples wishing to adopt, is likely to provide the best parents for this baby? This approach can be applied to the question of infertility. One example frequently cited of when it is wrong to assist reproduction is for a postmenopausal woman aged around 60 years.

There are two major problems with the analogy with adoption. The first is the nature of the judgements and the evidence on which they are based. What is the evidence that children brought up by a single mother are less happy (or whatever) than a child brought up by a healthy couple? Is the fertility clinic in a position to decide which of the couples or individuals will make the best parents? The second problem is more profound. This is to deny that the adoption model is the appropriate model in the first place.

Better to be born to this couple or individual than not to be born at all
There is a crucial difference between adoption and fertility treatment. For adoption we have the same baby whichever couple we choose as parents; in the case of fertility treatment it is a different baby in each case. For the child who would be born if we helped couple A, it is best that we help couple A. For the child who

---

Box 9.6 Examples of categories of people who might seek medical help in having a child

1. A single woman
2. A couple, one of whom has a serious life-threatening disease
3. A postmenopausal woman aged 50 years
4. A woman of 35 years who has undergone premature menopause
5. A couple, one of whom has had previous voluntary sterilization
6. A couple who are having marital difficulties and who believe that having a child will help secure their relationship
7. A couple who have suffered the death of a child
8. A same-sex couple
9. A couple who have a child that has been taken into care

Reproductive medicine

would be born if we helped couple B, it would be best that we help couple B. Asking whether it is in the interests of the potential child for us to help couple A or couple B does not make sense, as it is a different child who will be born depending on the decision we make. We could perhaps ask: is it in the best interests of the potential child 'b' to be born to parents B, or not to be born at all? But it is not possible for child 'b' to be born to couple A. The key point is that decisions about which couples to help are 'identity-altering' decisions (see Box 9.4).

In the case of the 60-year-old woman, what are the interests of the potential child? If we refuse help, the child will not come into existence. If we help, the child will be born to a mother aged 60 or 61 years. Which represents the best interests of the potential child? Although it might be preferable, if there were a choice, for the child to have a younger mother, there is no choice. On such a view, the criterion of the best interests of the potential child, which is given such a central place in most discussions about fertility treatment, is of little value. It would rule out assisting reproduction only in some rather extreme situations, for example when the potential child is likely to suffer either from a very serious genetic disorder or from very bad parenting, when it might be worse for the child to exist than never to exist.

Talk of interests of a potential child is meaningless

One response to the above arguments is to deny that it is meaningful to talk of the best interests of a potential child, or to compare life, in any state, with never existing. If this view is correct, then it means that the criterion of the best interests of the potential child is a meaningless concept. But this view faces a difficulty. Let us suppose, for the sake of argument, that if couple X had a child that child would suffer immensely (perhaps from some dreadful genetic condition). It makes sense to argue that we should prevent the couple from conceiving for the sake of the child that would come into existence if they were to conceive, i.e. for the sake of the potential child.

The interests of the potential parent(s)

Fertility clinics are often faced with couples who want IVF, although there are reasons for thinking that this would not be in their best interests – for example, another child would put great strain on the marriage, or the chance of success is very low (e.g. because of the woman's age). From the professionals' point of view it does not seem worth the risks or costs of the treatment, given the very low chance of success.

What should the professionals do? This situation, if we are considering only the interests of the couple, is similar to a situation frequently met with in medicine: a patient making a decision that the professionals believe is not in his or her best interests. One response to such situations is to provide the couple with relevant information and to explain the reasons for the professional opinion. However, if the couple, after due deliberation, still want to go ahead with fertility treatment, and will pay the costs, should such treatment be provided?

The interests of the state

The state has interests in the people who are born, even if the couple are paying for the entire costs of the fertility treatment. This may be significant, for example, if the child has profound impairments requiring considerable welfare provision. But the state's interests go further than this. When is it in the interests of society that a particular couple or individual should not be helped to conceive? Should a single mother, or a lesbian couple, or a woman aged 60, be allowed access to fertility treatment if the total costs are met by the couple or the individual? The starting point in a liberal society is that the state needs a good reason to interfere in individual liberty. It might be argued that in allowing fertility treatment to, for example, a lesbian couple, the state is condoning a form of family life that it should not condone. Reasons would need to be given as to not only why such family life is wrong, but also why it is the kind of wrong that justifies state interference.

Assisted reproduction and the law

The Human Fertilisation and Embryology Act 1990 (HFEA)

This Act, in addition to providing most of the key aspects of legislation in this area, set up the *Human Fertilisation and Embryology Authority*. This Authority regulates much of the provision for assisting reproduction, some of which is summarized in Box 9.7.

Box 9.7   The Human Fertilisation and Embryology Act 1990 (HFEA)

Areas covered by the act
1. Treatment that involves the use of donated genetic material (eggs, sperm or embryos), or stored genetic material, or embryos created outside the body (e.g. by IVF). Such treatments have to be *licensed*.
2. The storage of human eggs, sperm and embryos.
3. Research on human embryos.

The Human Fertilisation and Embryology Authority
This was set up by Parliament under the Act. It is funded partly by centres licensed to provide fertility treatment, and partly from taxation. The Authority has 19 members appointed by the Secretary of State for Health. The functions of the Authority include the following:
1. Inspecting and licensing centres involved in the areas covered by the Act (see above)
2. Keeping a confidential register of information about donors, patients and treatments
3. Publishing a code of practice
4. Giving information and advice to those seeking fertility treatment
5. Keeping the whole field under review.

Research on embryos
1. Research on human embryos more than 14 days old (i.e. from the appearance of the primitive streak) is illegal.
2. Research leading to the production of identical individuals by genetic replacement is illegal.

Reproductive medicine

3. It is illegal to attempt to produce embryos by combining the gametes of humans with animals.

Further points

1. Section 13(5) of the HFEA states that: 'a woman shall not be provided with treatment services unless account has been taken of the welfare of any child who may be born as a result of the treatment (including the need of that child for a father) and of any other child who may be affected by the birth'. The section is controversial not least because of the wide discretion it gives clinics to refuse individuals they considered 'unfit' parents. Guidance from the Authority on this section was revised in 2005. This advice gives more detailed guidance than previously as to when treatment should be refused, i.e. if the child is likely to be at risk of serious physical, psychological or medical harm (for further details see http://www.hfea.gov.uk). Most importantly, the new guidance explicitly states that parental age and the stability of the parental relationship are not issues that should be considered in assessing the welfare of the child. The HFEA has announced a review of the operation of the welfare test. There are several possible alternative views that might be taken (such as a maximum welfare principle and a reasonable welfare principle).
2. Under the Act a woman can be provided with treatment only if she (and any partner who is being treated with her) has been offered the opportunity to receive proper counselling.
3. A donor egg cannot come from a female embryo.
4. The current code of practice at the time of writing is the seventh edition.

The Surrogacy Arrangements Act 1985 (SAA)

Surrogacy is covered by the Surrogacy Arrangements Act 1985. This makes any commercial basis for surrogacy a criminal offence. Thus facilitators of commercial surrogacy would be committing an illegal act, and advertising for such arrangements is illegal. However, the Act specifically gives immunity to the actual parties themselves. The HFEA made amendments to the SAA stating: 'No surrogacy arrangement is enforceable by or against any of the persons making it ...'. Thus the surrogate mother (whatever the genetic relationships) will remain the child's mother if she wishes to be so.

Reform of the SAA is long overdue. Three areas in particular are problematic. First, the prohibition against commercialization has failed to prevent payments being made (typically of £10 000–15 000). Second, the HFEA's definition of motherhood and fatherhood does not adequately cover surrogacy arrangements. Third, the rules governing the transfer of legal parenthood are so complex that commissioning parents are reluctant to acquire a formal legal relationship with 'their' child. Whilst the government has accepted the need to reform the Act, it has so far failed to propose new legislation.

Anand K J S, Hickey P R 1987 Pain and its effects in the human neonate and fetus. New England Journal of Medicine 317:1321–1329

Benn S 1984 Abortion, infanticide, and respect for persons. In: Feinberg J (ed.) The problem of abortion. Wadsworth, Belmont, CA, pp. 135–144

Benschof J 1985 Reasserting women's rights. In: Late abortion and technological advances in fetal viability. Family Planning Perspectives. 17:160–164

Bolton Hospital NHS Trust v O [2003] FLR 1824

Dworkin R 1993 Life's dominion: an argument about abortion and euthanasia. HarperCollins, London

Englehardt T 1973 Viability, abortion, and the difference between a fetus and an infant. American Journal of Obstetrics and Gynecology 116:429–434

Feinberg J 1984 Potentiality, development and rights. In: Feinberg J (ed.) The problem of abortion. Wadsworth, Belmont, CA, pp. 145–150

Harris J 1997 Goodbye Dolly. The ethics of human cloning. Journal of Medical Ethics 23:353–360

Harris J 1998 Rights and reproductive choice. In: Harris J, Holm S (eds) The future of reproduction. Clarendon Press, Oxford, pp. 5–37

Holmes H B, Purdy L M (eds) 1992 Feminist perspectives in medical ethics. Indiana University Press, Bloomington, IN

Lockwood G M 2003 Infertility and early pregnancy loss. In: Waller D, McPherson A (eds) Women's health, 5th edn. Oxford University Press, Oxford, pp. 262–298

Petchesky R 1985 Abortion and women's choice. Northeastern University Press, Boston, MA

Purdy L M 1996 Reproducing persons: issues in feminist bioethics. Cornell University Press, Ithaca, NY

R (John Smeaton on Behalf of SPUC) v The Secretary of State for Health et al [2002] 2 FCR 193

Re M B (An Adult: Medical Treatment) [1992] 2 FLR 426 CA

Robertson J A 1994 Children of choice: freedom and the new reproductive technologies. Princeton University Press, Princeton, NJ

Royal College of Nursing of UK v DHSS [1981] AC 800

Royal College of Obstetricians and Gynaecologists 1996 Termination of pregnancy for fetal abnormality. RCOG, London

Royal College of Obstetricians and Gynaecologists 2006 Law and ethics in relation to court-authorised obstetric intervention. Ethics committee guideline no. 1. RCOG, London. Online. Available: http://www.rcog.org.uk/resources/Public/pdf/ethics_guideline_1_0906.pdf 24 Jun 2007

Singer P 1985 Technology and procreation: how far should we go? Technology Review Feb/Mar: 23–30

Singer P 1993 Practical ethics, 2nd edn. Cambridge University Press, New York

Singer P, Kuhse H 1987 The ethics of embryo research. Law, Medicine & Health Care 14:133–138

Strong C 1997 Ethics in reproductive and perinatal medicine. Yale University Press, New Haven, CN

Thomson J J 1971 A defence of abortion. Philosophy and public affairs, Princeton University Press.Reprinted in: Singer P (ed.) 1986 Applied ethics. Oxford University Press, Oxford, pp. 37–56

Tooley M 1983 Abortion and infanticide. Oxford University Press, Oxford

Warnock Committee 1984 Report of the Committee of Inquiry into Human Fertilisation and Embryology. Cmnd 9314. HMSO, London

Warren M A 1988 IVF and women's interests: an analysis of feminist concerns. Bioethics 2:37–57

Warren M A 1991 Abortion. In: Singer P (ed.) A companion to ethics. Blackwell, Oxford, pp. 303–314

Reproductive medicine

FURTHER READING

Abortion

Boonin D 2004 A defense of abortion. Journal of Moral Philosophy 1(3):378–382

Chambers J E 2003 Women's right to choose rationally: genetic information, embryo selection, and genetic manipulation. Cambridge Quarterly of Healthcare Ethics 12(4):418–428

Cohen A, Wellman C H 2005 Contemporary debates in applied ethics. Blackwell, Malden, MA

DeGrazia D 2003 Identity, killing, and the boundaries of our existence. Philosophy & Public Affairs 31:(4):413–442

Engelhardt H T Jr 2004 Moral knowledge: some reflections on moral controversies, incompatible moral epistemologies, and the culture wars. Christian Bioethics 10(1):79–103

Fischer J M 2003 Abortion, autonomy, and control over one's body. Social Philosophy and Policy 20(2):286–306

Frey R G, Wellman C H (eds) A companion to applied ethics. Blackwell, Oxford.

Gert B 2004 Moral disagreement and abortion. Australian Journal of Professional and Applied Ethics 6(1):1–19

Harris J, Holm S 2003 Abortion. In: LaFollete H (ed.) The Oxford handbook of practical ethics. Oxford University Press, Oxford, pp. 112–135

Hursthouse R 1991 Virtue theory and abortion. Philosophy & Public Affairs 20:223–246. Reprinted in Crisp R, Slote M (eds) 1997 Virtue ethics. Oxford University Press, Oxford, pp. 217–238

Kamm F M 1992 Creation and abortion: a study in moral and legal philosophy. Oxford University Press, New York
A complex but philosophically sophisticated analysis of abortion and creating people.

LaFollete H (ed.) 2003 The Oxford handbook of practical ethics. Oxford University Press, Oxford

Little M 2003 The morality of abortion. In: Frey R G, Wellman C H (eds) A companion to applied ethics. Blackwell, Oxford, pp. 313–325

McDonagh E L 1996 Breaking the abortion deadlock: from choice to consent. Oxford University Press, New York

Outka G 2002 The ethics of human stem cell research. Kennedy Institute of Ethics Journal 12(2):175–213

Scott R 2005 Prenatal testing, reproductive autonomy, and disability interests. Cambridge Quarterly of Healthcare Ethics 1491:65–82

Shannon T A 2004 Reproductive technologies: a reader. Rowman & Littlefield, Lanham, MD

Sherwin S 1996 Abortion through a feminist ethics lens. In: Munson R (ed.) Intervention and reflection: basic issues in medical ethics. Wadsworth, Belmont, CA, pp. 93–97

Thomson J J 1971 A defence of abortion. Philosophy & Public Affairs 1:47–66. Reprinted in: Singer P (ed.) 1986 Applied ethics. Oxford University Press, Oxford, pp. 37–56

Thomson J J 1996 Abortion: whose right? Boston Review 20:3
A defence of abortion by one of the most influential philosophers to write on the topic.

Warren M A 1973 On the moral and legal status of abortion. In: Mappes T A, DeGrazia D (eds) Biomedical ethics. McGraw-Hill, New York, pp. 456–461
A philosophical examination of the status of the fetus.

Assisted reproduction

Glover J 1984 What sort of people should there be? Pelican, Harmondsworth

Glover J 1989 Fertility and the family: the Glover report on reproductive technologies to the European Commission. Fourth Estate, London

Harris J, Holm S (eds) 1998 The future of human reproduction: ethics, choice and regulation. Oxford University Press, Oxford
A collection of essays. The introduction by Harris provides a useful overview of ethical issues in assisted reproduction.

Lauritzen P 1993 Pursuing parenthood: ethical issues in assisted reproduction. Indiana University Press, Bloomington, IN

Overall C 1993 Human reproduction: principles, practices, policies. Oxford University Press, Toronto

Peterson M M 2005 Assisted reproductive technologies and equity of access issues. Journal of Medical Ethics 31(5):280–285

Purdy L M 1996 Reproducing persons: issues in feminist bioethics. Cornell University Press, London

Robertson J 1994 Children of choice: freedom and the new reproductive technologies. Princeton University Press, Princeton, NJ

An excellent examination of a wide range of issues associated with assisted reproduction and the new genetics, with an extensive review of the associated literature. Robertson is a legal theorist who writes regularly and accessibly on medical ethics.

Tong R, Kaplan J 1996 Controlling our reproductive destiny: a technological and philosophical perspective. MIT Press, Cambridge, MA

Warnock M 2002 Making babies: is there a right to have children? Oxford University Press, Oxford

Prenatal screening

Paintin D (ed.) 1997 Medical and ethical issues: antenatal screening and abortion of fetal abnormality. Birth Control Trust, London

Maternal–fetal relations

Hornstra D 1998 A realistic approach to maternal–fetal conflict. Hastings Center Report 28:7–12

Mackenzie C 1995 Abortion and embodiment. In: Komesaroff P (ed.) Troubled bodies: critical perspectives on postmodernism, medical ethics and the body. Melbourne University Press, Melbourne pp 38–61

Mathieu D 1996 Preventing prenatal harm. Georgetown University Press, Washington, DC

An excellent overview of the issue of prenatal harm that covers the literature comprehensively. Especially good on involuntary caesarean sections.

Sterilization

Cartwright W 1994 The sterilisation of the mentally disabled: competence, the right

to reproduce and discrimination. In: Grubb A (ed.) Decision making and problems of inclusion. John Wiley, New York, pp. 67–88

Sills E S, Strider W, Hyde H J et al 1998 Gynaecology, forced sterilisation and asylum in the USA. Lancet 351:1729–1730

Other issues

Brazier M 2003 Medicine, patients and the law, 3rd edn. Penguin, London

Fuscaldo G, Savulescu J 2005 Spare embryos: 3000 reasons to rethink the significance of genetic relatedness. Reproductive Biomedicine Online 10(2):164–168

Savulescu J 2001 Procreative beneficence: why we should select the best children. Bioethics 15:413–426

Savulescu J 2002 Education and debate: deaf lesbians, 'designer disability,' and the future of medicine. British Medical Journal 325:771–773

Savulescu J 2002 Is there a 'right not to be born'? Reproductive decision making, options and the right to information. Archives of Disease in Childhood. Fetal and Neonatal Edition 87(2):F72–F74

Savulescu J 2004 Embryo research: are there any lessons from natural reproduction? Cambridge Quarterly of Health Care Ethics 13(1):68–75

Savulescu J 2007 In defence of procreative beneficence: response to Parker. Journal of Medical Ethics (in press)

Savulescu J, Harris J 2004 The creation lottery. Cambridge Quarterly of Health Care Ethics 13(1):90–95

Spriggs M, Savulescu J 2002 Saviour siblings. Journal of Medical Ethics 28(5):289

Children

The way we think about children is fraught with tensions. On the one hand we want to be protective, and on the other we want to encourage increasing autonomy. We value family relationships, wishing to give parents the right to determine the care of their children without state interference. We want the state, however, to protect children when their parents do not act in their best interests. Doctors are caught up in these tensions. In this chapter we will focus on two key issues for doctors who have child patients: consent to treatment and suspicion of abuse.

From the legal point of view, a person becomes adult, on his or her 18th birthday. Until that time a person is a minor. This chapter is concerned with the law as it relates to doctors caring for patients aged less than 18 years.

THE CHILDREN ACT 1989

Overview of the Act

The Children Act 1989, which came into force in 1991, articulates a number of general principles (Box 10.1), as well as providing specific legal procedures. It also provides a 'welfare checklist' (Box 10.2) to help guide the courts, i.e. factors that, when relevant, should be considered, by the court in coming to a decision.

Although the Children Act 1989 remains the principal statute concerning children, it has been supplemented by several subsequent Acts. Of these, the Children Act 2004 is one of the most important. The 2004 Act makes radical changes to the system of children's services, with the intention of providing a better integrated service for the protection of children. The Act provides for a national database that will enable local authorities, the NHS, and other agencies to share information on suspected abuse and neglect, with the aim of achieving early intervention. The Act also sets out the powers and duties of the Children's Commissioner. The role of the Commissioner is to act as a champion for children, his or her general function being to promote an awareness of the rights, views, welfare and interests of children.

The Act addresses issues of potential conflict in the care of children, such as:

- care arrangements if parents split up
- decision-making where those with responsibility for the care of the child cannot come to an agreement (e.g. with respect to schooling or medical treatment)
- arrangements to protect a child from harm, either in an emergency or in the longer term.

> **Box 10.1**   Some general principles of the Children Act 1989
>
> - The child's welfare is paramount.
> - The child is a person, not an object of concern: children of sufficient maturity should be listened to (although not necessarily be given full power of autonomy).
> - Children should be brought up by parents, or wider family, without the interference of the State, unless placed at risk.
> - Family links should be maintained if a child is placed out of the home.
> - Cooperation, negotiation and partnership should be the aim when conflicts do arise.
> - Avoid delay when legal processes are required.

> **Box 10.2**   The Children Act 1989: welfare checklist
>
> The following should be taken into account by courts in guiding their decisions:
> - The wishes and feelings of the child
> - The child's physical, emotional and educational needs
> - The likely effect on the child of a change in circumstances
> - The age, sex and background of the child, and any characteristics the court considers relevant
> - Any harm the child has suffered or is at risk of suffering
> - The capability of parents and others to meet the child's needs
> - The range of powers open to the courts.

The Act is a key piece of legislation relevant to England and Wales. Scotland has its own Act: the Children (Scotland) Act 1995 (see below).

The specific issue order

The specific issue order is an order giving directions (from the court) for the purpose of determining a specific question. It is of value where there is dispute between relevant people as to what should be done. Effectively, the court says, 'Go and do it this way'. This order is of particular relevance to doctors when those with parental responsibility are refusing consent for the child to receive treatment that the doctor thinks is strongly in the child's best interests. The court will decide whether treatment should be given. This order is rarely used if the child is over 16 years old.

Other types of order under the Children Act of particular relevance to doctors

The emergency protection order enables a child at urgent risk of harm to be taken to a safe place. A care order enables a local authority to take over the care of a child and gives that authority parental responsibility (see below). A child assessment order is appropriate when there is suspicion of harm but lack of evidence; otherwise, it is appropriate to go directly to a care order. Medical assessment may be part of the assessment directed by the court.

Parental responsibility

Parental responsibility is a key concept in the Children Act. Doctors need to understand about parental responsibility because it is critically important to the question of who can give consent for medical assessment and treatment of a child not yet old enough and mature enough to give his or her own consent.

There are some general points about parental responsibility:

- More than one person may have parental responsibility for a child (typically both parents will have such responsibility).
- Many actions or decisions, including consent to medical examination and treatment, can be carried out by just one person with parental responsibility, and there is no duty for that person to consult anyone else with parental responsibility before acting (or giving consent to treatment).
- Parental responsibility cannot normally be transferred or surrendered.

Those with parental responsibility have a duty to ensure that the child receives essential medical assistance and adequate full-time education, among other things. They have the right to make decisions on major issues such as day-to-day care and schooling. The law relating to who has parental responsibility is summarized in Box 10.3.

THE CHILDREN (SCOTLAND) ACT 1995

The Children (Scotland) Act 1995 applies to Scotland. This Act, like the Children Act 1989, was a major piece of social legislation that affects many areas of common and statute law concerning children. A key aim of the Act was to move towards a more child-centred approach. The Act is based on three principles:

1. The welfare of the child is paramount.
2. The views of the child must be taken into account where practicable; a child aged 12 years and over is presumed to form a view.
3. A court, or hearing, should make an order concerning a child's future only if it is convinced that making an order is better than not making it.

The Children (Scotland) Act 1995 makes more explicit reference to children's views than does the Children Act 1989. The Scottish Act has a similar set of orders to protect children and resolve disputes to the English Act.

The Scottish Act defines parental responsibilities and rights in more detail than the English Act. Under the Scottish Act a parent has a responsibility towards a child up to the age of 16 years to:

1. safeguard the child's health and welfare and development
2. provide direction and guidance
3. maintain personal relations and direct contact with the child on a regular basis (if not living with the child).

The responsibility to provide guidance lasts until the child is 18 years old.
A parent has a right to:

1. have a child live with him or her, or regulate where a child will live
2. control, direct or guide the child's upbringing
3. maintain personal relations and direct contact (if the child is not living with the parent).

CHILDREN

Box 10.3   Who has parental responsibility?

1. The mother of the child.
2. The father of the child if he is married to the mother, either at the time of insemination or at the time of the birth of the child (or at both times).
3. If the father of the child is not married to the mother of the child at the time of insemination or birth then he has no automatic parental responsibility, but he may acquire it:
   - by marrying the mother (thus the married parents of a child will both have parental responsibility)
   - by a written agreement with the mother (this is to allow fathers in long-term relationships without marriage to acquire parental responsibility, but only with the agreement of the mother)
   - by court order (e.g. residence and parental responsibility orders)
   - if the father is appointed the child's guardian following the mother's death
   - by registering as the father (with the child's mother) on the child's birth certificate (this provision applies in England, Wales and Scotland).

In the situations described above, once acquired, parental responsibility continues if the person is named on the birth certificate, except in unusual circumstances of which the most important is that the child is adopted – in which case the original parent(s) cease to have parental responsibility and the adopting parents acquire parental responsibility.

   NB1: Parental responsibility, once acquired, remains even when the parents divorce.

   NB2: The law presumes that a child born to a married woman is the child of her husband.

   Where a husband does not deny paternity, and no other man asserts that he is the father, the husband is considered in law to be the father (whatever the biological fact).

How people other than parents may acquire parental responsibility

1. Adoption – in which case the original parent(s) cease to have parental responsibility.
2. Guardian – parents with parental responsibility may (without involving a court) appoint a guardian to acquire parental responsibility for their child on their death.
3. A person obtaining a residence order normally acquires parental responsibility – this might be when a child is effectively given over to the care of a grandparent. The parent(s), however, do not lose parental responsibility.
4. A local authority named in a care order (again the parent(s) do not lose parental responsibility).
5. An applicant granted an emergency protection order, but only for the duration of the care order.

   NB1: Step-parents (by marriage or civil partnership) do not automatically have parental responsibility. They may acquire it by making a parental responsibility agreement or by obtaining a parental responsibility order or a special guardianship order, or by a residence order, or by adopting the child.

> **NB2:** A person (e.g. an unmarried father) may be a parent without having parental responsibility. There are some legal consequences that arise from the status of being a parent (e.g. responsibility for child support). However, in the context of consent to medical treatment the key legal issue is that of parental responsibility.
>
> **NB3:** In the case of couples undergoing fertility treatment (licensed under the Human Fertilisation and Embryology Act) and involving donated gametes, the legal parents of the child are normally the couple and not the gamete donors.
>
> **Scotland**
> Parental responsibility under the Children (Scotland) Act 1995 is allocated in the same way as under the Children Act 1989.

THE FAMILY LAW REFORM ACT 1969

The Family Law Reform Act 1969 is relevant to consent to treatment for patients aged 16 and 17 years in England and Wales. It is not relevant in Scotland (see below). The Family Law Reform Act 1969 states: '...the consent of a minor who has attained the age of sixteen years to any surgical, medical or dental treatment ... shall be as effective as it would be if he were of full age [i.e. aged 18 years or above]; and ... it shall not be necessary to obtain any consent for it from his parent or guardian'. The implications of this are considered below.

THE GILLICK CASE

Victoria Gillick had four daughters under the age of 16 years. She wrote to her health authority seeking assurance that none of her daughters would be given contraception, or abortion advice or treatment, without her knowledge and consent, until they reached 16 years of age. The health authority gave no such assurance. Mrs Gillick went to court arguing that the Department of Health and Social Security's advice (stating that doctors could, under certain circumstances, give contraceptive advice and treatment to children under 16 years without the parents' knowledge) was unlawful. The case went to the House of Lords (Gillick v West Norfolk and Wisbech Area Health Authority [1985]). The Lords decided, by three to two, against Mrs Gillick. Lord Scarman said: '... the parental right yields to the child's right to make his own decisions when he reaches a sufficient understanding and intelligence to be capable of making up his own mind on the matter requiring decision' (see Brazier 2003).

This case has given rise to the concept of *'Gillick competence'*, i.e. when a child achieves sufficient understanding and intelligence to enable him (or her) to understand fully what is proposed.

A Gillick-competent child aged less than 16 years may give consent to medical treatment (although refusal of consent may be overridden – see below).

THE AGE OF LEGAL CAPACITY (SCOTLAND) ACT 1991

This Act, relevant only in Scotland, gives statutory power to mature minors under the age of 16 years to consent to treatment. The Act states (Section 2(4)):

'A person under the age of 16 years shall have legal capacity to consent on his own behalf to any surgical, medical or dental procedure or treatment where, in the opinion of a qualified medical practitioner attending him, he is capable of understanding the nature and possible consequences of the procedures or treatment'. The Act effectively does through statute what the Gillick case has done through common law in England and Wales. The Act does not affect a parent's ability to give consent on behalf of a person aged less than 16 years.

With regard to people aged 16 and 17 years, it is common law rather than the Family Law Reform Act 1969 that is relevant in Scotland. In Scotland, a person aged 16 years and above is presumed to have the ability to make medical decisions and give consent to procedures.

CONSENT TO TREATMENT AND MINORS

In the light of the Children Act, the Family Law Reform Act and the Gillick case, we can now turn to the tricky issue of consent to treatment and minors. Three points are worth emphasizing:

1. In general, the law allows increasing autonomy to the minor with increasing age, maturity and understanding. This is, of course, perfectly reasonable, but it does result in uncertainty.
2. Despite allowing considerable autonomy to older minors (in particular those over 16 years of age), it is probably the case (but this is not altogether clear) that, from a legal point of view, the patient's refusal of treatment should be overridden in order to prevent serious harm. This is in contrast with the competent 18-year-old (adult) who can refuse treatment even if harm or death is likely (see Chapter 6).
3. Those with parental responsibility (see above) have the legal right to give consent on behalf of minors for medical treatment. But such proxy consent is limited. A minor should not, at least from a legal point of view, be allowed to come to serious harm because the parent refuses consent for the appropriate treatment.

Box 10.4 summarizes the law on consent with regard to minors.

As with adult patients it is generally the case that consent is needed before a doctor can treat a patient who is a minor. Without consent, treatment (or indeed any 'touching'; see Chapter 6) is a battery. Consent can be given *either* by the minor (if competent) *or* by at least one person with parental responsibility. However, if consent is refused the legal position is more complex than it is with regard to adults. Both those with parental responsibility and doctors are legally obliged to act in the minor's best interests. The difficulties arise when there is disagreement as to what these are. A number of points are relevant in deciding what to do in difficult situations:

1. If a 16–17-year-old with capacity *refuses consent* for the treatment that the doctors consider on reasonable grounds to be appropriate, then the doctors can proceed with the treatment as long as someone with parental responsibility gives consent (i.e. it would not be a battery to proceed). This is because, although the Family Law Reform Act 1969 allows 16–17–year-olds to give consent for treatment, it does not take away the ability of those with parental responsibility to give proxy consent.

Box 10.4 Summary of the law in England and Wales on consent and children

Minors (less than 18 years old) and consent
- The law is complex and not always clear.
- Do not allow a person under 18 years to come to serious harm on the grounds that the minor and the parents refuse consent for necessary and urgent treatment.

16–17-year-olds (governed by the Family Law Reform Act 1969)
- Are presumed to have capacity to give consent to medical procedures unless the contrary is shown.
- If they have capacity, they can give consent.
- If the patient refuses consent then those with parental responsibility, or a court, can give consent to treatment that is in the child's best interests (see text).

Under 16 years old and Gillick competent (governed by common law)
- Children under 16 years old are presumed not to have capacity to consent unless they satisfy health professionals that they do have such capacity.
- However, the common law case of Gillick established that a child aged less than 16 years who does have capacity (i.e. is Gillick competent) can give consent for medical treatment.
- The criteria for judging capacity (Gillick competence) are not well specified. The key wording in the Gillick case was that children have capacity when they reach a sufficient understanding and intelligence to enable them to understand fully what is proposed (see text).
- It is unlikely that the courts would consider children of 13 years or less to be Gillick competent in most situations, although there is no clear legal guidance on this matter.
- If the patient refuses consent, the legal situation is as for 16–17-year-olds above.

Children who are not Gillick competent
- At least one person with parental responsibility should normally give consent.
- Those with parental responsibility are under a legal obligation to act in the child's best interests.
- If all those with parental responsibility refuse consent for a procedure that the doctors think is strongly in the child's best interests, then the doctors should involve the courts (specific issue order; see text).
- In an emergency, if parental consent is not forthcoming and there is no time to involve the courts, act to save the child from death or serious harm.

Court decisions have tended to support the view that the refusal of beneficial treatment by a minor (even if aged 16–17 years) can be overridden in the interests of that minor. Most doctors, however, would be reluctant to enforce treatment on a competent 16–17-year-old, even with consent from someone with parental responsibility, unless in an emergency to prevent death or serious harm.

2. A Gillick-competent minor, even if less than 16 years old, may give valid consent to treatment. It would therefore be lawful for a doctor to proceed with treatment (e.g. an operation) that the doctor believes to be in the child's best interests, and for which the Gillick-competent child has given consent.

The problem is that the law gives little guidance on the assessment of Gillick competence. If a doctor were to operate on a child less than 16 years old with the child's consent but without parental consent, she could find herself having to defend her assessment that the child had been competent to give consent. In the case of children aged less than 16 years (and therefore not covered by the Family Law Reform Act), doctors would, in our view, be wise to obtain parental consent for the procedure.

3. Consent from just one person with parental responsibility is sufficient. If there is disagreement between those with parental responsibility, i.e. one (or more) gives consent and one (or more) refuses consent, then the doctor can proceed (because consent has been given by one person with parental responsibility). The doctor might, of course, be found negligent if the treatment decision, or the manner in which it was carried out, failed the 'Bolam test' (see Chapter 4).

4. If all those with parental responsibility refuse consent, and if the minor either lacks Gillick competence or also refuses consent, then the doctor can potentially proceed in one of three ways:

   - Give treatment despite lack of consent. This is advisable only when treatment is needed to prevent serious harm or death, *and* there is not sufficient time to apply for a court order (see below).
   - Not give treatment. This is lawful providing that failure to treat does not expose the minor to significant harm. It is in keeping with the Children Act to accord those with parental responsibility considerable say in decisions concerning the minor. Parents, for example, may normally refuse whooping cough vaccination for their children. The legal risk in taking this option is that, if the doctor were subsequently sued on the grounds that it had been negligent not to treat the child, it would not be a defence that consent was refused from all those with parental responsibility. In practice it may be best, if treatment does not need to be given urgently, for the doctor to come to a reasonable decision on management with those with parental responsibility — there may be a good reason for refusal of consent. If the failure to treat is unlikely to result in long-term harm then it may be best to respect the refusal of consent. However, if the doctor believes that failure to treat puts the minor at significant and unnecessary risk, then the option below (a court order) should be sought.
   - Apply to the court for a 'specific issue order' (see above). These are designed exactly for this kind of situation. The court will decide whether or not the refusal of consent by those with parental responsibility should be overridden. Such an order may be given within a matter of hours (by the duty magistrate or judge). The courts have almost always overridden parental refusal when the consensus of medical opinion is that the child's health is at serious risk without treatment (e.g. when Jehovah's Witness parents refuse essential blood transfusions). The court has powers other than a specific issue order that could be used, such as wardship. In any case, the first step, for the doctor, is to contact the legal department, or the relevant social worker, of the appropriate hospital.

5. Occasionally a child will be brought to the general practitioner or to hospital by someone without parental responsibility, for example by a childminder, schoolteacher or step-parent. Under some circumstances

(see Box 10.3) even the child's father may lack parental responsibility. Under these circumstances, if a person with parental responsibility can be contacted for consent, without undue delay in treatment, he or she should be contacted. The more invasive the treatment, the more important this is. However, the duties of those who have the care of the child at any one time, whether or not they have parental responsibility, include doing what is reasonable in all circumstances to safeguard and promote the welfare of the child. Furthermore, a parent may specifically delegate authority to another (e.g. a childminder) to consent to medical treatment. However, in most circumstances the doctor may not be able to verify this without contacting someone with parental responsibility. The child should not be allowed to come to harm on the grounds that there is no-one with parental responsibility who can give consent to the medical care. In such circumstances the *de facto* carer can probably give consent, and, indeed, the doctor herself could be regarded as a *de facto* carer.

The principles outlined above are broadly relevant to Scotland as well as to England and Wales. The legal background is different, however, as outlined above, and in Scotland more weight is given to respecting the minor's autonomy. There is uncertainty as to the extent to which Scottish law allows those under 18 years the absolute right to refuse medical treatment.

Those aged 16 and 17 years who lack capacity (The Mental Capacity Act 2005)

If a person aged less than 16 years lacks capacity, then both those with parental responsibility and doctors should treat that person in his or her best interests. The doctor should, however, seek parental consent and if this is not forthcoming proceed as outlined above. The legal position with regard to 16–17-year-olds is slightly different because the Mental Capacity Act 2005 (MCA) (see Chapter 6) applies to any person aged 16 years and above who lacks capacity. The doctor can treat either with the consent of a person with parental responsibility or under the protection of Section 5 of the MCA (see Chapter 6, p. 84). The MCA obliges doctors to consult with parents (see p. 91) but it does not oblige doctors to obtain parental consent. There is thus less legal necessity for doctors to obtain a specific issue order, in the event that no valid consent is forthcoming, for those who lack capacity aged 16 years or over compared with those aged less than 16 years.

CHILD ABUSE

Protecting children from abuse and exploitation is a responsibility of all capable adults. In addition to this general responsibility, doctors have professional duties and responsibilities. The doctor may become professionally involved in three ways:

1. A member of the public may tell a doctor that she suspects, or has evidence of, child abuse.
2. A doctor may become suspicious of abuse in the course of his work (for example, from the nature of injuries to a child, or from what a patient tells him).
3. A doctor may be asked by the local authority to help in the investigation of child abuse (e.g. by examining a child suspected of being a victim of abuse).

The Children Act 1989 provides the main legal structure for protecting children from abuse. The Children (Scotland) Act 1995 contains provisions regarding child abuse that are broadly similar to those of the English Act. Some of the key principles of the Children Act 1989 are:

- when abuse is suspected, the prime responsibility is to the child
- agencies should cooperate in the best interests of the child
- the prime duty to investigate suspected child abuse lies with the local authority. A doctor is obliged to assist such investigations where appropriate.

Types of abuse

Box 10.5 lists the main types of child abuse.

What to do if abuse is suspected

Box 10.6 describes some features that should alert doctors to the possibility of child abuse. The investigation and management of suspected abuse requires specialist expertise. We discuss only the initial step here. If a

---

Box 10.5 Types of child abuse (based on Jones 1996)

Physical abuse
Actual, or likely, physical injury, or failure to prevent injury or suffering, to a child by a person having care of the child. (This definition includes Munchausen syndrome by proxy.)

Neglect
Actual or likely persistent or severe neglect of a child, or failure to protect a child from exposure to danger, or extreme failure to carry out aspects of care, resulting in significant impairment of the child's health or development.

Emotional abuse (psychological maltreatment)
Actual or likely persistent or severe psychological ill-treatment or rejection, or absence of affection, resulting in a severe adverse effect on the child.

Sexual abuse
Actual or likely occurrence of a sexual act(s) perpetrated on a child by another person, without that child's full consent. Children cannot generally give consent freely because of their dependent condition. Exploitation (and therefore abuse) has occurred if the activity was unwanted when first begun and/or involved misuse of conventional age or authority differentials. Sexual acts include indirect acts such as genital exposure and the production of pornography.

> **Box 10.6** Some features that may raise suspicion for doctors (based on Jones 1996)
>
> **NB:** A finding should not normally be used in isolation but in the context of history and other findings
>
> **Physical abuse**
> - Physical findings discrepant with account given
> - Conflicting or unrealistic explanation of cause of injury
> - Delay in reporting injury
> - Previous episodes of abuse to child or sibling
> - Child's own account
> - Some injuries particularly suggestive, e.g. human bite marks, bloodshot ear, finger–thumb marks (from pinching)
>
> **Sexual abuse**
> - The most common presentation is the child's own statement (usually first to a friend or adult).
> - There are often no other features, i.e. no behavioural changes or physical injuries.
> - Sudden unexplained behavioural changes, or inappropriately sexualized behaviour, should raise possibility of sexual abuse.
> - Physical clues to abuse include genital injuries, sexually transmitted diseases and pregnancy.

member of the public reports suspicion of abuse to a doctor, that doctor should:

1. Write down as much detail as possible, e.g. name and details of child; details of the person who is reporting the suspicion; the precise grounds for the suspicion, trying to clarify the facts on which the suspicion is based; details of the suspected perpetrator.
2. Advise the person to report directly to social services at the local authority.
3. Report direct to social services if the member of the public does not herself report it – and check that a report has been made.

If a doctor becomes suspicious of child abuse he is obliged to report these suspicions to the local authority. In the case of abuse other than sexual abuse, this should normally be done after letting the relevant adult know that this is what will be done.

For example, if injuries to a child seem inconsistent with the story given by the parents, the parents should be told that the explanation is not consistent and that the local authority will be contacted.

In the case of suspected child sexual abuse it is not necessarily appropriate for the doctor to discuss her suspicions before reporting them to the local authority, as the perpetrator may respond by trying to silence the child.

REFERENCES

Brazier M 2003 Medicine, patients and the law, 3rd edn. Penguin, London

Gillick v West Norfolk and Wisbech Area Health Authority 1985. 3 All ER 402

Jones D 1996 In: Hope R A, Fulford K M W, Yates A (eds) Oxford practice skills manual. Oxford University Press, Oxford, pp. 93

FURTHER READING

General

Aikewn W, La Follette H (eds) 1980 Whose child?: parental rights, parental authority and state power. Littlefield, Adams, Totowa, NJ

Alderson P 1993 Children's consent to surgery. Open University Press, Milton Keynes
This excellent book focuses on involving children in decision-making about surgery, but it is relevant more broadly to children's involvement in medical decisions about their care.

Alderson P 2000 Young children's rights. Jessica Kingsley, London

Buchanan A E, Brock D W 1990 Deciding for others: the ethics of surrogate decision making. Cambridge University Press, Cambridge, pp. 215–266

Dworkin G 1988 The theory and practice of autonomy. Cambridge University Press, Cambridge (Chapter 6 'Consent, representation and proxy consent' was originally published in Gaylin W, Macklin R (eds) 1982 Who speaks for the child? The Hastings Center, New York, pp. 191–208)

Goldworth A, Silverman W, Stevenson D K, Young E W D 1995 Ethics and perinatology. Oxford University Press, New York
An examination of the ethical issues that arise around the time of birth involving fetuses and neonates.

Murray T 1996 The worth of a child. University of California Press, Berkeley, CA

Nelson H L, Nelson J L 1995 The patient in the family: an ethics of medicine and families. Routledge, New York

Ross L F 1998 Children, families, and health care decision-making. Clarendon Press, Oxford

Children and the Law

Bainham A 2005 Children: the modern law, 3rd edn. Family Law. Jordan Publishing, Bristol

Hendrick J 1993 Child care law for health professionals. Radcliffe Medical Press, Oxford

Hendrick J 1997 Legal aspects of child health care. Chapman & Hall, London

Child Abuse

British Medical Association 2004 Doctors responsibilities in child protection cases. BMA, London

Department of Health 1991 Working together [addendum: Child Protection: Medical Responsibilities]. HMSO, London

Department of Health 1995 Child protection and child abuse: messages from research. HMSO, London

Department of Health 1999 Working together to protect children – government guidance on inter-agency co-operation. HMSO, London

HM Government 2006 Working together to safeguard children: a guide to inter-agency working to safeguard and promote the welfare of children. The Stationery Office, London

Children

11 Mental health

Most countries have legal mechanisms that are designed specifically for people with mental disorder (Koch et al 1996). In England and Wales the major statute is the Mental Health Act 1983, and in Scotland the Mental Health (Care and Treatment) (Scotland) Act 2003. These Acts have two main functions: they enable the state to enforce hospital admission for the assessment and treatment of patients with mental disorder that go beyond the powers of common law; and they provide mechanisms, including appeal mechanisms, designed to ensure that such powers are not misused. This raises the question of why powers are needed that go beyond the common law? Under common law (see Chapter 6) a competent patient can refuse treatment. This provides legal protection for individual patient autonomy. However, if a patient is not competent then he can be treated in his best interests. Why is anything more needed for patients with mental disorder? If, despite the mental disorder, the patient is competent, should he not have the same right to refuse treatment as any other competent patient? On the other hand, if the patient is not competent he can be treated under common law in his best interests.

JUSTIFYING A MENTAL HEALTH ACT

One problem with relying entirely on common law is that it is not envisaged that any restraint used to treat an incompetent patient will be needed for a prolonged period of time. For example, a patient suffering an acute confusional state, or a hypoglycaemic attack, may resist treatment. It would be perfectly reasonable for health professionals to enforce the initial treatment under common law. In practice, the patient will soon cease to resist treatment. The mental state will either improve so that the patient is competent to agree (or not) to further treatment, or the patient will remain incompetent but cease to resist treatment (for example because of becoming comatose). By contrast, in the case of psychiatric illness (severe depression or schizophrenia, for example) the patient may remain ill and incompetent for several weeks, during which time he is continually resisting treatment. Not only would such persistent restraint be beyond what is envisaged under powers within the common law, but also clear procedures to protect patients from abuse of such powers would be lacking. This is one reason for justifying specific mental health legislation.

A second reason, which is more controversial, is to widen the justification for overriding refusal beyond the traditional legal concept of incapacity (incompetence). As is discussed in Chapter 6, the legal concept of capacity (to consent to or to refuse treatment) has focused on whether a patient has the cognitive ability to understand and weigh up the key issues relevant to the decision. Mental illness can affect the process of decision-making other than through its effect on cognitive ability. A person suffering from moderate depressive illness may have good cognitive abilities. For example, she may be able to understand, believe and weigh up all the issues relevant to a decision about treatment. However, the illness may affect her values. She may refuse treatment because she thinks herself worthless. Once treated, and no longer suffering from depressive illness, her values may change such that she is then pleased that her refusal was overridden.

There are two approaches that may justify the overriding of refusal of treatment in such circumstances. The first is to argue that the patient does not have the capacity to refuse treatment because the illness interferes with her normal values in a way that is relevant to the decision. On such a view, respecting the patient's autonomy is to respect what that person wants when free from depressive illness. The second is to argue that it is right to override the patient's refusal on the combined grounds that it is in her best interests to do so and that she is suffering from a mental illness. English law takes this second approach, at least with regard to the treatment of the mental illness itself. A person can be treated for the mental disorder under the Mental Health Act without reference to the question of whether she is competent to refuse treatment. The problem with this approach is that it opens the door to overriding patients' refusals of treatment even when they are competent to refuse. Either it assumes that the presence of mental illness necessarily results in lack of capacity, which is false; or it discriminates between those who are mentally ill and those who are physically ill. The alternative is to take the first approach and allow a patient's refusal of treatment to be overridden only if the patient lacks the capacity to refuse. This would ensure consistency between mental health law and common law. But, as the example of moderate depressive illness suggests, it would require a more sophisticated account to be given than the common law currently uses, of how people might lack capacity.

THE PROTECTION OF THE PATIENT OR THE PROTECTION OF OTHERS

There are two principal reasons for enforcing hospital treatment on a mentally disordered person. The first is for the sake of the person himself. The second is for the protection of others. The Mental Health Act tries, in one piece of legislation, to address these two quite distinct issues as though they can be approached in the same way. One justification for this is that, in practice, a mentally disordered person may pose a risk to both himself and others. A problem, however, is that the grounds that justify enforced hospital admission in the two situations are rather different.

The question of competence (capacity) is central to overriding refusal for the sake of the person himself. The main method by which society protects itself from those who are dangerous to others is through the criminal law. It may be inappropriate to use the criminal law in the case of some mentally ill people, because as a result of their mental illness they are not responsible for their dangerous acts. The central issue, therefore, in the case of dangerousness to others, is not that of competence but of responsibility. Perhaps because of these differences the Mental Health Act makes little use of the concepts of either capacity or responsibility. The result is that it can be argued that the Act discriminates against the mentally ill in two ways. In the first place, as we have seen, it enables a competent but mentally disordered patient's refusal of treatment to be overridden. In the second place it gives society much wider powers forcibly to restrain, for the protection of others, mentally disordered people compared with those without mental disorder. For example, mentally disordered people, if they are considered to be dangerous, may be kept in a secure place for an indefinite period. Those without mental disorder cannot be kept in a secure place, however dangerous they are thought to be, if they have either not yet committed a crime, or have committed a crime and have served their prison sentence.

THE MENTAL HEALTH ACT 1983

The most important aspects of the Mental Health Act (MHA) (Department of Health and Welsh Office 1999, Jones 2001) are concerned with the issue of compulsory detention in hospital. It should be noted that mental health law in England is currently under review (see below for reform proposals). There are two key facts about the MHA:

1. The Act is relevant only for a person with a mental disorder.
2. The Act is concerned only with the treatment (or assessment) of the mental disorder, and not with the treatment of an independent physical disorder. Box 11.1 describes a case to illustrate these two points.

Box 11.1   Clinical case – blistering skin condition

Mr Jones is suffering from a blistering skin disorder. His consultant strongly advises treatment, as the disorder could lead to serious infection. Mr Jones refuses the treatment. His consultant contacts the on-call psychiatrist, asking him to 'put Mr Jones under the Mental Health Act' in order to allow enforcement of the treatment.

Analysis
Is the use of the Mental Health Act (MHA) appropriate? Mr Jones' consultant says that Mr Jones is making a grave error in refusing treatment. However, he does not think that Mr Jones is suffering from a mental disorder.

The MHA is not an appropriate way of enforcing treatment in a patient who is not suffering from a mental disorder. Furthermore, even if Mr Jones did have a mental disorder, the MHA could not be used to enforce treatment of the skin disorder. It could be used only, if at all, to enforce treatment of the mental disorder. Treatment of the skin condition could be enforced only under common law. A key issue would be whether Mr Jones had legal capacity (was competent) to refuse consent for the treatment of the skin disorder (see Chapter 6). A mental disorder (such as severe depression) might cause Mr Jones to lack capacity to refuse (or give consent to) treatment, and it may then be legally valid to treat Mr Jones under common law in his best interests. However, if treatment for the skin disorder were not urgent it would be preferable first to treat the mental disorder, so that Mr Jones would then be competent to consent to (or refuse) treatment for the skin condition.

Mental disorder

A key term in the MHA is 'mental disorder' (Box 11.2). There are four things to note:

1. The three important exclusions from mental disorder (see Box 11.2).
2. The two categories of mental disorder concerned with learning disability (mental impairment) and the category of psychopathic disorder meet the legal definition of mental disorder only when 'associated with abnormally aggressive or seriously irresponsible conduct'.
3. The term 'mental illness' is not defined in the Act, although its scope has been clarified to some extent by use, and by subsequent guidelines. In practice it would rarely be considered appropriate to detain a person suffering from a 'neurotic' disorder alone (e.g. agoraphobia or obsessive–compulsive disorder).
4. The final category (see Box 11.2) allows considerable scope for inclusion under 'mental disorder'. However, a patient whose mental disorder fitted this category alone could not be detained under Section 3 (Box 11.3). Furthermore, the category does not include the three important exclusions, and it cannot be used to justify compulsory admission simply on the grounds that a person is making a bad decision.

Compulsory detention in hospital

There are three necessary conditions for compulsory detention in hospital (although the precise details of these depend on which section of the Act is relevant; see Box 11.3):

1. The patient is suffering from a mental disorder.
2. The nature and degree of the mental disorder make it appropriate for the patient to receive treatment in a hospital.
3. It is necessary, either for the health or safety of the patient or for the protection of others, that she should be detained in hospital.

Together, these three necessary conditions are sufficient. The powers under the MHA relevant to compulsory detention and treatment are summarized in Box 11.3. Sections 2 , 3, 4 and 5 are particularly important.

Applications under the MHA are made either by the nearest relative or by an approved social worker (approved under Section 13 of the MHA as having particular expertise in the area of mental health). In general the latter is preferred, so as to protect the longer-term relationship of the relative with the patient.

The MHA places some restrictions on specific types of treatment. Thus psychosurgery can be undertaken only with the valid consent of the patient and a second medical opinion. Drug treatment for mental disorder for longer than 3 months, and electroconvulsive therapy, can be imposed on a patient without consent only if supported by a second medical opinion.

Enforcing treatment outside hospital

The focus of the MHA is on hospital treatment. However, over the past two decades there has been a substantial move towards the treatment of

---

Box 11.2 The key term 'mental disorder' in the Mental Health Act

Five 'types' of mental disorder are distinguished in the MHA. One purpose in distinguishing these is that different types feature separately in some parts of the Act.

1. Mental illness

This is not defined further in the Act, although there are guidelines (from the Department of Health) suggesting that this is either sustained cognitive impairment or, essentially, psychosis (delusions, hallucinations, disordered thinking).

2. Severe mental impairment

'A state of arrested or incomplete development of mind which includes severe impairment of intelligence and social functioning and is associated with abnormally aggressive or seriously irresponsible conduct on the part of the person concerned …'. In other words, this is severe learning disability coupled with behavioural problems. The behavioural problems need not be caused by the 'mental impairment' (they need only be associated with it).

3. Mental impairment

'A state of arrested or incomplete development of mind (not amounting to severe mental impairment) which includes significant impairment of intelligence and social functioning and is associated with abnormally aggressive or seriously irresponsible conduct on the part of the person concerned …'. Again, this is learning disability coupled with behavioural problems.

4. Psychopathic disorder

'A persistent disorder or disability of mind (whether or not including significant impairment of intelligence) which results in abnormally aggressive or seriously irresponsible conduct on the part of the person concerned'. Again, there must be behavioural problems. These stipulations for behavioural problems are to some extent repeated in the grounds for detention, as they are what constitutes the 'danger to themselves or others'.

5. 'Any other disorder or disability of mind'

Something of a catch-all.

Three important exclusions

By themselves the following are not sufficient to count as mental disorder (and therefore not enough to come under the Act):

1. Dependence on drugs and alcohol
2. Promiscuity (included because some people used to be detained in hospital because of sexually promiscuous behaviour)
3. Sexual deviancy.

---

psychiatric disorder in the community. Guardianship orders (Sections 7–10 of the MHA) enable the appointed guardian to require a patient to reside at a specified place, to attend a specified place for medical treatment, and to allow, for example, a doctor access to the patient. However, most of the guardian's powers are not enforceable and rely on the cooperation of the patient. There has been much debate over the issue of whether, and how, treatment of mental disorder can be enforced outside hospital. This has been partly in response to

Box 11.3 Summary of the powers under the Mental Health Act (MHA) to detain and treat patients in hospital without consent

Admission for assessment (Section 2)
Grounds
1. Suffering from a mental disorder 'of a nature or degree which warrants the detention of the patient in a hospital for assessment (or for assessment followed by medical treatment) for at least a limited period'.
2. Ought to be detained in the interests of his own health or safety, or with a view to the protection of other persons.

Authorization
The application must be made by the nearest relative or approved social worker (ASW) and supported by a recommendation by two registered medical practitioners. In practice one of the doctors is normally the general practitioner and one a psychiatrist of specialist registrar or consultant status.

Length of detention
Not more than 28 days.

Appeal
An appeal against detention can be made by, or on behalf of, the patient within the first 14 days. The appeal is heard by the Mental Health Review Tribunal.

Notes
a. On the whole this section is for patients in whom the diagnosis is uncertain and a period of assessment is required (otherwise Section 3 would be used). However, assessment can probably also cover assessment of response to treatment.
b. The assessment can be followed by medical treatment – which is not part of the assessment.
c. Deterioration in a patient's mental health is sufficient grounds – danger to self or others is not the only criterion.
d. The Code of Practice states that the danger of harm to others can include 'serious persistent psychological harm'.

Admission for treatment (Section 3)
Grounds
1. Suffering from mental illness, severe mental impairment, psychopathic disorder or mental impairment.
2. This is of a 'nature or degree which makes it appropriate for him to receive medical treatment in a hospital'.
3. In the case of psychopathic disorder or mental impairment, treatment in hospital is likely to alleviate or prevent deterioration of his condition (further legal cases have clarified that 'likely to' does mean that it is likely and not merely possible).
4. It is necessary for the health or safety of the patient or for the protection of other persons that he receive such treatment, and it cannot be provided unless he is detained under this section.

Authorization
As for Section 2.

Length of admission
Up to 6 months, and can be renewed after this, initially for a further 6 months and subsequently for a year at a time.

Notes
a. The admission for treatment must not be nominal, i.e. it must not simply be in order to be able to then put the patient on leave of absence for treatment out of hospital.
b. Unlike Section 2 it is not possible to use this section for people who suffer from 'any other disability of mind …'.

Appeal
This can be made within the first 6 months, in the second 6 months, and then annually. Review by the Mental Health Review Tribunal is automatic if there has been no appeal either in the first 6 months or in any 3-year period.

Emergency admission (Section 4)
The purpose of this section is to arrange emergency compulsory admission when there is no senior psychiatrist available within the time needed. It needs only the general practitioner (and applicant, e.g. social worker). The use of this section should be kept to a minimum.

Grounds
As for Section 2.

Length of time
72 hours.

Detention of a patient already in hospital (Section 5 subsection 2)
A person may be a voluntary patient in hospital and her condition may then change so that it is thought that she should stay in hospital (and she is no longer willing to do so). In this case the patient may be detained in hospital (for up to 72 hours). This can be done quickly without a second medical opinion (i.e. this does not need the general practitioner). For longer detention, Section 2 or 3 should subsequently be used. The relevant doctor is the consultant (or one nominated deputy). This section is used almost solely for patients in a psychiatric hospital, although in theory it could be used for patients in a general hospital (e.g. if a patient with an acute confusional state were inappropriately trying to leave hospital). In this case the relevant consultant would be the patient's consultant (not a psychiatrist). However, such patients would normally be prevented from harming themselves under common law.

   Section 5 subsection 4 allows a senior nurse to detain the patient for up to 6 hours without a doctor.

the perceived need to protect the public from dangerous attacks by mentally disordered people in the community who have stopped taking their medication.

   Furthermore, many doctors, nurses and relatives of patients are dissatisfied with 'revolving door admissions'. These arise when a patient has a chronic mental illness (for example schizophrenia) that is well controlled with medication. If the patient stops taking the medication after discharge he may subsequently relapse and require compulsory treatment in hospital. On discharge from hospital the cycle is repeated. The legal consequence of these debates are the supervised community treatment order (SCT) as part of the MHA 2007 (see p. 174).

Further issues covered by the Mental Health Act

In addition to the areas already described, the MHA covers many other aspects of the care of people with mental disorder. These include: the powers of police to take a person who appears to be mentally disordered to a place of safety and the admission to hospital of mentally disordered people who come before the court.

The Mental Health Act Commission is set up to give second opinions under the MHA, to examine complaints, to check the working of the Act, and to make recommendations (to the Secretary of State) as to what should be put in the Code of Practice. Mental Health Review Tribunals review the justification for individual patients being detained under the MHA. There is one tribunal for each health region.

Reform of the Mental Health Act 1983: the Mental Health Act 2007

There have been several attempts by the government to reform the MHA, but these have been strongly opposed by an unusual alliance between the medical (psychiatric) profession and groups representing patients with mental disorder. Much of the driving force behind the government's wish to reform the MHA is due to concerns about public safety. As we have seen (p. 168) those without mental disorder cannot be kept secure, however dangerous they are thought to be, if they have either not (yet) committed a crime or have served their prison sentence. It is difficult for a government to change this legal position, partly because the civil liberties underlying such limits on forcibly keeping people secure are protected by European legislation, and partly because the protests from those concerned to maintain our civil liberties are likely to be politically powerful.

So what can a government that wishes to lock away those who are thought to be dangerous do? One answer is to increase the scope of mental health legislation. A current presumption that is central to mental health legislation is that it aims to enable people to benefit from medical (psychiatric) care. Thus if a person who suffers from a mental disorder (within the meaning of the MHA) is not treatable (for example because the person has an intractable severe personality disorder) then under the current MHA that person cannot be kept secure against his will. One proposed change to the Act is to allow a person to be kept forcibly secure even if there is no effective treatment. A second change is to alter the definition of 'mental disorder' to allow more people to be included within it. In essence, what is at issue is what to do with people who are thought to be dangerous because of their personalities and proclivities (for example paedophiles who have shown evidence of violent behaviour). The government wants to keep such people securely locked up beyond what is currently possible, but does not think that it can change the criminal law to extend its powers. The solution: call such people mentally disordered and put pressure on doctors to lock them up, under a new Mental Health Act, potentially for ever. Changing mental health legislation to enable this to happen is thought to be politically easier than changing criminal law.

The Mental Health Act 2007 is the government's third and successful attempt in 8 years to reform the MHA 1983. The new Act does not replace the 1983 Act but instead introduces several important amendments. The proposed amendments include the following:

- A new supervised community treatment order (SCT) for suitable patients following an initial period of detention and treatment in hospital. This will allow professionals to enforce treatment on patients after they have been discharged from hospital and make it easier to readmit such patients involuntarily to hospital.
- A new single definition of mental disorder, i.e. any disorder or disability of mind.
- Replaces the treatability test with a new test, namely the appropriate treatment test. This new test will apply to all longer-term powers of detention. Under the 1983 Act a patient could be detained only if he could be treated; under the new proposals he can be detained if his condition is treatable. This is a subtle distinction. The political purpose is to increase the number of people who can be detained, particularly those who are thought to be dangerous and have personality disorder. A person might have personality disorder of a type for which some psychological treatment is appropriate but which in this person's case is not effective. Under the 1983 Act such a person could not be detained because he did not pass the treatability test, but he might pass the appropriate treatment test because there is an 'appropriate treatment', i.e. a treatment is available that is appropriate to the patient's mental disorder.
- Further information on the Act is available at http://www.opsi.gov.uk.

The Mental Health (Care and Treatment) (Scotland) Act 2003

This Act is the key statute in Scotland relating to the management of people with mental disorder. It is summarized in Box 11.4.

CRIME AND MENTAL ILLNESS

It has long been established in law that mental disorder can affect criminal responsibility. Mental disorder can affect three main aspects in the court's procedure in dealing with a person accused of a crime:

1. The question of whether the person is *fit to plead*
2. The question of whether the person is (fully) responsible for the crime
3. The sentence.

Fitness to plead

In order to stand trial, in English law, a person must be in a fit state to defend himself. Essentially, the test follows the framework for capacity in general (see Chapter 6). If a person is found on a 'trial of facts' to have done the act with

Box 11.4   The Mental Health (Care and Treatment) (Scotland) Act 2003

The Act came into force in October 2005. It covers a wide range of issues but broadly can be summarized under four headings:

1. Principles, roles and responsibilities

The Act sets out some principles that most people performing functions under the Act have to consider. These include: the present and past wishes and feelings of the patient; the views of the patient's named person, carer, guardian or welfare attorney; the importance of the patient participating as fully as possible; the importance of providing the maximum benefit to the patient; the importance of providing the appropriate services to the patient and the needs and circumstances of the patient's carer. The Act also sets out principles relating to the way the functions must be discharged, i.e. involving the minimum restriction on the freedom of the patient and encouraging equal opportunities. In addition the Act defines the nature, powers and duties of a number of organizations and individuals involved in mental health law (e.g. Mental Welfare Commission).

2. Compulsory powers

The Act comprehensively reforms and modernizes the legal framework for compulsory detention and treatment. In so doing it sets out clear criteria that must be met before compulsion can be authorized as well as detailed procedures that must be followed. The forms of compulsion are emergency detention (72 hours), short-term detention (28 days; this can be extended), compulsory treatment orders (6 months; this may also be extended), and other powers in relation to entry, removal and detention. In keeping with the community care philosophy of the Act, compulsory treatment orders can include a requirement that patients will attend for outpatient treatment or for assistance from social services (Section 66). There are also measures to ensure compliance with the terms of such orders (allowing the patient to be taken into custody (Sections 112 & 113). The Act incorporates the greater part of the Mental Health (Patients in the Community) Act 1995.

3. People with mental disorder within the criminal justice system

The Act substantially reforms the law relating to people with mental disorder who enter the criminal justice system and how they are subsequently cared for. For example, the courts are given new options in how they deal with people with mental disorder (such as an assessment order, treatment order, and a compulsion order).

4. Rights, safeguards and duties

The Act provides additional rights for people accessing mental health services and increased safeguards. These include giving all people with mental disorder the right of access to independent advocacy services; the right for patients to nominate a named person (who has the right to be kept informed of the patient's status in certain circumstances); and the right for patients to make an advance statement regarding how they wish to be treated or not treated in the event of their becoming unable (due to their mental disorder) to make their views known. Note that the advance statement only covers treatment for the mental disorder and not other illnesses or conditions requiring treatment. Additionally the Act includes a number of safeguards for treatment of mental disorder; for example, it is not possible to give ECT to a patient, even in an emergency, if the patient is able to make a treatment decision and refuses treatment. For further information about the Act see http://www.scotland.gov.uk/Publications.

which he is charged but is not fit to plead, then the judge would normally require that he receive psychiatric treatment, in the case of violent crimes in a secure hospital environment.

Responsibility for the crime

In English law, for a person to be found guilty of a crime two aspects have to be proved: that it was this person who actually carried out the criminal act; and that the person had the state of mind necessary to be held responsible for the crime. The first aspect is known as the *actus reus* ('guilty act') and the second as the *mens rea* ('guilty mind').

The precise *mens rea* required for a person to be found guilty varies from crime to crime. For example, to be guilty of murder a person must have had 'specific intent', i.e. must have had the intention to kill (or cause serious physical harm to) the victim. To be found guilty of *manslaughter* it is necessary only to establish that the person showed gross negligence. For some road traffic offences it is not necessary to establish any *mens rea* at all.

Insanity – the McNaughten rules

The McNaughten rules provide the main legal guidelines for establishing that someone is 'not guilty by reason of insanity'. They are essentially criteria for fully absolving a person of responsibility for a crime on grounds of mental disorder. They state (see, for example, Gelder et al 2006, p. 747):

> To establish a defence on the ground of insanity, it must be clearly proved that, at the time of committing the act, the party accused was labouring under such a defect of reason, from disease of the mind, as not to know the nature and quality of the act he was doing, or, if he did know it, that he did not know what he was doing was wrong.

Diminished responsibility

In English law diminished responsibility may be pleaded only as a defence to the charge of murder; if the defence is successful but the accused is found guilty, the crime is 'reduced' from murder to manslaughter. The criteria for diminished responsibility are much less stringent than those for insanity.

The Homicide Act 1957 (Section 2) states:

> " Where a person kills or is party to a killing of another, he shall not be convicted of murder if he was suffering from such abnormality of mind (whether arising from a condition of arrested or retarded development of mind or any inherent causes or induced by disease or injury) as substantially impaired his mental responsibility for his acts and omissions in doing or being party to the killing.

Murder carries with it a mandatory sentence of life imprisonment, but in the case of manslaughter the judge has considerable discretion in determining the sentence.

The sentence

Even when a mentally disordered person is found guilty of a crime, the judge, in most situations, although not in the case of murder, has considerable discretion with regard to sentencing. A judge may consider that the presence of mental disorder, although not being such as to exonerate the person from responsibility for the crime, does justify a less severe sentence. In addition, the Mental Health Act gives powers to the court to require that a mentally disordered offender found guilty of a crime be treated in a psychiatric hospital, rather than sent to prison.

REFERENCES

Department of Health and Welsh Office 1999 Mental Health Act 1983: Code of Practice. The Stationery Office, London

Gelder M, Harrison P, Cowen P 2006 The shorter Oxford textbook of psychiatry, 5th edn. Oxford Universtiy Press, Oxford

Jones R 2001 Mental Health Act manual, 7th edn. Sweet & Maxwell, London

Koch H-G, Reiter-Theil S, Helmchen H (eds.) 1996 Informed consent in psychiatry: European perspectives on ethics, law and clinical practice. Nomos Baden, Baden

FURTHER READING

General

Bloch R, Chodoff P, Green S A 1999 Psychiatric ethics, 3rd edn. Oxford University Press, Oxford

Green S, Bloch S 2006 An anthology of psychiatric ethics. Oxford University Press, Oxford
This is a companion to their Psychiatric Ethics and provides selected readings

Dickenson D, Fulford B 2001 In two minds: a casebook of psychiatric ethics. Oxford University Press, Oxford
Clinical cases with ethical analysis

Fulford B, Thornton T, Graham G 2006 Oxford textbook of philosophy and psychiatry. Oxford University Press, Oxford
A large book covering not only ethical issues in psychiatry but also broader philosophical issues

Griffiths A 1995 Philosophy, psychology and psychiatry. Cambridge University Press, Cambridge
Edited series of essays from many authors covering issues, both in ethics and philosophy more broadly, raised by psychiatric practice

Radden J 2007 The philosophy of psychiatry: a companion. Oxford University Press, New York
An edited collection of essays, again including not only ethical but also other philosophical aspects of psychiatry

Radden J 2007 Divided minds and successive selves: ethical issues in disorders of identity and personality. MIT Press, Cambridge, MA
A rich analysis of the ethical issues

The concept of disease and mental illness

Boorse C 1997 A rebuttal on health. In: Humber J F, Almeder R F (eds.) Defining disease. Humana Press, Totowa, NJ, p 7–8
An excellent overview of Boorse's classic naturalistic theory of disease, with a response to his critics. Also contains other important approaches to disease

Fulford K W M 1989 Moral theory and medical practice. Cambridge University Press, Cambridge

Reznek L 1987 The nature of disease. Routledge & Kegan Paul, London

Svensson T 1995 On the notion of mental illness. Avebury, Aldershot

Szasz T S 1984 The myth of mental illness. HarperCollins, London

Mental illness and crime

Elliott C 1996 The rules of insanity. State University of New York, New York

Misuse of psychiatry

Chodoff P 1999 Misuse and abuse of psychiatry: an overview. In: Bloch S, Chodoff P, Green S A (eds.) Psychiatric ethics, 3rd edn. Oxford University Press, Oxford, p 49–66

Psychotherapy

Holmes J, Lindley R 1991 The values of psychotherapy. Oxford University Press, Oxford

Neurology

Zeman A, Emanuel L 2000 Ethical dilemmas in neurology. W B Saunders, London

MENTAL HEALTH

End of life

ENDING LIFE AND THE LAW

The legal position relevant to end-of-life decisions in a clinical context is summarized in Box 12.1.

Active euthanasia (mercy killing) is illegal (murder): the case of Cox

The key case in determining that voluntary active euthanasia is illegal (murder) was that of Dr Cox (Box 12.2). The judge, in directing the jury, said: 'Even the prosecution case acknowledged that he [Dr Cox] ... was prompted by deep distress at Lillian Boyes' condition; by a belief that she was totally beyond recall and by an intense compassion for her fearful suffering. Nonetheless ... if he injected her with potassium chloride for the primary purpose of killing her, or hastening her death, he is guilty of the offence charged [*attempted murder*] ... neither the express wishes of the patient nor of her loving and devoted family can affect the position'.

Intending relief of distress in the patient's best interests, but foreseeing death, is normally legal

In the Cox case the judge drew a clear distinction between intending death and foreseeing death. The former is potentially murder, the second may be good practice. The judge said: 'It was plainly Dr Cox's duty to do all that was medically possible to alleviate her [*Lillian Boyes'*] pain and suffering, even if the course adopted carried with it an obvious risk that, as a side effect of that treatment, her death would be rendered likely or even certain. There can be no doubt that the use of drugs to reduce pain and suffering will often be fully justified notwithstanding that it will, in fact, hasten the moment of death. What can never be lawful is the use of drugs with the primary purpose of hastening the moment of death'.

Intending death, as the means to relieve suffering, is potentially murder

In the Cox case the judge made it clear that there is an important legal distinction between relieving distress while the patient lives (even though it is

Box 12.1 Summary of the law relating to medical decisions at the end of life

Active euthanasia (mercy killing) is illegal (see also Box 12.6)

To take an active step, such as injecting potassium chloride, with the *intention* of shortening the patient's life is murder, and therefore a criminal offence. This is the case even if the patient competently requests to be killed, and even if, because of the patient's distress, pain, etc., it is in his or her best interests to die. Thus active euthanasia, whether voluntary or not, is illegal.

Passive euthanasia is not necessarily illegal (see also Box 12.6)

It is not normally illegal for a doctor to withhold treatment (such as ventilation) if the grounds for doing so are the patient's best interests. Thus, a doctor may withhold life-prolonging treatment if it is judged better for the patient to be allowed to die (as a result of the natural course of the illness) than to be given such treatment. The decision to withhold such treatment could be challenged in the courts. The courts would have to decide whether the doctor had been negligent in judging that withholding treatment had been in the patient's best interests. The test would normally be the Bolam test (see Chapter 6). The law therefore accepts that in some circumstances continued life is worse than death.

Withdrawing treatment is legally equivalent to withholding treatment

From the legal perspective, withdrawing treatment (e.g. stopping artificial ventilation) is considered passive, not active, treatment. The law places withdrawing treatment in the same category as withholding treatment, and not in the category of killing (i.e. not in the category of active euthanasia). A doctor may therefore withdraw such treatment on the same grounds as she may withhold treatment.

Intending relief of distress, but foreseeing death, is normally legal

To take an active step, such as the injection of morphine, with the *intention* of relieving the patient's distress, but with the *foreseen result* that it is likely to shorten life, is normally legal. The doctor's legal duty is to act in the patient's best interests. It would, however, be illegal to relieve distress if shortening life were the means to relieving distress. This would come under the category of active euthanasia (see above).

Assisting suicide is a criminal offence

Suicide was illegal until the Suicide Act 1961. The decriminalization of suicide (under the Suicide Act 1961) means that, even if a person's intention to commit suicide is discovered, the law cannot prevent her from ending her life (Re Z (An Adult: Capacity) [2004]).

Although attempting, or committing, suicide, however, is not illegal, it is a criminal offence for anyone (not just a doctor) to assist suicide (or a suicidal attempt) (s.2(1) of the Suicide Act 1961). Thus, if a patient committed suicide by taking an overdose of tablets that the doctor had left by the bedside for that purpose, the doctor could be found guilty of assisting suicide. If a patient takes an overdose of tablets prescribed by the doctor for normal therapeutic purposes, the doctor would not be guilty because she had not intended to assist suicide. Such a doctor might, in unusual circumstances, be found negligent in having provided the patient with such an opportunity.

A competent patient who refuses life-saving treatment is not committing suicide

A competent patient can refuse any, even life-saving, treatment. The law does not consider such refusal as suicide (nor as attempted suicide). A doctor is therefore not guilty of assisting suicide in acceding to the patient's refusal, or withdrawal, of treatment. Indeed, the doctor would be committing a battery to give the treatment in the light of the patient's competent refusal.

The impact of the Human Rights Act 1998 (HRA)

The law on euthanasia and assisted suicide has been challenged in several high-profile cases involving the HRA 1998. In summary these establish that:

1. The HRA does not confer a right to die nor to assistance in suicide (Pretty v UK [2002]).
2. Choosing the manner of one's death could be included as an aspect of the right to respect for private life, but the interests of the state and others could nevertheless justify an interference with that right (Pretty v UK [2002]).
3. General Medical Council guidelines that set out good practice for doctors in withdrawing and withholding treatment (e.g. artificial hydration and nutrition) do not conflict with Article 3 (prohibition of inhuman or degrading treatment) (Burke v UK [2006]). For example, withholding or withdrawing treatment in the patient's best interests (e.g. to enable a comfortable death) can be lawful and not contrary to Article 3.

Box 12.2   The case of Dr Cox (R v Cox [1992])

Lillian Boyes was a 70-year-old woman with very severe rheumatoid arthritis, the pain of which seemed to be beyond the reach of analgesics. She was expected to die within a matter of days or weeks. She asked her doctor, Dr Cox, to kill her. Out of compassion for his patient, and because this is what she wanted him to do, Dr Cox injected a lethal dose of potassium chloride. He was charged with attempted murder. The reason for not charging him with murder was that, given her condition, Lillian Boyes could have died from her disease and not from the injection.

Dr Cox was found guilty of attempted murder.

End of life

foreseen that life will be shortened) and relieving distress *through* shortening life. He said: 'Of course … to hasten the death not merely alleviates suffering, it brings it to an end. A dead person suffers no more. But that is not what I mean by alleviation of suffering. Alleviation of suffering means that easing of it for so long as the patient survives; not the easing of it in the throes of, and because of, deliberate purpose of killing'.

Withholding and withdrawing treatment are not necessarily illegal

In the Bland case (Box 12.3) Lord Goff said: '… the law draws a crucial distinction between cases in which a doctor decides not to provide, or to continue

> **Box 12.3** The Case of Bland (Airedale NHS Trust v Bland [1993])
>
> In 1989, 21-year-old Anthony Bland was seriously hurt when crushed by overcrowding at Hillsborough football stadium. Attempts to resuscitate Bland resulted in his being permanently unconscious and with no prospect of ever regaining consciousness (permanent/persistent vegetative state). After Bland had been in this state for about 3 years, the hospital Trust applied to the court for a ruling as to whether it would be lawful to discontinue Bland's life support (artificial hydration and nutrition), which would inevitably lead to his death. The case went to the House of Lords.
>
> The judgment is important in medical law in three respects:
>
> 1. It clarified the legal position with regard to a doctor withholding or withdrawing treatment from a patient who is in a permanent state of unconsciousness.
> 2. It established that nutrition and hydration, i.e. what might be called basic care, are part of 'medical treatment'.
> 3. It made a significant contribution to the legal position with regard to advance directives.

to provide, for his patient treatment or care which could or might prolong his life, and those in which he decides, for example by administering a lethal drug, actively to bring his patient's life to an end … the former may be lawful …' (but not the latter).

What this added to the Cox decision was clarification that, even if the doctor intends the death of her patient by withholding or withdrawing treatment, then it may be lawful if so doing is in the best interests of the patient. The British Medical Association (BMA) Guidelines (1999) state that there is no ethical distinction between withdrawing and withholding treatment.

The competent patient

See Box 12.1. A competent patient may refuse any treatment, whatever the likely consequences. It would be a battery for a doctor to impose treatment against a competent patient's wishes. A recent case involved a competent patient who wished life support to be withdrawn. Her doctors were unwilling to carry out her wishes. The court confirmed that she had the right to demand withdrawal of treatment and that the doctors had either to comply with her wishes, or to transfer her care to doctors who would comply with her wishes (Re B [2002] Adult: refusal of medical treatment).

The incompetent patient

In the case of an incompetent patient, a doctor's duty of care is to treat in that patient's best interests. How does the law tackle the situation where one management plan (e.g. withdrawing treatment) will result in a shorter life? In deciding best interests, does the law allow us to balance life against death? Until the important case of Wyatt v Portsmouth Hospitals NHS Trust [2005] the answer to this question was relatively straightforward: that in making decisions about non-treatment and the withdrawal of treatment the duty to prolong life was the guiding principle. However, this sanctity of life principle was subject to the so-called 'intolerability test'. According to this test (established in Re J (a minor) Wardship: Medical Treatment [1991]) the doctor or court should consider 'whether the quality of life that the child would endure if given the treatment would be so afflicted as to be intolerable'. In the Wyatt case the Court of Appeal agreed that the intolerability test was a valuable guide in establishing the patient's best interests, but it emphasized that it was just that, i.e. just one of several approaches to establishing what was the only relevant test, namely, the patient's best interests. Despite the Court of Appeal's statement that the intolerability test is a 'valuable guide', it is interesting to note that in a subsequent High Court case (Re NHS Trust v MB [2006]) the judge said:

> **"** I avoid reference to the concept of 'intolerability'. It seems to me that it all depends on what one means by 'intolerable' and that the use of the word really expresses a conclusion rather than provides a test. If it is correct to say, or once it has been concluded, that life is literally intolerable, then it is hard to see in what circumstances it should be artificially prolonged. If conversely, it is 'tolerable' then it is hard to see in what circumstances it should be permitted, avoidably to end.

In relation to those aged 16 years and over the interpretation of best interests is now governed by s.4 of the Mental Capacity Act 2005 (unless a valid advance decision applies; see Chapter 6). Particularly relevant in this context is s.4(5), which states that 'where the determination [*of best interests*] relates to life-sustaining treatment [*the decision-maker*] must not, in considering whether the treatment is in the best interests of the person concerned, be motivated by a desire to bring about his death'. Essentially this section enshrines the double-effect doctrine (see p. 185). This section can be interpreted as extending the double-effect doctrine to withholding and withdrawing treatment. According to one commentator, by attempting to give statutory effect to the sanctity of life principle the provision 'fails to ensure a coherent moral and intellectual shape to the law'. Indeed, in practice it may 'result in a real dilemma in some cases: either a doctor will act unlawfully by not treating a patient in his best interests or he will act unlawfully by not according with the sanctity principle' (Coggon 2007).

As regards those aged under 16 years, who are not covered by the Mental Capacity Act 2005, the Wyatt case makes it clear that in making end-of-life decisions the best interests test must be applied. In applying this test, medical, emotional and other relevant welfare issues must be taken into account. This will involve a balancing exercise in which all relevant issues are considered.

Persistent states of unconsciousness

Following devastating brain injury patients may be unconscious with no prospect of regaining consciousness – a persistent/permanent vegetative state (PVS). Patients in such a state require assistance in order to remain alive. Such assistance will include, at a minimum, artificial nutrition and hydration. It may also include mechanical ventilation and other life support measures. The question arises as to whether it is lawful to withdraw the life support measures, allowing the patient to die. Unlike in the case of Re J, life to the patient is not 'intolerable'. The patient, it is presumed, is having no conscious experience, nor is ever likely to have. This was the situation in the case of Bland (Box 12.3). The Lords judged that life support could be stopped, allowing Bland to die. The principle on which the judgment was based has been called the principle of 'not against the best interests'. Although it is not in the best interests of the patient for treatment to be stopped, it is also not against those best interests. The BMA (1996) has published guidelines on treatment decisions in the case of PVS that have influenced the courts. Under the Mental Capacity Act (s.15) doctors must obtain permission from the Court of Protection before discontinuing life support in the case of patients in persistent states of unconsciousness.

The Scottish case of Law Hospital NHS Trust v Lord Advocate [1996] followed the precedent set in the Bland case.

Are hydration and nutrition medical treatments?

A further issue that arose in the case of Bland was whether the provision of basic care (intravenous fluid and nutrition) can be withdrawn using the same principles as for withdrawing medical care, such as ventilation. The answer given was that such basic care should be considered in a similar way to medical care.

The ethical principles embedded in English law

English law looks at end-of-life issues mainly from the perspective of what is a doctor's duty of care to her patients. That duty of care is primarily to act in the patient's best interests. However, there are three ethical principles, each contentious, that are adopted to some extent by the law: a qualified principle of sanctity of life; the doctrine of double effect; and the moral difference between acts and omissions.

THREE MORAL PRINCIPLES RELEVANT TO END-OF-LIFE DECISIONS

In Box 12.4 we describe a number of cases (some hypothetical, some real) that test moral intuitions with regard to killing.

The principle of the sanctity of life

There are differing versions of the principle (or doctrine) of the sanctity of life. The most extreme form is called *vitalism*. According to vitalism, human life is of absolute value: it is an absolute good. Whenever possible, human life should be maintained, and it is always wrong to take human life (Gormally 1985). This view would seem to commit us to putting enormous resources into trivial extensions of human life. It would also commit us to maintaining a person's life no matter what burden it is to that person.

A less extreme form of the sanctity-of-life principle is one that sees life as a basic but not an absolute good. By denying that life is an absolute good, it is meant that preserving life does not necessarily outweigh all other basic goods. By asserting that life is a basic good, it is meant that the value of life cannot be

---

Box 12.4   Some cases, both hypothetical and real, to test principles relevant to end-of-life issues

---

Case 1: The trapped lorry driver – a case of mercy killing

A driver is trapped in a blazing lorry. There is no way in which he can be saved. He will soon burn to death. A friend of the driver is standing by the lorry. This friend has a gun and is a good shot. The driver asks this friend to shoot him dead. It will be less painful for him to be shot than to burn to death.

• *Should the friend shoot the driver dead?*

Case 2: The wreck of the whale-ship *Essex*

In 1820 the whale-ship *Essex* sank after being rammed by a sperm whale. The crew distributed themselves between three lifeboats. Captain Pollard and six other men took one boat. Eighty days after the wreck, and separated from their companions in the other boats, three of Pollard's crew had died from starvation and dehydration. Those who survived had done so only through eating the dead bodies of their companions. The four survivors had no food. They agreed to cast lots to decide who should be killed in order to provide food for the rest. The alternative was almost certain death for them all. (The classic account of the ordeal was written by Owen Chase [1999], first mate of the *Essex*. Further information is given in Philbreck [2000].)

Case 3: Self-defence (based on Anscombe; see Glover 1977)

a. Someone who is trying to kill you attacks you. The only way you can adequately defend yourself is by hitting your assailant so hard that there is a high risk of killing him.

   • *Would it be wrong for you to defend yourself in his way?*

b. Someone, you are reliably informed, is looking for you in order to kill you.

   • *Would it be wrong for you to seek this person out and poison him in order to prevent him from killing you?*

Case 4: Sacrificing one to save five: organ donation and the runaway train

a. Organ donation – one healthy person is killed in order to use her organs to save the lives of five people with various types of organ failure.

b. The runaway train – a runaway train is approaching the points on the railway line. If the points are not switched, the train will kill five people who are on that line. If the points are switched, the train will go along a different line where there is one person (different from the five) who will be killed. There is no way of preventing these deaths, but the one thing you can do is to switch the points.

• *Is there a moral difference between killing the organ donor in the first case and switching the points in the second case, and if so, why?*

---

accounted for completely in terms of a person's experiences and beliefs. There is therefore a value to a person's simply being alive, no matter what state that person is in, even, for example, if he is in a state of permanent unconsciousness.

The moral distinction between foresight and intention: the doctrine of double effect

The doctrine of double effect was developed in mediaeval Catholic theology. The core of the doctrine can be summarized as two moral claims (Glover 1977,

p. 87). The first is that performing a bad act in order to bring about good consequences is always wrong. The second is that performing a good act, which one foresees will lead to bad consequences, may sometimes be right. In order for both of these claims to be held consistently, a moral distinction must be made between intending an outcome and foreseeing an outcome.

Consider the following situation. A pregnant woman suffers from carcinoma of the uterus. The only effective treatment that will save the mother's life involves surgical removal of the uterus, with the inevitable result that the fetus will die. Can it be morally right to carry out an operation that will, inevitably, kill the fetus?

Those who hold a broadly consequentialist morality (see Chapter 1) are likely to argue in favour of surgery on the grounds that removing the uterus has the better (foreseeable) consequences. Many non-consequentialist ethical theories (see Chapter 1) require the evaluation of acts independently of outcomes. According to many such theories, some acts are morally wrong even if, overall, they bring about better consequences than the alternative acts. One act that is widely held as wrong, in this sense, is the act of killing. Can a moral theory that considers killing a fetus wrong nevertheless defend surgical removal of the uterus in the example given above? The doctrine of double effect is intended to provide such a defence.

According to this doctrine, it may be right to remove the uterus despite the inevitable result that the fetus will die, if, and only if, four conditions hold:

1. The action (saving the mother's life) is good in itself.
2. The intention is solely to produce the good effect (i.e. the intention is to save the mother, and in no way is the intention to kill the fetus).
3. The good effect is not achieved through the bad effect (i.e. the saving of the mother is not achieved directly through killing the fetus: killing the fetus is a 'side effect' of the action taken to save the mother).
4. There is sufficient reason to permit the bad effect (i.e. the good of saving the mother provides sufficient grounds to justify the bad result – the death of the fetus).

The doctrine does not justify an intended good action if the unintended foreseeable result is worse than the good achieved.

At the core of the doctrine of double effect is the claim that there is a moral distinction between *foreseeing* a result and *intending* a result. Thus, it may be forbidden on moral grounds to bring about a bad result if that result is intended (even if as a means to a better overall outcome), but not forbidden to bring about the same result if the result is foreseen but not intended.

There are two main criticisms of the doctrine of double effect. The first is that it is conceptually confused; the second is that, although clear, it is morally wrong.

The argument that the doctrine of double effect is conceptually confused

Consider the pair of cases involving killing one person to save five (see Box 12.4, cases 4a & 4b). This pair provides one of the strongest *prima facie* examples in support of the doctrine of double effect. Most people's intuition is that it is wrong to kill the 'organ donor' in order to save the five organ recipients.

On the other hand, it would be right to switch the rail points in order to save the five people, with the foreseeable result that one person will die. The doctrine of double effect appears to provide the grounds in support of this intuition. However, we could argue that in removing the organs we do not intend the death of the donor. It is unfortunately the case that the organs do not regenerate, so that in removing them the donor dies. His death is foreseeable, but it is not intended.

The argument that the doctrine of double effect is morally wrong

The doctrine of double effect is part of a moral theory that considers some acts as always wrong, if carried out intentionally, whatever the consequences. Killing is the key example of such an act. Such theories seem problematic to many in the face of counter-examples such as the 'trapped lorry driver' (see Box 12.4, case 1). In this example, shooting the trapped driver is an act of killing that is not morally permissible if the doctrine of double effect is right. In this case the doctrine seems to give priority to the purity of the intention of the bystander at the expense of the suffering of the lorry driver.

The moral distinction between acts and omissions

According to the acts–omissions distinction, 'in certain contexts, failure to perform an act, with certain foreseen bad consequences of that failure, is morally less bad than to perform a different act which has the identical foreseen bad consequences. It is worse to kill someone than to let them die' (Glover 1977, pp. 92–93).

The distinction is relevant in English law (see above). It accords with common intuitions. Acting to kill a patient, even for good reasons, may seem wrong, whereas omitting to act, for example by withholding life-saving treatment, may seem the right thing to do. The moral distinction between active and passive euthanasia rests principally on the distinction between acts and omissions.

Box 12.5 describes two pairs of cases, one of which (Robinson and Davies) provides intuitive support in favour of the moral distinction between acts and omissions. The other pair (Smith and Jones) provides support against such a distinction.

Arguments against the acts–omissions distinction

1. The cases of Smith and Jones (see Box 12.5) provide a 'controlled experiment': everything is kept the same, except that Smith *acts* whereas Jones *omits to act*. The distinction between an act and an omission seems morally irrelevant in this pair of cases.
2. We are just as responsible for omissions as we are for acts. Essentially, when faced with a problematic situation we could pursue two or more paths. If we choose one path, whether this is to act or to omit to act, both are 'active' choices, and both carry equal moral weight.
3. It is not always conceptually clear when something is an act or an omission. Is switching off a ventilator an act or an omission? At first sight it appears to be an act, but suppose the ventilator needs to be switched off for a few seconds to correct some electrical fault. If the responsible person intentionally fails to switch it back on (an omission), is it meaningful to consider this different from switching it off (an act)?

Box 12.5   Two pairs of cases to test the acts–omissions distinction

The cases of Robinson and Davies
This pair of cases is based on an article by Foot (1967) and discussed in Glover (1977, p. 93).

Robinson does not give £100 to a charity that is helping to combat starvation in a poor country. As a result, one person dies from starvation who would have lived had Robinson sent the money.

Davies does send £100 but also sends a poisoned food parcel for use by a charity distributing food donations. The overall and intended result is that one person is killed from the poisoned food parcel and another person's life is saved by the £100 donation.

Is there a moral difference between what Robinson and Davies do? If there is, is this because Davies acts to kill, whereas Robinson only omits to act?

The cases of Smith and Jones (Rachels 1975)
Smith sneaks into the bathroom of his 6-year-old cousin and drowns him, arranging things so that it will look like an accident. The reason Smith does this is that the death of his cousin results in his coming into a large inheritance.

Jones stands to gain a similar large inheritance from the death of his 6-year-old cousin. Like Smith, Jones sneaks into the bathroom with the intention of drowning his cousin. The cousin, however, accidentally slips and knocks his head and drowns in the bath. Jones could easily have saved his cousin, but instead stands ready to push the child's head back under. However, this does not prove necessary.

Arguments in favour of the acts–omissions distinction

1. It seems from the Robinson–Davies pair of cases (see Box 12.5) that if we do not believe there to be a moral difference between acts and omissions, we must either be incredibly guilty about all the good we fail to do, or we must be less censorious about people who carry out evil acts. (See Glover 1977, Chapter 7, for a detailed analysis and criticism of the acts–omissions distinction.)
2. A conceptually clear – if complex – account can be given of the distinction (Stauch 2000). The law operates the distinction, and in practice there is no difficulty in classifying Cox (see Box 12.2) as having actively killed a patient, whereas doctors who withdraw life support, for good reasons, as acting legally in omitting to provide burdensome treatment.

EUTHANASIA

Arguments concerning euthanasia are often muddled by insufficient clarity over terms (Box 12.6). Voluntary active euthanasia remains illegal in the UK despite three debates over its legalization in the House of Lords. In the Netherlands it can be carried out legally under certain conditions. The debate over whether or not it should be legalized in the UK is unlikely to go away. Doctors will play an important part in such debate. Box 12.7 summarizes some arguments for and against voluntary active euthanasia.

> **Box 12.6** Euthanasia and suicide: terminology
>
> - Euthanasia comes from the Greek *eu thanatos*, meaning good or easy death.
> - Euthanasia: X intentionally kills Y, or permits Y's death, for Y's benefit.
> - Active euthanasia: X performs an action which itself results in Y's death.
> - Passive euthanasia: X allows Y to die. X withholds life-prolonging treatment or withdraws life-prolonging treatment.
> - Voluntary euthanasia: Euthanasia when Y competently requests death himself, i.e. a competent adult wanting to die.
> - Non-voluntary euthanasia: Euthanasia when Y is not competent to express a preference, e.g. Y is a severely disabled newborn.
> - Involuntary euthanasia: Death is against Y's competent wishes, although X permits or imposes death for Y's benefit.
> - Suicide: Y intentionally kills herself.
> - Assisted suicide: X intentionally helps Y to kill himself.
> - Murder: X intentionally kills Y.

'DO NOT RESUSCITATE' ORDERS, AND OTHER LIMITATIONS TO TREATMENT

A 'do not resuscitate' (DNAR) order is a specific example of a limitation of treatment. The BMA, UK Resuscitation Council, Royal College of Nursing guidelines (2001) state that it is appropriate to consider a DNAR decision in the following circumstances:

1. CPR is unlikely to be successful ('futile').
2. CPR is not in accord with the recorded, sustained wishes of the patient who is mentally competent.
3. Where CPR is not in accord with a valid advance directive (living will).
4. Resuscitation is likely to be followed by a length and quality of life that would not be in the best interests of the patient to sustain.

The first criterion ('futility') is, in practice, a major reason for patients to be considered as 'not for resuscitation'. The data from case series studies suggest that patients with organ failure (such as renal failure) are very unlikely (chance less than 1%) to survive a cardiac arrest even if resuscitation is attempted. If resuscitation is 'futile' then doctors do not need to offer resuscitation and a DNAR order can be made without the patient's permission (Doyal & Wilsher 1993) (Fig. 12.1). Such practice is consistent with other areas of medicine where 'futile' treatment is not offered.

The difficulty with the concept of 'futility' is that it can have several different meanings. The concept of 'futility' combines the *probability* of a successful outcome with an *evaluation* of what counts as a successful outcome. The evaluation of a successful outcome itself combines both length and quality of life. Different patients are likely to evaluate these issues differently. What probability of success is so low as to make resuscitation futile? Some patients might want to take the chance of the resuscitation being successful, however small. Attempting resuscitation under these circumstances would certainly be

Box 12.7 Some arguments for and against voluntary active euthanasia

For
Consistency
- *Suicide is accepted* and no longer illegal. Some suicidal acts are rational. However, those who are most disabled will be unable to take their own life without assistance. The more disabled a person is by disease and illness, the more she requires the assistance of others to die.
- *From passive to active euthanasia.* Withdrawing and withholding life-prolonging treatment (passive euthanasia) is widely accepted and practised. The slow death after treatment is withdrawn may cause more suffering for the patient than would a more rapid death. Therefore, active euthanasia may be preferable.
- *From painkillers to lethal injections.* It is widely accepted that painkillers or sedatives should sometimes be given, particularly to terminally ill patients, even if it is foreseen that life may thereby be shortened. If we reject the doctrine of double effect (see text), then this practice provides grounds for allowing the use of purely life-shortening drugs in those circumstances.

Appeal to principles
Euthanasia can be justified by appeal to two principles:
- *Mercy/beneficence.* Euthanasia is often described as 'mercy killing'. The suffering associated with some diseases is so great that it outweighs the benefits of continuing to live. If active euthanasia will result in less suffering, it is preferable to perform passive euthanasia in these cases. Even with modern pain control and other palliative care measures, patients can still suffer near the end of life (for example from persistent breathlessness or psychological pain).
- *Autonomy.* Respect for patient autonomy should include respecting their wish for active euthanasia, at least when the patient's grounds for preferring death to continuing illness are reasonable.

Against
Palliative care obviates the need for euthanasia
One of the main arguments for euthanasia is relief of suffering. Great advances have been made in palliative care, and many argue that this obviates the need for euthanasia (House of Lords Select Committee on Medical Ethics 1994).

Manipulation or exploitation by others
Those who are severely disabled and ill are the most vulnerable. There may be coercion or pressure on an ill (especially an elderly) person to ask for euthanasia. Even if no-one is putting pressure on patients to choose euthanasia, they may want to die to spare relatives the burden of looking after them. Views differ as to whether euthanasia in such circumstances is highly undesirable, or a laudable respecting of autonomy.

Slippery slope objections
If active voluntary euthanasia were legalized this might be the first step on a slippery slope which would take us to non-voluntary mercy killing of people with severe learning disability; and then what? From a public policy perspective we need laws prohibiting euthanasia to protect vulnerable innocents. This argument has a *logical*

version and an *empirical* version (see Chapter 2). The logical version is that we are logically committed to extending euthanasia to those who cannot consent, or who are vulnerable to pressure to consent. The empirical version holds that, as a matter of psychological fact, when we loosen the constraints on killing, undesirable practices will result.

Contrary to the aims of medicine
The aims of medicine include the promotion of health and life. Patients would not trust doctors if active euthanasia were made legal.

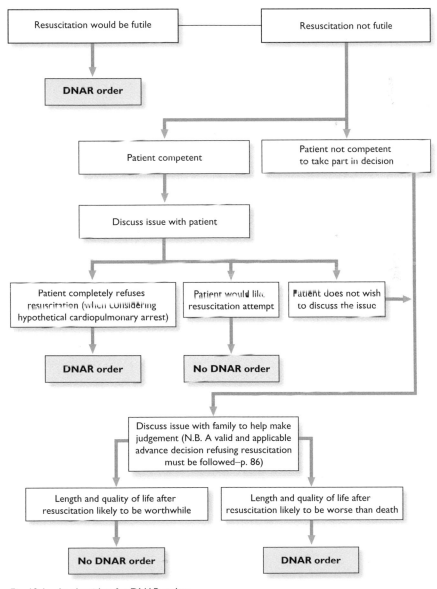

Fig. 12.1   An algorithm for DNAR orders.

disheartening for the resuscitation team, but it could be argued that such considerations must not be decisive. It might be argued, therefore, that a competent patient should normally be given the opportunity to decide whether or not to be considered as 'not for resuscitation', even where the doctors consider resuscitation to be 'futile'. Three reasons against this position can be given:

1. In practice, the possible outcomes following resuscitation fall into three categories, not two: immediate death; some prolongation of life in a state similar to that prior to the cardiac arrest; and some prolongation of life in a state that is worse than that prior to the cardiac arrest. This latter state may be worse than death. If, therefore, the patient is to decide on her resuscitation status, she would need to know all these probabilities. This argument, it could be said, leads to the conclusion that the patient needs to be given all this information, not that the decision should be taken out of her hands.
2. For many, perhaps most, patients a discussion of the issue of resuscitation will be too burdensome. Even the hypothetical question: 'Would you like to be involved in decisions about resuscitation' could upset patients who are already very ill. This, however, sounds like the arguments used 30 years ago to justify not informing patients of a poor prognosis.
3. Resuscitation costs money, and other resources. In addition to the cost of the resuscitation itself is the cost of expensive care subsequently. For example, if the patient survives the resuscitation itself she may then need treatment on an intensive care unit – treatment that was not needed before the arrest. In deciding whether to offer resuscitation to a person for whom it is unlikely to be successful, or for a person whose length of life is in any event short, these costs must be taken into account. The cost-effectiveness of resuscitation should be considered in just the same way as the cost-effectiveness of any healthcare intervention (see Chapter 13).

Legal considerations, and the involvement of family members

The legal position with regard to DNAR orders follows from the considerations summarized above (see Box 12.1 and accompanying text), and in the light of the law on consent (see Chapter 6). The key points are the following:

- Resuscitation is a treatment, like any other.
- If the patient is incompetent to discuss the issue, the doctor must treat in the patient's best interests.
- The patient's best interests may be served by withholding resuscitation.
- A doctor is not obliged to provide futile treatment, even at the patient's request.
- A competent adult patient can refuse resuscitation. In the light of valid refusal or advance decision (see p. 86) it would be battery to give resuscitation, even though the patient would be incompetent at the time of resuscitation (s.25 and 26 of Mental Capacity Act 2005).
- Not resuscitating is an example of withholding treatment (see Box 12.1).
- A Lasting Power of Attorney (see p. 86) may authorize a proxy to make decisions about the carrying out or continuation of life-sustaining

treatment. In the absence of such a power, although family members and carers must be consulted they do not have the right to demand or refuse such treatment (see Chapter 6).

- When the patient is a minor, the law is more complex (see Chapter 10).
- In theory, a person who attempts resuscitation could be liable for damages if the resuscitation were carried out negligently and resulted in injury. If without resuscitation the person would have died, the risk of a doctor incurring such liability is very small. The Resuscitation Council (2000) has published guidance on this issue.

ORGAN TRANSPLANTATION

The clinical situation

In March 2000 more than 5000 people in the UK were on the national transplantation waiting list. It has been estimated that over the 5-year period from 1995 to 1999 about 1000 people died while awaiting transplant of heart, lung or liver. In 1999, 16% of renal transplants were from living donors. This proportion has been steadily increasing (BMA 2000). An audit, carried out in England in 1989–1990 (BMA 2000) suggested that of 24 023 deaths in intensive care, 3266 had a possible diagnosis of brainstem death and might therefore have been suitable for donation. Only 1232 (37.7%) became donors. The reasons why 2034 potential donors did not become actual donors included: the tests for brainstem death were not carried out (39% of the 2034 potential donors); refusal by relatives (27%); medical contraindication to donation (22%); relatives not asked about donation (6%); heart stopped beating before brainstem death completed (4%); organs offered but not retrieved, for example because of lack of suitable recipients (2%). Although organs from either dead or living donors currently account overwhelmingly for the organs used in transplantation, other sources may become important. Animal organs have been used; mechanical hearts are under development; and it may become possible to use cloning techniques to produce human organs independently of people. These developments may alter the ethical and legal framework in which organ transplantation takes place.

The legal framework

New legislation has come into force governing transplantation, namely the Human Tissue Act 2004. Similar legislation has been introduced in Scotland – the Human Tissue (Scotland) Act 2006.

The Human Tissue Act 2004 was passed in the wake of 'scandals' involving the retention of body parts and organs from dead children without their parents' knowledge or permission. It repeals and replaces several Acts (including the Human Organ Transplants Act 1989 and the Human Tissue Act 1961). The Act sets out a new legal framework for the storage and use of tissue from the living, and for the removal, storage and use of tissue and organs from the dead. It also sets up a new body, the Human Tissue Authority, to advise and oversee compliance with the Act. This includes operating a licensing scheme and issuing Codes of Practice (there are currently six), which are designed to give practical guidance to those carrying out the Act's activities.

Consent provisions

The Act makes consent a fundamental principle. The Code of Practice (Code 1) describes consent as 'a positive act' that needs to be obtained for the removal, storage and use of human tissue or organs, and the storage and use of whole bodies for certain scheduled purposes. The consent requirements differ depending on whether tissue is taken from the living or the dead.

From the living, consent is needed for storage and use of tissue for:

- obtaining scientific or medical information that may be relevant for any other person (now or in the future)
- research in connection with disorders, or the functioning, of the human body
- public display
- transplantation.

In relation to the deceased, consent is required in certain circumstances after a coroner's post-mortem examination (as long as the coroner has no further interest), and for the removal, storage and use for the so-called 'scheduled purposes', namely:

- anatomical examination
- determining the cause of death
- establishing the efficacy of a drug or other treatment
- obtaining scientific or medical information, which may be relevant to any other person
- research in connection with disorders of the functioning, of the human body
- transplantation
- public display
- clinical audit
- education or training relating to human health
- performance assessment (presumably assessment of the performance of the health services)
- public health monitoring
- quality assurance.

Despite the central role of consent, there are several circumstances in which consent is unnecessary. Thus, in relation to the living, consent is not needed for storage and use of tissue for:

- clinical audit
- education or training relating to human health (including training for research into disorders, or the functioning, of the human body)
- performance assessment
- public health monitoring
- quality assurance
- research, provided that the research is ethically approved by the appropriate authority and that the tissue is anonymized.

As regards the deceased, consent is not needed for:

- carrying out an investigation into the cause of death under the authority of a coroner

- keeping material after an autopsy
- keeping material in connection with a criminal investigation or following a criminal investigation.

We will focus on transplantations from dead and living donors. For full details of all the Act's other provisions covering, for example, post-mortem examinations, anatomical examinations, removal, storage and disposal of human organs and tissue, and donation of allogeneic bone marrow and peripheral blood stem cells for transplantation, see http://www.hta.gov.uk/.

Organ transplants from the dead

The Human Tissue Act 2004 adopts an opt-in system under which the deceased's objections prevent others from opting-in on his behalf. According to s.1 of the Act the removal, storage and use of organs for transplantation from the dead are lawful if there is 'appropriate consent'. For adults (i.e. aged 18 years or over) consent can be obtained in three ways:

1. From the deceased himself (as evidenced, for example, by a donor card or by registration on the NHS organ donor register). However, the consent need not be in writing, in which case the Code of Practice (Code 1) requires every effort to be made to establish any known wishes of the deceased person.
2. If there is no prior decision by the deceased, consent can come from a nominated representative (who can be appointed orally or in writing). If made orally, the nomination must be made before two witnesses present at the same time.
3. In the absence of (1) or (2), consent can be obtained from a 'qualifying relative'. Qualifying relationships are ranked in a hierarchy headed by the spouse or partner, then parent or child (of any age), brother or sister, grandparent or grandchild, niece or nephew, stepfather or stepmother, half-brother or half-sister, friend of long standing (s.27(4)).

As regards children (a child is defined in the Act as being under 18 years of age), there are again three options. Thus consent can be obtained:

1. from the deceased child (providing she was 'Gillick' competent; see p. 158)
2. from a person with parental responsibility (if there is no prior decision by the deceased child)
3. from the highest ranking qualifying relationship (as set out in s.27(4)).

Note that the Code of Practice states that, even in a case where a child has given consent to the use of his or her body or any tissue, it is essential to discuss this with the child's family and to take their views and wishes into account (Code 1, para 60–65). The Code also advises that in some cases it may be advisable to discuss with the person who had parental responsibility for the deceased child whether the child was indeed competent to make the decision (Code 2, para 43).

Other aspects of the Act worth noting are the following:

- Section 5 makes it a criminal offence to take organs without appropriate consent (unless the person reasonably believes he had such consent).
- The Act authorizes the removal of organs for transplantation, but it does not make it obligatory.

- The deceased's family does not have a legal right of veto. This means that the deceased's wishes must be respected. So, if she has made it clear that she wants to donate, relatives cannot object. Similarly, if the deceased had made it clear that she does not wish to donate, this too must be respected.
- Although consent is central, the Act fails to define or indicate what information should be provided. However, both Code 1 (Consent) and Code 2 (donation of organs, tissue and cells for transplantation) provide detailed guidance on what information must be disclosed.

Organ donations from the living

Live donations are governed mainly by s.33 of the Human Tissue Act 2004 (HTA), but also by the common law.

The key common law issues focus on non-regenerative donations (e.g. kidney), when two important legal principles concerning consent apply. The first is that it is not lawful to consent to a procedure that causes death or serious injury. Thus, for example, it would be unlawful for a parent to donate his or no heart to a child, or for a surgeon to carry out such a procedure. It would probably be unlawful for a surgeon to remove both kidneys for transplant (e.g. where a parent requested it), even though the parent could remain alive on dialysis. Lesser injuries or risks, however, may be lawful, such as donating one kidney. The second is that valid legal consent must be obtained. In this context that means that the donor must fully understand the processes involved. Particularly problematic is the issue of live donations by children and incompetent adults.

Doctors should treat incompetent adult patients in their best interests (see Chapter 6). Can organs for transplant ever be taken from a donor who lacks capacity to give consent? This issue has arisen in the case of bone marrow transplantation (Re Y [1996], Stauch et al 2006, p. 574). This case involved Miss Y, aged 25 years but with a severe learning disability and living in care. Her sister, aged 36, who suffered from a preleukaemic bone marrow disorder, sought a court declaration that it would be lawful for Miss Y to have blood tests with a view to possible bone marrow extraction for donation, in order to treat the disorder, despite the fact that Miss Y did not have the capacity to give consent. The judge said that such tests (and subsequent transplantation) would be illegal unless in the best interests of Miss Y; the interests of Miss Y's sister had no weight. In fact, the judge allowed that Miss Y's best interests were served by the tests going ahead, because there were reasons to suppose that Miss Y would get better care if her sister lived. Donation from an incompetent adult would require a court's approval except in the most unusual circumstances.

According to Pattinson (2006, p. 444) the decision in Re Y [1996] would almost certainly be permitted under the Mental Capacity Act 2005 (see p. 84). Whether live donations are lawful ultimately turns on whether they are in the best interests of the incompetent adult (as defined by the MCA 2005; see Chapter 6).

There is no case on the specific issue of live donations by children and young people aged less than 18 years. The lawfulness of using children as living donors is therefore uncertain. However, it seems that before the removal of a solid organ from a child, whether competent or not, it is good practice for court approval to be obtained. That said, many legal commentators (e.g. Herring 2006, Jackson 2006) assert that in theory a Gillick-competent young person could consent to organ donation, although in practice such procedures are very rare (unlike skin or blood donations, which are more common).

Section 33 of the HTA states that it is an offence to remove or use 'transplantable material' (i.e. human organs, part organs, and bone marrow) from a living person unless each of several conditions is met, namely:

- no payment or reward has been given
- regulations required by the Act have been satisfied
- appropriate consent has been obtained

As with donations from the dead, the Codes of Practice (Codes 1 and 2) provide guidance about the information that should be given to prospective living organ donors. The Act distinguishes between various types of donation, in particular between donations to a person within a specific group ('directed'), such as to family members, and non-specific donation ('non-directed'), such as so-called 'altruistic' donations (for detailed guidance on the significance of the distinctions, see http://www.hta.gov.uk).

Finally, the Act's provisions about consent need to be mentioned briefly as these supplement the common law.

For a *competent* adult, consent simply means her consent (for the legal definition of competence, see Chapter 6).

If the adult is *incompetent* and no decision about the removal of transplantable material was made while he was competent, then donations can be carried out in specified circumstances set out in the Human Tissue Act 2004 (Persons who Lack Capacity to Consent to Transplants) Regulations 2006. Briefly, these Regulations permit the transplantation of organs or part of organs if it is in the best interests of the person lacking capacity to do so and approval has been given by at least three members of the Human Tissue Authority.

As regards *children*, the Act states that the child herself can consent (if Gillick competent) and that such consent cannot be overridden by a person with parental responsibility. Again, however, the Code of Practice states that even if a child is competent, and as such the decision to consent must be the child's, it is good practice to consult the person with parental responsibility and involve him and/or her in the child's decision-making process (Code 2, para 33). Note, too, that, even if a child is competent, when the transplantable material is an organ or part of an organ three members of the HTA must give their approval. As regards donations involving incompetent children, consent can be obtained from a person with parental responsibility (providing it is in the child's best interests). Finally, it is worth noting that despite the Act allowing donations by children, the Code states that in practice they will be living donors only in extremely rare circumstances (Code 2, para 30).

Given all this complexity, it would be wise, for a surgeon contemplating the removal of a solid organ for transplantation from a competent child (with the child's consent), to go both to court (in order to find out whether it is lawful to carry out the transplantation) and to the HTA (in order to verify that the child's consent is valid).

The legal definition of death

Doctors have traditionally diagnosed people as dead on the basis that they are pulseless, apnoeic, with fixed pupils and no heart sounds. Most organs will be suitable for transplant only if they are removed while being perfused with oxygenated blood. In practice, this means that the donor would have to be on a ventilator and have a beating heart at the time of organ removal. In order to enable transplantation, and to develop criteria for when a person on a ventilator might be diagnosed as dead, the concept of brain death or brainstem death was developed. From the legal point of view, death is now equated with irreversible loss of brainstem function.

In 1976 the Medical Royal Colleges put forward criteria for establishing brain death. These include that:

- the patient is in deep coma with no spontaneous respiration
- there is an absence of various possible reversible causes for such coma (such as drug intoxication, hypothermia or electrolyte imbalance)
- all brainstem reflexes are absent.

Tests have to be carried out twice (typically 24 hours apart). The doctor diagnosing brain death must be a consultant and the opinion of one other doctor (not necessarily a consultant) must be sought. The official time of death is the time of completion of the second set of tests. The concept of brain death was accepted as the legal definition of death in Re A [1992]. The Department of Health (1998) has produced guidelines for its diagnosis.

The allocation of organs for donation

There are insufficient organs for all those who could benefit to do so. Decisions therefore have to be made as to who should have priority for the organs that are available. United Kingdom Transplant (UKT) has developed guidelines to help such allocation. These are different for different organs. The guidelines are available from the UKT website (www.uktransplant.org.uk). The factors that are taken into account in allocating the organs are: the chance of success of the transplant, for example as predicted from the degree of compatibility between donor and recipient; the age of the donor (those under 18 years are given priority); the difference in age between the donor and the recipient (partly on the grounds of most effective use of the organ); and the proximity of the centre that is the source of the donor and the centre undertaking the transplant.

Ethics and the transplantation of organs

It will be clear from the discussion of the legal framework for organ transplantation that a large number of ethical issues are raised. Box 12.8 lists several such issues.

Box 12.8 Some ethical issues that arise in organ donation

The definition of death
The concept of brain death or brainstem death (Medical Royal Colleges 1976) is crucial in organ transplantation. Value judgements enter into the criteria for death. For example, if the definition of death were to be changed to the irreversible lack of conscious experience, organs for donation could be removed from people in a persistent vegetative state under the conditions that now allow organs to be used from people with brainstem death (for discussion of definitions of death see, for example, Singer 1995).

Incompetent donors
The legal standard allows organ donation only either where the donor can give consent or where donation is in the donor's best interests. Is it right to give no weight to the recipient's interests?

Markets in organs
The Human Tissue Act 2004 prohibits (as did previous legislation) the commercial dealing in human organs, of any kind, except for 'expenses and loss of earnings incurred by the donor'. Are markets in organs necessarily unethical?

How should scarce organs be allocated
In the UK there is an elaborate process of allocation. Is the method of allocation right? Should those under 18 years old, for example, be given priority over those aged more than 18 years? And if they should, would it not be consistent to give higher priority to, say, a 22-year-old over a 40-year-old?

Opting in and opting out
Organs for donation are scarce. Their supply depends in part on the consent procedure. Should organs be available only from cadavers if the person gave explicit consent when alive, or should the presumption be the other way round? In other words, should a system of 'opting in' or 'opting out' be adopted? In the UK people may 'opt in', e.g. through carrying a donor card, although the system is complicated by the powers given to relatives (see text).

Some countries (e.g. Austria and Belgium) operate an 'opting out' system. The arguments in favour of an 'opting out' system include the expectation that it would lead to more organs becoming available for transplantation than an 'opting in' system. Empirical data on this issue are not clearcut (see BMA 2000). Furthermore, most surveys suggest that the majority of people are happy for their organs to be used for transplantation after their death, although only a minority bother to fill in donor cards (BMA 2000, Lamb 1990).

Should a person be allowed to refuse consent for their organs to be used after their death?
An organ may save someone's life. Removing an organ from someone after their death does them no harm. We do not have property rights over our bodies after our death. Even if a person does not want their organs to be used after their death, it could be argued that this should not preclude the use of the organ. On this view, saving someone's life should take precedence over whatever interest a person can have over how their body is used after their death.

What power of veto should relatives have?

Under the HTA relatives do not have the legal right to veto a deceased's wishes. Should they have such power?

Should donors be allowed to donate conditionally?

Suppose a donor said: you may use one of my kidneys (in the case of a live donor), or you may use both my kidneys after my death, but only if the recipient is Jewish, a woman, white, etc. Should such conditional donations be accepted?

REFERENCES

Airedale NHS Trust v Bland [1993] 1 All ER 821 HL

British Medical Association 1996 Treatment decisions for patients in PVS. BMJ Books, London

British Medical Association 1999 Withholding or withdrawing life-prolonging treatment – guidance for decision making. BMJ Books, London

British Medical Association 2000 Organ donation in the 21st century: time for a consolidated approach. BMJ Books, London

British Medical Association, UK Resuscitation Council and Royal College of Nursing 2001 Decisions relating to cardiopulmonary resuscitation. Journal of Medical Ethics 27:310–316(followed by several commentaries). Online. Available:http://www.bma.org. uk/ap.nsf/Content/cardioresus 19 Jun 2007

Burke v UK (Application No. 19807/06) 11 July 2006

Chase O 1999 Haverstick I, Shepard B (eds) The wreck of the whaleship *Essex*. Harvest, San Diego

Coggon J 2007 Ignoring the moral and intellectual shape of the law after Bland: the unintended side-effect of a sorry compromise. Legal Studies 27(1):110–125

Department of Health 1998 Code of Practice for the diagnosis of brain stem death – including guidelines for the identification and management of potential organ and tissues donors. HSC 1998/035. Department of Health, London

Doyal I, Wilsher D 1993 Withholding cardiopulmonary resuscitation: proposals for formal guidelines. British Medical Journal 306:1593–1596

Foot P 1967 The problem of abortion and the doctrine of double effect. The Oxford Review. Discussed in Glover J (ed.) 1977

Causing death and saving lives. Penguin, Harmondsworth, pp. 93 & 97

Glover J 1977 Causing death and saving lives. Penguin, Harmondsworth

Gormally L 1985 Against voluntary euthanasia. In: Gillon R, Lloyd A (eds) The principles of health care ethics. John Wiley, Chichester, pp. 761–774

Herring J 2006 Medical law and ethics. Oxford University Press, Oxford

House of Lords Select Committee on Medical Ethics 1994 Report of the Select Committee on Medical Ethics, Vol. 1. HMSO, London

Jackson E 2006 Medical law: text and materials. Oxford University Press, Oxford

Lamb D 1990 Organ transplants and ethics. Routledge, London

Law Hospital NHS Trust v Lord Advocate [1996] 2 FLR 407

Medical Royal Colleges 1976 Diagnosis of brain death. British Medical Journal ii:1187–1188

Pattinson S 2006 Medical law and ethics. Sweet & Maxwell, London

Philbreck N 2000 In the heart of the sea. HarperCollins, London

Pretty v UK [2002] 35 EHRR 1 (European Court of Human Rights) Application No. 2346/02

Rachels J 1975 Active and passive euthanasia. New England Journal of Medicine 292:78–80 (Reprinted in: Singer P (ed.) 1986 Applied ethics. Oxford University Press, Oxford)

R v Cox [1992] 12 BMLR 38 (Active euthanasia (mercy killing) is illegal)

Re A [1992] 3 Med L R 303

Re B [2002] EWHC 429 (Adult: refusal of medical treatment)

Re J [1990] (A Minor) (Wardship: Medical Treatment) 3 All ER 930, Court of Appeal

Re NHS Trust v MB [2006] EWHC 507

Re Y [1996] (Adult patient) (Transplant: bone marrow) 35 BMLR 111 Family Division

Re Z [2004] (An adult) (Capacity). EWHC 2817

Resuscitation Council (UK) 2000 The legal status of those who attempt resuscitation. Resuscitation Council, London

Singer P 1995 Rethinking life and death. Oxford University Press, Oxford

Stauch M 2000 Causal authorship and the equality principle: a defence of the acts/omissions distinction in euthanasia. Journal of Medical Education 26:(4):237–241

Stauch M, Wheat K, Tingle J 2006 Text, cases and material on medical law. Taylor & Francis, Abingdon

Wyatt v Portsmouth NHS Trust & Anor 2005 EWHC 693 (Fam)

FURTHER READING

General

Brock D W 1993 Life and death: philosophical essays in biomedical ethics. Cambridge University Press, Cambridge

Dworkin R 1993 Life's dominion. Vintage Books, New York
Addresses euthanasia and abortion.

Glover J 1977 Causing death and saving lives. Penguin, Harmondsworth

McMahan J 2002 The ethics of killing: problems at the margins of life. Oxford University Press, New York

Rachels J 1986 The end of life. Oxford University Press, Oxford

Singer P 1994 Rethinking life and death. Text Publishing, Melbourne

Euthanasia and physician-assisted suicide

Battin M, Rhodes R, Silvers A (eds.) 1998 Physician assisted suicide: expanding the debate. Routledge, New York

Dworkin G, Bok S, Frey R G 1998 Euthanasia and physician-assisted suicide: for and against. Cambridge University Press, New York

Emanuel L (ed.) 1998 Regulating how we die: the ethical, medical, and legal issues surrounding physician-assisted suicide. Harvard University Press, Cambridge, MA

Keown J 1995 Euthanasia examined. Cambridge University Press, Cambridge

Weir R F (ed.) 1997 Physician-assisted suicide. Indiana University Press, Bloomington, IN

Cardiopulmonary resuscitation and futility

British Medical Association 2007 Withholding and withdrawing life-prolonging medical treatment: guidance for decision-making, 3rd edn. BMA, London

British Medical Association, UK Resuscitation Council and Royal College of Nursing 2001 Decisions relating to cardiopulmonary resuscitation. Journal of Medical Ethics 27:310–316(followed by several commentaries). Online. Available:http://www.bma.org.uk/ap.nsf/Content/cardioresus19 Jun 2007

Lee R 1996 Death rites: law and ethics at the end of life. Routledge, London
A collection of essays on law and ethics.

Woods S 2006 Death's dominion: ethics at the end of life. Open University Press, Milton Keynes
This covers a broad spectrum of clinical decisions at the end of life.

Zucker M B, Zucker H D 1997 Medical futility. Cambridge University Press, Cambridge

Organ transplantation

Price D 2000 Legal and ethical aspects of organ transplantation. Cambridge University Press, Cambridge

Shelton W 2001 The ethics of organ transplantation. JAI Press, Amsterdam
An edited collection of essays.

Trzepacz P, Dimartini A 2000 The transplant patient: biological, psychiatric and ethical issues in organ transplantation. Cambridge University Press, Cambridge

End of life

13 | Resource allocation

Healthcare systems throughout the world face the problem of how the resources available should best be allocated. No system has sufficient funds to provide the best possible treatment for all patients in all situations. On average, three new pharmaceutical products are licensed each month in the UK. Almost all have some benefit over existing drugs. Many are expensive. When is the extra benefit worth the extra cost? Both managed care systems in the USA and publicly funded systems such as the British National Health Service face this fundamental issue. In this chapter we focus on the question of how decisions about slicing the healthcare cake should be made. The question of how large should such a cake be is a political issue of great importance. Table 13.1 shows just how different is the size of the cake between different wealthy countries.

There are a number of theories that address the question of how to distribute health resources fairly. We will consider two: cost-effectiveness analysis, in particular QALY theory, and needs theory. No theory addresses all the factors that may be relevant.

COST-EFFECTIVENESS ANALYSIS AND QALY THEORY

The acronym *QALY* stands for quality-adjusted life year; QALYs are the invention of philosophically minded economists. QALY theory is the most thoroughly worked approach to cost-effectiveness analysis and the only one that we will consider here. Three alternative approaches are: saved young life equivalents (SAVEs) (Nord 1992), healthy-years equivalents (HYEs) (Mehrez & Gafni 1989) and disability-adjusted life years (DALYs) (Anand & Hanson 1997, Murray 1994).

❝ The essence of a QALY is that it takes a year of healthy life expectancy to be worth 1, but regards a year of unhealthy life expectancy as worth less than 1. Its precise value is lower the worse the quality of life of the unhealthy person (which is what the quality adjusted bit is all about)' (Williams 1985).

The general idea is that a beneficial healthcare activity is one that generates a positive number of QALYs, and an efficient healthcare activity is one where the cost per QALY is low. The lower the cost per QALY, the higher the priority of that healthcare activity. In this way, the resources available purchase the greatest number of QALYs. QALY theory is a direct descendant of utilitarianism (see Chapter 2). Indeed, the founder of utilitarianism (Jeremy Bentham) thought of the idea of a 'felicific calculus' – a calculus of happiness.

Table 13.1 National expenditure on health (data for year 1998, from OECD 2001)		
Country	Proportion of GDP (%)	Per capita purchasing power ($)
Australia	8.6	2085
Canada	9.3	2360
Denmark	8.3	2132
Finland	6.9	1510
France	9.4	2043
Germany	10.3	2361
Greece	8.4	1198
Ireland	6.8	1534
Italy	8.2	1824
Netherlands	8.7	2150
New Zealand	8.1	1440
Norway	9.4	2452
UK	6.8	1510
USA	12.9	4165

GDP, gross domestic product.

The central argument in favour of QALYs is as follows. The purpose of health care in general is to increase both the quantity and the quality of life. Both quantity and quality are important to us, and if choices have to be made we trade these two factors against each other. If we call the combination of quantity and quality the overall welfare for a patient then, in allocating resources within health care, we should maximize the amount of welfare. If, therefore, we have a specified amount of money to spend on health care, it should be so allocated as to buy the maximum amount of welfare. QALYs are, in effect, units of welfare.

Some examples of the cost per QALY of different kinds of health care are given in Table 13.2.

What is wrong with QALYs?

The main criticisms of QALYs boil down to three concerns:

1. That *welfare* is not the only value to be put into the equation.
2. That QALYs are *unjust* because they do not take into account who is experiencing them.
3. That the *calculation of quality is problematic*. Either such calculation is not possible, or it is so subjective and dependent on the way in which it is calculated that it renders the theory unworkable.

Welfare is not the only value

Many believe that there is an important distinction between needs and benefits. For example, a person who has been severely injured in a car accident

Table 13.2   Some estimates of cost per QALY for various healthcare interventions

Intervention	Cost/QALY (£ sterling)	Reference
Cervical cancer screening (targeted call of unscreened women aged 20–59 years)	200	Waugh et al 1996
Thrombolytic therapy following acute myocardial infarction in men with previous infarction aged 35–39 years, compared with no therapy	1300	Fenn et al 1991
Thrombolytic therapy following acute myocardial infarction in women aged 45–49 years	2000	Fenn et al 1991
Breast cancer screening programme	6800	Forrest 1986
Decreasing cervical cancer screening interval, from 5 to 3 years, in women aged 20–59 years	7600	Waugh et al 1996
Coronary artery bypass graft for patients with mild angina and double vessel disease compared with medical management	26 000	Williams 1985
Hospital dialysis for end-stage renal disease in people aged 55–64 years, compared with no treatment	45 000	Ludbrook 1981

The authors are grateful to Dr A Briggs and Dr A Gray for these data. The costs have been corrected for inflation from the original articles to reflect 1996 prices.

needs medical care, whereas a smoker would benefit only from antismoking advice. Even if the QALY calculation favours the antismoking advice, the accident victim should have priority for the resources.

A second argument against considering welfare as the only value can be understood in the context of terminal care. However, much such care enhances the quality of life, the cost per QALY is likely to be high because the length of life is short. The assumption behind QALYs is that a person's good can be found by adding the good at each moment of life. Is this the case? Many people feel that the manner in which a person's life ends is of considerable importance: that there is a sense in which the whole life of a person is a unity, and not simply an addition of each slice of life. Seen from this perspective, good terminal care might increase total welfare in a way that cannot be calculated by summing time slices equally. Although this is a problem with QALYs, it may be overcome by other approaches to cost-effectiveness analysis (e.g. healthy-years equivalents).

QALYs are unjust

The second main criticism is that QALYs take no account of justice. To see why this might be the case, consider chronic disease. Other things being equal, a person with arthritis will have a lower quality of life than someone without. Suppose that two people, one with arthritis and one without, are in need of life-extending treatment – for some reason unconnected with the arthritis. Both would get the same life extension for the same cost. However, the cost per

QALY would be greater for the person with arthritis because the quality of life is less. This leads to what John Harris (1985) has called 'double jeopardy'. First of all a person has some handicap. Then she becomes in further need of medical help. Because she has the first handicap she is less entitled, from the QALY perspective, to further medical help. To overcome this problem, Nord (1992) has suggested replacing QALYs by 'saved young life equivalents' (SAVEs).

A separate issue of justice is what is known as the distribution problem. The QALY approach maximizes total welfare without regard to how such welfare is distributed. Should resources be used preferentially to give a great benefit to relatively few people, or relatively little benefit to a large number of people? Is the QALY answer (to do whatever maximizes welfare overall) the right one?

The problem with calculating quality of life

If QALYs are to be used in practice then there has to be a method for calculating quality of life. Because the whole purpose of QALYs is to help choose between different ways of spending healthcare money, quality of life cannot be just one person's view of quality of life. In practice, the kind of question that has to be answered is: what is the quality of life of being unable to walk and confined to a wheelchair? Or, what is the quality of life of having severe facial scarring? There is no single answer to these questions, as the answer will depend both on how the question is asked and on who answers it. With regard to the first issue, there are several different ways of approaching this question (Brookes 1996, Edgar et al 1998, EuroQol Group 1990, Rosser & Kind 1978). With regard to the second issue there is a difference between the answers given by healthy people and those with a disability or illness. People with serious health problems tend to rate their quality of life surprisingly highly. Furthermore, the correlation between quality of life and disease severity is not very strong (Fitzpatrick 1996).

Age and QALYs

Because QALYs are the product of quality and length of life, the cost per QALY will rise in inverse proportion to life expectancy. In practice, QALYs will tend to disadvantage the elderly because they have a shorter life expectancy in general than do younger people. Does this mean that QALYs are *ageist*, i.e. that they unjustly discriminate against the elderly?

The argument that QALYs are not ageist

QALY theory does not *explicitly* discriminate against the elderly. The old are not discriminated against because they are old. A young person with a short life expectancy would be treated in exactly the same way as an old person with the same life expectancy (assuming quality of life and cost are the same). Further arguments about age and resource allocation are considered below in the section on needs theories.

The case in favour of QALYs being ageist

1. It is irrelevant that QALYs do not *explicitly* discriminate against old age. It is inevitable that, however impartially the theory is expressed,

it will *in fact* discriminate against the old. Consider a parallel example. Suppose that, for some technical reason, an operation is more expensive when performed on a woman than on a man (or vice versa). Would it be unjust if we denied the operation to a woman who was in exactly the same state as a man to whom we offer the operation? QALYs could lead to this happening, even though the sex of the patient is not mentioned explicitly.

2. Imagine two people both in need of life-saving treatment and at the same cost. One is aged 30 and the other is 40 years old. Both are equally desirous of living. According to QALY theory, if the resources available are sufficient for only one person to be treated, that should be the person with the longer life expectancy (usually the younger person) because the cost per QALY will be less. Is this just, or does justice require that we value both lives equally?

The fair-innings argument

Some have argued that, far from being ageist, QALY theory is not 'ageist' enough. QALY theory is concerned with life expectancy. Lockwood (1988, p. 50) argues that younger people should have priority over older people, irrespective of life expectancy. He outlines the argument as follows:

" To treat the older person, letting the younger person die, would thus be inherently inequitable in terms of life lived: the younger person would get no more years than the relatively few he had already had, whereas the older person, who has already had more than the younger person, will get several years more.

A variant on Lockwood's position is the *fair-innings* argument, which states that all should have equal priority up to a certain age (e.g. 70 years) after which priority should become lower. Harris (1985) has argued that the value of life can only sensibly be taken to be that value that those alive place upon their lives. Consequently if you and I are of different ages but value our lives equally, then it is unfair to give you priority simply because you are younger.

NEEDS THEORY

Needs theory is based on the view that some patients have a special claim on resources that rests not on the maximization of overall welfare but on their greater need for treatment. The most thoroughly worked-out version of needs theory is that of John Rawls, who emphasizes the value of *fairness*.

Rawls' approach

Rawls (1972) proposed a general theory of distributive justice, i.e. of how money and other goods should be distributed within a society. Rawls' approach has been applied to health care by Daniels (1985).

Rawls rejected the utilitarian principle of maximizing total welfare. He also rejected the libertarian 'free for all', where all individuals should own whatever goods they can legally secure for themselves. He favoured developing a theory of social justice based on what rational individuals would choose. In order to ensure impartiality he constructed a device: the veil of ignorance.

Veil of ignorance

The veil of ignorance can be seen as a kind of thought experiment. This involves your imagining that you are situated in some ethereal place, looking down on a vast array of different societies. Each of these societies distributes wealth among its citizens in a different way. In some societies there are enormous differences between rich and poor. In others goods are distributed almost equally. Some societies are, overall, well off; others are badly off. From your ethereal place you can see exactly what each society is like. The thought experiment requires that you choose to join one of these societies without knowing who, in that society, you will be. You might be among the richest, or among the poorest, or at any point in between. Not only do you not know who you will be, you do not know what attributes you will have. You may have high or low intelligence. You may have one kind of personality or another. You may be male or female. The question is: which society would you choose to join?

The 'difference principle'

Rawls, perhaps because he is not a gambler, argues that it is rational to choose that society in which the worst-off groups are maximally well off. This may not be the society with least difference between rich and poor, because some inequality may lead to the worst off being better off. The idea that justice is best achieved by the worst-off groups being maximally well off is known as the 'difference principle'. Rawls outlines this principle as follows: 'The intuitive idea is that the social order is not to establish and secure the more attractive prospects of those better off unless doing so is to the advantage of those less fortunate' (Rawls 1972, p. 975).

Applying Rawls to health care: hernia treatments versus kidney treatment

For the money available, either 100 otherwise healthy people with hernias can be treated or one very sick person with severe and debilitating renal disease. Assume that each hernia treatment provides one unit of benefit (e.g. one QALY) and the kidney treatment provides 50 units.

QALY theory would favour treating those with hernias. Rawls' theory might favour treating the person with renal disease, i.e. the person who is worst off.

Problems with Rawls' approach

There are two major problems with Rawls' approach:

1. Need, or maximizing the welfare of the worst off, is not the only value that should be taken into account. When there is a clash between this value and other values it is unclear that need should have the priority that Rawls' theory gives it.
2. It is not clear that behind a veil of ignorance people would choose the difference principle. Many might wish to gamble on not being one of the worst off, if they expected to be better off.

With regard to the first point, a strict application of the difference principle might lead to enormous health resources being used to produce very small gains for the very badly off. Although it may be reasonable to give some preference to the worst off, it seems unreasonable to give the degree of preference required by the difference principle. If the very badly off have only a little to gain from treatment (or at very high cost), whereas the moderately badly off have much to gain, many of us would choose (behind the veil, if necessary) to put the limited resources into those who are moderately badly off.

Ageism and needs theory

The usual way of considering the question of the allocation of resources between young and old is as a distribution problem between different individuals. Daniels (1985), using an adaptation of the veil of ignorance approach, argues that we should see the issue of age and the allocation of resources not as a question of distribution between people, but as of one of distribution through the life of a single individual. Daniels considers two 'insurance' schemes: the first involves providing better treatment for younger people at the cost of some reduction in resources for the old; the second provides identical quality of care at all ages, with the result that the health care for the young is not so good as on the first scheme. Daniels believes that it is more prudent to choose the first scheme, because this gives the maximum chance of living to old age.

RESPONSIBILITY FOR BRINGING CONDITION ON ONESELF

If a patient's behaviour or lifestyle has contributed to her ill health, should she, therefore, be at a lower priority for health care? This issue is not addressed by either QALY or needs theories.

Some examples of when patients' behaviour or lifestyle may contribute to their ill health, or to their need for health care, are given in Box 13.1. Perhaps most patients have contributed to some extent to their health problems.

Arguments in favour of responsibility affecting priority

An argument in favour of responsibility affecting healthcare priority can be made in two stages:

1. That the person is responsible, at least to some extent, for bringing the problem on herself
2. That such responsibility is a reason for reducing priority for health care.

Although there may be many situations in which it is impossible to assess responsibility, that is by no means always the case. The fully informed person who elects for sterilization, or the sportsperson who knows of the risk of soft tissue injury, makes choices in knowledge of the health risks. In many other walks of life we expect people to accept the consequences of the choices they make: why should medicine be any different? Would it not be unfair on the person who takes care of his health to be denied treatment because another, responsible for his ill health, took priority (perhaps on the grounds of being

> **Box 13.1** Examples of patients' behaviour contributing to the need for health care
>
> 1. Lung disease or heart disease in someone who smokes
> 2. Liver failure in someone who drinks large amounts of alcohol
> 3. Tattoo that the patient now wants removed
> 4. Reversal of sterilization
> 5. Soft tissue injury from sport
> 6. Accident in someone engaging in risky behaviour, for example hang-gliding or cycling along a busy road
> 7. Accident due to person's own careless driving
> 8. Heart disease in obese person
> 9. Respiratory infection in someone who travelled in a crowded train
> 10. Renal disease in someone with diabetes who has not controlled their diabetes carefully

more ill)? At the very least, if resources are scarce the issue of responsibility should be given some weight, even if the weight is small compared with other factors such as clinical need, or ability to benefit.

Arguments against responsibility affecting priority

The arguments against responsibility affecting priority can be directed at either stage 1 or stage 2 of the argument given above. An extreme position relevant to stage 1 would be to deny that people are responsible for anything. A less extreme view is that, although we are free to choose different things in life, people have little effective choice over most of the factors that affect health, or at any rate cannot reasonably be blamed for what they have done. Consider a smoker. Upbringing, peer group pressure, and perhaps genetic factors predisposing to addictive behaviour, may combine to make her vulnerable to smoke. Furthermore, she may have become addicted to smoking when a teenager. Would it be right to hold her responsible for the health consequences of her smoking as an adult, 20 years later? More generally, attributing responsibility is too imprecise. Some factors affecting responsibility are given in Box 13.2.

With regard to stage 2, it might be argued that, even if a person is responsible, this should have no influence over priority. Access to health care, and priority, should depend on factors such as clinical need, not responsibility. The central importance of health to our lives justifies health care being different from many walks of life where we do expect people to accept the consequences of their own behaviour.

SOCIAL FACTORS, DEPENDANTS AND PRIORITY

Are dependants, for example children or frail elderly parents, grounds for increasing a person's priority for health care? Caring for dependants is only one example of how we can benefit others. Should a person's value to society more generally be a relevant factor in deciding priority for health care?

Box 13.2 Some factors affecting responsibility for ill health

Knowledge and education
Did the person know, at the relevant time, that sniffing fabric cleaner can cause liver disease? Has the person been properly educated about 'safe sex'?

Social and biological setting
Was the healthier behaviour a reasonable possibility given, for example, the financial and social pressures under which the person lived? Was the healthier behaviour a reasonable possibility given the person's maturity and intelligence, or other biological factors, such as genetic predisposition to addiction?

Probability of ill health
Was the chance of the bad (unhealthy) consequence sufficiently high, given what the person did voluntarily, to view it as the person's responsibility? In other words, was he simply unlucky?

Arguments in favour of social factors being taken into account

Consequentialist perspective

According to the consequentialist perspective (see Chapter 2) we should consider all the consequences of our actions. If treating person A in preference to person B results in the best overall consequences, that provides a good reason in favour of treating A. These overall consequences include those contributions to society that A or B would make. If A would make a greater contribution to society then that will be a factor in favour of A having a higher priority.

Public money for public benefit

If health care is provided using public money then it is essentially a good that society provides for individuals. If choices have to be made regarding priority, it is reasonable for public money to be spent in a way that maximizes public good. This may be achieved by giving priority to those who, as a consequence of the healthcare provision, will benefit society.

Arguments against social factors being taken into account

Argument from principle

Priority for health care should be decided on clinical factors. Doctors, or health managers, should not make judgements about patients' 'social worth'. There are other ways in which society rewards people for what they contribute (e.g. by the level of income or through various honours). The provision of health care should not be one of these ways.

Argument from practice

Even if it is not wrong in principle to give higher priority to those of higher 'social worth', it is too difficult in practice to judge such worth. For example, we may not know of the good that one patient does in supporting other people.

THE BOUNDARIES OF HEALTH CARE

Many things affect people's health that are not part of health care, such as enforcing speed limits, or maintaining high standards for building construction. In deciding on the allocation of healthcare resources, one issue is whether a particular activity or intervention should be funded from healthcare resources at all, however cost-effective it is. Some examples of activities that might not be considered as appropriate for health care are given in Box 13.3. This is a heterogeneous group of activities. Some require health professionals (e.g. in-vitro fertilization, cosmetic surgery); others have an impact on health, but are not carried out primarily by health professionals (e.g. the provision of traffic-calming measures).

Attempts to define health care have shown how difficult this is (New 1997, New & Le Grand 1996). Klein (1997) argues that there is no satisfactory way of determining general criteria for what should be funded from healthcare resources. There are two different questions that a society needs to answer:

1. Is this an activity that individuals should 'fund themselves'?
2. Is this an activity that the state should fund, but not as part of health care?

FAIR PROCEDURE FOR MAKING ALLOCATION DECISIONS

Each theory of resource allocation highlights some relevant values, and each has some strengths and some weaknesses. There seems to be no one theory that should determine the use of resources. For these reasons, much recent work has focused not on the theories but on the process by which decisions should be made. Daniels & Sabin (1997; Daniels 2000, p. 92) specify four conditions in order to implement what they call 'accountability for reasonableness' in allocation decisions:

  " 1. (Publicity) Decisions regarding coverage for new technologies (and other limit-setting decisions) and their rationales must be publicly accessible.
    2. (Reasonableness) The rationales for coverage decisions should aim to provide a *reasonable* construal of how the organisation should provide "value for money" in meeting the varied health needs of a defined population under reasonable resource constraints.
    3. (Appeals) There is a mechanism for challenge and dispute resolution regarding limit-setting decisions, including the opportunity for revising decisions in light of further evidence or arguments.

Box 13.3 Some examples of valuable activities that might not be appropriately funded from the healthcare budget

- Treatments, such as in-vitro fertilization, to assist reproduction
- Cosmetic surgery
- Long-term nursing care for the elderly
- Health education in schools
- Provision of traffic calming measures (e.g. 'sleeping policemen')
- Reversal of sterilization

4. (Enforcement) There is either voluntary or public regulation of the process to ensure that conditions 1–3 are met.

In practice, such procedures usually involve setting up a group of people, from a variety of backgrounds, to decide issues of resource allocation (Crisp et al 1996, Hope et al 1998, Martin & Singer 2000), and this raises the question of who should be involved in this process and how should they be chosen. Such a group, even when provided with good evidence concerning both the cost and the effectiveness of a healthcare intervention, frequently faces problematic ethical choices. If the group is to behave in a responsible way it needs to provide reasons for its decisions. It cannot avoid considering the values highlighted by the theories of allocation discussed above.

One issue of importance is whether and how the public should be involved in the process of decision-making. There are two principal reasons for involving the public: first, in most healthcare systems public money provides a substantial portion of the resources; and second, the purpose of medicine is to help patients. Because the public are the patients of the future, their perspective is important.

Involving the public, however, is by no means straightforward. Four questions arise: Who are the relevant public? How is the opinion of the relevant public to be ascertained? How are the inevitable wide variations in public opinion to be accommodated? How much weight should be given to the public's opinion?

A number of different methods have been developed for assessing the public's views (Kneeshaw 1997). The research suggests that the majority believe that the young should have priority over the old, and that people with family responsibilities should have priority over those without. The British public seem split, roughly evenly, on the question of whether those who bring a condition on themselves should therefore have a lower priority.

RATIONING AND THE LAW

If a health authority or other healthcare provider were challenged in the courts on a decision about the allocation of resources, then it would need to be able to explain its decision in two ways:

1. Was the *procedure* for making the decision reasonable?
2. Were the *grounds* for making the decision reasonable?

Two legal challenges to resource allocation decisions

Decisions about the allocation of resources can be legally challenged through actions in either public or private law. The legal framework of the National Health Service (NHS) imposes a number of specific legal obligations on the Secretary of State for Health. The National Health Service Act 2006 (which came into force in March 2007) is a new consolidating Act (i.e. one that brings all relevant provisions into a single Act). It primarily covers the structure and operation of the NHS and therefore includes most, but not all, of health legislation since 1977. This means that the NHS Act 1977 and much subsequent legislation is repealed and replaced. The obligations in the NHS Act 2006 nevertheless remain the same as in the 1977 legislation and include the promotion of a comprehensive health service designed to secure an improvement (a) in the physical and mental health of the people, and (b) in the prevention, diagnosis and treatment of illness. One potential way of involving the courts in decisions of resource allocation is to claim that, in not funding a particular treatment or service, the NHS has failed in its statutory duty. The procedure involved is a part of public law and is known as judicial review. If the claim succeeds, the court will strike down the decision to refuse treatment.

The second (private action) approach is to use civil law to claim that some person or institution has been negligent in making the decision. If such a claim were to succeed, the claimant (e.g. patient) would be compensated for the loss suffered. The decision, however, would not be reversed – although a successful claim would be likely to affect future decisions about resource allocation.

From an analysis of the relevant cases, Montgomery (2003) concluded: '… judicial review is unlikely to be successful if it is based on an attack on the substance of the decision. Applications will be stronger if they allege that the process by which the decision was taken was flawed'. In general, the courts have not been sympathetic to private claims, and in particular to negligence claims. One of the reasons, Montgomery believes, why courts have been reluctant to become involved in rationing decisions is to ensure that authorities make decisions based on the best use of resources, rather than on satisfying those most likely to complain.

Although the general principle that the courts will not intervene in issues of resource allocation in the NHS still seems to hold, there have been two cases where health authorities have been held to be liable for failure to provide services. One case involved β-interferon for sufferers of multiple sclerosis. This is an expensive drug that has some beneficial effect for some patients, although that benefit is not great. A sufferer challenged the decision by a health authority to refuse to pay for the drug, and the challenge was successful on the grounds that the authority had failed to follow guidance issued by the Department of Health (R v North Derbyshire Health Authority [1997]).

The second case concerned three transsexuals who wanted gender reassignment surgery. Such surgery had been given a low priority by the authority and was not funded. The Court of Appeal found that the health authority's policy was flawed. In particular, the authority had failed to assess the effectiveness of various forms of treatment accurately (North West Lancashire Health Authority v A, D and G [1999]).

In a third case, R (on the application of Ann Marie Rogers v Swindon NHS Trust [2006], much of the media coverage implied that the courts appeared willing to challenge policy decisions about resource allocation and decisions about treatment in the case of individual patients. It remains the case that the courts are unwilling to override Trust decisions with regard to funding. They come down heavily, however, on poor reasoning such as that demonstrated by the minutes of the Swindon PCT meetings.

As to the impact of the Human Rights Act 1998 on access to treatment, several Articles could be invoked by patients refused treatment (especially life-saving treatment). These include Article 2 (right to life), Article 3 (protection from torture or inhuman or degrading treatment), Article 8 (right to private life) and Article 14 (protection from discrimination). According to Herring (2006), Article 14 is potentially the most promising approach if used by a patient alleging discrimination on the basis of, for example, age or disability.

The impact of European law may also be relevant to the allocation of health resources. Could a patient who faces a lengthy delay in obtaining treatment seek it in another EEC country and require payment for it from the NHS? This is essentially what happened in R (on the application of Watts v Bedford PCT and Secretary of State for Health [2004]). The decision in this case suggests that a patient would succeed in such a claim only if the waiting time in the UK amounted to 'undue delay'.

REFERENCES

Anand S, Hanson K 1997 Disability-adjusted life years: a critical review. Health Economics 16:685–702

Brooks R for the EuroQol Group 1996 EuroQol: the current state of play. Health Policy 37:53–72

Crisp R, Hope T, Ebb D 1996 Rationing in general practice: the Asbury draft policy. British Medical Journal 312:1528–1531

Daniels N 1985 'Just health care'. Studies in philosophy and health policy. Cambridge University Press, Cambridge

Daniels N 2000 Accountability for reasonableness in private and public health insurance. In: Coulter A, Ham C (eds) The global challenge of health care rationing. Open University Press, Buckingham, pp. 89–106

Daniels N, Sabin J 1997 Limits to health care: fair procedures, democratic deliberation and the legitimacy problem for insurers. Philosophy & Public Affairs 26:303–350

Edgar A, Salek S, Shickle D, Cohen D 1998 The ethical QALY: ethical issues in healthcare resource allocations. Euromed Communications, Haslemere

EuroQol Group 1990 EuroQol: a new facility for the measurement of health-related quality of life. Health Policy 16:199–202

Fenn P, Gray A M, McGuire A 1991 The cost–effectiveness of thrombolytic therapy following acute myocardial infarction. British Journal of Clinical Practice 45:181–184

Fitzpatrick R 1996 Patient-centred approaches to the evaluation of health care. In: Hope R A, Fulford K W M, Ersser S (eds.) Essential practice in patient-centred care. Blackwell Science, Oxford, pp. 229–240

Forrest P 1986 Breast cancer screening. HMSO, London

Harris J 1985 The value of life: an introduction to medical ethics. Routledge, London

Herring J 2006 Medical law and ethics. Oxford University Press, Oxford

Hope T, Hicks N, Reynolds D J M et al 1998 Rationing and the health authority. British Medical Journal 317:1067–1069

Klein R 1997 Defining a package of health care services: the case against. In: New B (ed.) Rationing, talk and action in health care. King's Fund & BMJ Publishing, London, pp. 85–93

Kneeshaw J 1997 What does the public think about rationing? A review of the evidence. In: New B (ed.) Rationing: talk and action in health care. King's Fund & BMJ Publishing, London, pp. 58–76

Lockwood M 1988 Quality of life and resource allocation. In: Bell J M, Mendus S (eds) Philosophy and medical welfare. Cambridge University Press, Cambridge, pp. 33–55

Ludbrook A 1981 A cost–effectiveness analysis of the treatment of chronic renal failure. Applied Economics 13:337–350

Martin D K, Singer P A 2000 Priority setting and health technology assessment: beyond evidence-based medicine and cost–effectiveness analysis. In: Coulter A, Ham C (eds) The global challenge of health care rationing. Open University Press, Buckingham, pp. 135–145

Mehrez A, Gafni A 1989 Quality-adjusted life years, utility theory, and healthy-years equivalents. Medical Decision Making 9:142–149

Montgomery J 2003 Health care law. Oxford University Press, Oxford

Murray C J L 1994 Quantifying the burden of disease: the technical basis for disability-adjusted life years. Bull of the World Health Organization 72:429–445

New B 1997 Defining a package of health care services the NHS is responsible for. In: New B (ed.) Rationing, talk and action in health care. King's Fund & BMJ Publishing, London, pp. 79–84

New B, Le Grand J 1996 Rationing in the NHS: principles and pragmatism. King's Fund, London

Nord E 1992 An alternative to QALYs: the saved young life equivalent (SAVE). British Medical Journal 305:875–877

North West Lancashire Health Authority v A, D and G [1999] Lloyds Law Reports Medical, pp. 399

Organisation for Economic Co-operation and Development 2001 OECD health data 2001: a comparative analysis of 30 OECD countries. OECD, Paris (CD-ROM)

R v North Derbyshire Health Authority [1997] Med LR 327

R (on the application of Ann Marie Rogers v Swindon NHS Trust [2006] EWCA 392

R (on the application of Watts v Bedford PCT and Secretary of State for Health [2004] EWCA 166

Rawls J 1972 A theory of justice. Oxford University Press, Oxford

Rosser R, Kind P 1978 A scale of valuations of states of illness: is there a social consensus? International Journal of Epidemiology 7:347–358

Waugh N, Smith K, Robertson A 1996 Costs and benefits of cervical screening III. Cost/benefit analysis of a call previously unscreened women. Cytopathology 7:249–255

Williams A 1985 The value of QALYs. Health and Social Service Journal 94(Suppl): 3–5 (quoted by Lockwood M 1988 Quality of life and resource allocation. In: Bell J. Mendus S (eds) Philosophy and medical welfare. Cambridge University Press, Cambridge, pp. 36)

FURTHER READING

Battin M, Rhodes R, Silvers A (eds) 2002 Medicine and social justice. Oxford University Press, New York
A collection of papers with perspectives from both sides of the Atlantic.

Bell J N, Mendus S 1988 Philosophy and medical welfare. Cambridge University Press, Cambridge
Although now quite old, this remains a useful collection of good essays. It is particularly strong on the philosophical issues raised by QALYs.

Coulter A, Ham C (eds) 2000 The global challenge of health care rationing. Open University Press, Buckingham
An edited collection of practical and theoretical papers covering a wide range of contemporary issues in healthcare rationing.

Daniels N 1985 Just health care: studies in philosophy and health policy. Cambridge University Press, Cambridge
A thorough and seminal application of Rawlsian theory to the distribution and healthcare resources.

Edgar A, Salek S, Shickle D, Cohen D 1998 The ethical QALY: ethical issues in healthcare resource allocations. Euromed Communications, Haslemere
This provides an up-to-date European perspective on QALYs in practice. It covers the measurement of QALYs, ethical and technical difficulties with QALYs, and contains a number of short summaries of healthcare rationing in various European countries, including some from the former Eastern Europe.

New B 1997 Defining a package of health care services the NHS is responsible for. In: New B (ed.) Rationing, talk and action in health care. King's Fund & BMJ Publishing, London, pp. 79–84
This is a collection of articles (some previously published, others written for this book) with wide coverage of issues, especially practical issues and from a UK perspective. It does not cover the basic philosophical theories.

Newdick C 2005 Who should we treat? Oxford University Press, Oxford
A clear account of the political and legal context on resource allocation in the UK NHS.

Nord E 1999 Cost–value analysis in health care: making sense of QALYs. Cambridge University Press, Cambridge
An alternative to measuring patients' quality of life is proposed (cost–value analysis). This book provides a thoughtful critique of QALYs. The Journal of Medical Ethics published an interesting and lively debate between Harris on the one hand and Singer and colleagues on the other:

Harris J 1987 QALYfying the value of human life. Journal of Medical Ethics 13:117–123
Harris argues against QALY theory.

Singer P, McKie J, Kuhse H, Richardson J 1996 Double jeopardy and the use of QALYs in health care allocation. Journal of Medical Ethics 21:144–150

Singer and colleagues reply to Harris.

Harris J 1995 Double jeopardy and the veil of ignorance – a reply. Journal of Medical Ethics 21:151–157

Harris defends his original position.

McKie J, Kuhse H, Richardson J, Singer P 1996 Double jeopardy, the equal value of lives and the veil of ignorance: a rejoinder to Harris. Journal of Medical Ethics 22:204–208

The debate then continued in three adjacent articles:

Hope T 1996 QALYs, lotteries and veils: the story so far. Journal of Medical Ethics 22:195–196

Summary of the debate.

Harris J 1996 Would Aristotle have played Russian roulette? Journal of Medical Ethics 22:209–215

McKie J, Kuhse H, Richardson J, Singer P 1996 Another peep behind the veil. Journal of Medical Ethics 22:216–221

Research

14

HISTORY OF THE REGULATION OF RESEARCH

The regulation of research focuses on safeguarding individuals who take part in medical research from either harm or failure to respect autonomy. The central concern is to ensure that the interests of society, or the enthusiasm of the researcher, do not override the interests of the individual. The differences in the history of the regulation of research and of clinical practice account for much of the tension that can arise between a medical researcher and a research ethics committee. They also account for the differences in standards of consent between research and clinical practice, differences that may not always be ethically justified.

The appalling experiments carried out by some Nazi doctors led to the first internationally agreed guidelines on research involving people: the Nuremberg Code (1949). This code consisted of ten principles, which were incorporated by the medical profession into the Declaration of Helsinki, first published by the World Medical Association in 1964 and last updated in 2000.

Principle 13 of the Declaration of Helsinki (World Medical Association 2004) states:

> " The design and performance of each experimental procedure involving human subjects should be clearly formulated in an experimental protocol. This protocol should be submitted for consideration, comment, guidance, and where appropriate, approval to a specially appointed ethical review committee, which must be independent of the investigator, the sponsor or any other kind of undue influence.

Ethical review bodies are called *research ethics committees* in the UK and *institutional review boards* in North America. Research is regulated in a number of ways. These include professional guidance issued by various bodies such as the Royal College of Physicians (1996), General Medical Council (GMC 2000) and Medical Research Council (MRC 2007); the common law; and various statutes such as the Human Rights Act 1998, the Human Tissue Act 2004 and the Mental Capacity Act 2005.

As we shall see below, the general principles that apply to the law of consent to treatment also apply to research. Thus, for consent to be legally valid it must be voluntary, i.e. obtained without duress or undue influence, and informed, i.e. following full and detailed disclosure.

Research is also regulated by a centralized system of research ethics committees (RECs), and all medical research involving humans as participants (subjects) should be scrutinized by such a committee. The duties of these committees include maintaining ethical standards of practice in research and protecting participants from harm.

Since 2001 the conduct of research has also been regulated by the Research Governance Framework for Health and Social Care. Now in its second edition (Department of Health 2005), the framework is designed to ensure that the procedures and powers of ethics committees are less fragmented and more effective in producing high-quality and ethically sound research than in the past. Also important in regulating research is the guidance on standard operating procedures (SOPs; Department of Health 2004) issued by the Central Office for Research Ethics Committees (COREC) (which is currently within the National Patient Safety Agency).

If research involves the clinical trial of a new medicine involving human participants, researchers must follow the requirements of The Medicines for Use (Clinical Trials) Regulations 2004. The regulations are lengthy and detailed, and aim to standardize the regulation of medical research throughout the EU, including the ethical review of research protocols. There are several key regulations covering the factors that RECs must consider before approving a clinical trial. These include, for example, the anticipated risks and benefits of the trial and its design, the procedure for obtaining consent, and the suitability of the protocol. Most significantly, the regulations introduce new criminal sanctions. Sixteen principles of good practice are also identified (which largely repeat those contained in various international codes and guidance).

The Research Governance Framework (Department of Health 2005) makes it quite clear that neither RECs, nor reviewers, are responsible for giving legal advice. Nor are they liable for any of their decisions in this respect. Rather, the responsibility for not breaking the law rests with researchers and health and social care institutions.

ETHICAL PRINCIPLES RELEVANT TO MEDICAL RESEARCH

The autonomy of the research participant

One approach to the ethics of research would be to give almost exclusive weight to respecting participant autonomy (the 'libertarian position'). On this view, if a potential research participant is fully informed, competent and not coerced, then that person has a perfect right to take part in even very dangerous research. In defence of this position, libertarians might point out that we allow people to take considerable risks, for example in the pursuit of dangerous sports. This position is *not* that endorsed in the guidelines for research ethics (Box 14.1), which emphasize that research participants should not normally be put at more than minimal risk of harm.

The risk of harm to the research participant

A different ethical perspective emphasizes the duty of the researcher to ensure that the potential participant is not put at risk of harm through taking part in

Box 14.1 Summary of international and national guidelines on research ethics

1. Research participants should not be put at more than minimal risk of harm as a result of taking part in research. Guidelines suggest that some balancing between risk of harm and other considerations, such as the potential value of the research and whether it can be carried out without exposure to harm, is appropriate. However, even if the research is likely to lead to enormous benefit to others, the risk to participants should be small. The only possible exception is in some therapeutic research.

2. Potential research participants should be fully informed about both the purpose of the study and what will be involved in taking part, including an honest account of risks and benefits.

3. It is difficult or even impossible to carry out some research with individual consent from participants, for example some research using data from case notes or clinical databases. Ethics committees need to be satisfied that such research is of sufficient value to justify the breach of autonomy (confidentiality) and that the research cannot be carried out satisfactorily in any other way.

4. No coercion must be brought to bear on people to take part in research. Care must be taken to ensure that the potential participant does not feel an obligation to take part. It must be made clear to patients that their clinical care (outside the research study) will not be affected by their refusal to take part in research.

5. Payments may be made to patients only to offset reasonable costs, and must not be such as to act as inducement for the person to take part in the research.

6. Patients who are not competent to give consent for research may still be eligible to take part in research. Ethics committees will need to be satisfied that:
   - the risk of harm is very low, probably lower than the risk that is acceptable in the case of competent participants
   - the research aims cannot be achieved by other means
   - the research is of considerable value, and
   - a relevant person (usually a close relative) gives valid consent.

the research. Almost exclusive concern for such risk gives rise to what might be called the paternalistic position. Thus, the (somewhat caricatured) paternalist would consider research that involves more than minimal harm unethical, even if the potential participant gives fully informed consent, and even if the participant wishes, perhaps from altruistic motives, to take part in such research. On the other hand, the paternalist would be little concerned with research that involved no risk of harm but did take place without the consent of the participants, for example research that involved collecting information from patients' medical notes without consent.

The consequences of the research

Consequentialist approaches to ethics see the consequences of our choices as being of crucial importance (see Chapter 1). An important aspect of a consequentialist approach to research is that the benefits and harms both to participants *and* to those in the future are to be considered. On the consequentialist view, the risk of harm to research participants may be justified by the good to people in the future who will benefit from the research. Some consequentialist perspectives would give equal weight to the interests of research participants and those in the future who might benefit from the research. The Declaration of Helsinki and national guidelines reject this position. The interests of research participants are given much greater weight than the interests of people in the future.

The general presumption of research ethics guidelines is that participating in research is potentially harmful, or at least burdensome. However, at least for some therapeutic research, participants may benefit simply from participating in the research, because, for example, the standard of clinical care is often better within a funded research project (Chalmers & Lindley 2001).

CONTRASTING THESE ETHICAL APPROACHES

These different approaches are contrasted, in somewhat caricatured form, in Box 14.2. Each approach highlights different values, and the national and international guidelines on research ethics make use of all three approaches. The importance of consent and confidentiality reflect respect for the autonomy of the participant. Central to the guidelines is the general prohibition on putting the participant at more than minimal risk, reflecting the duty not to harm. The consequentialist approach informs the view that the potential for the research to benefit people in the future is a necessary condition for the research to be undertaken. Some guidelines suggest that the greater the expected value of the research, the greater the risk of harm to the participants that can be justified. However, no guideline allows significant risk of harm to the research participants for the sake of those in the future.

Box 14.2 A comparison of three different ethical approaches to research				
	Research where participants knowingly expose themselves to high risk	Low-risk research where participants do not know they are taking risks	Low-risk research where participants are fully informed	Poor-quality research that is of little value but where participants are fully informed
Libertarian (rights based)	Yes	No	Yes	Yes
Paternalistic (duty based)	No	Yes	Yes	No
Utilitarian (consequentialist)	Yes	Yes	Yes	No

KEY ETHICAL CONSIDERATIONS IN CARRYING OUT RESEARCH

Box 14.3 summarizes the main ethical issues that need to be considered when designing a study involving people as research participants.

Scientific validity

The Declaration of Helsinki (Principle 11) states:

" Medical research involving human subjects must conform to generally accepted scientific principles, be based on a thorough knowledge of the scientific literature, other relevant sources of information, and on adequate laboratory and, where appropriate, animal experimentation (World Medical Association 2004).

Box 14.3 Some key issues in assessing the ethical aspects of a research protocol

Scientific validity
- Are the aims worthwhile?
- Is the method appropriate to the aims?

Safety
- Are the procedures safe, and are all reasonable precautions being taken?
- Is the degree of risk for participants acceptable?

Consent procedure
Informed
- Is the information clearly written, honest, sufficient, and balanced?

Voluntary (absence of coercion)
- Is it clear to participant that refusal to take part will not affect clinical care?
- Is the relationship between researcher and participant free from potential coercion?
- Is the payment such as to encourage participation 'against the person's better judgement'?
- Is the researcher under undue pressure to recruit participants?
- Is there sufficient time after being given information for the person to decide whether to participate?

Competent
- Are the potential participants competent to decide whether or not to take part?
- Is such competence being assessed, when relevant?
- If potential participants are not competent, are they either excluded or is the recruitment procedure adequate?

Confidentiality
- Have participants given consent for confidential data to be accessed in the research?
- Are the safeguards to prevent those not involved in the research from having access to confidential data adequate?

Research that is scientifically poor may be considered unethical for two reasons: it will not benefit people in the future and so any risk of harm to participants cannot be justified; and it may harm people in the future because the results are misleading.

The risk of harm

The Declaration of Helsinki (Principle 5) states:

" In medical research on human subjects, considerations related to the well-being of the human subject should take precedence over the interests of science and society' (World Medical Association 2004).

A central ethical position taken by international and national guidelines is that research participants must be protected from being at much risk of harm, even if the benefit of the research to people in the future is considerable. The term 'minimal risk' is often used to describe an acceptable level of risk. The Royal College of Physicians (1990a) describes minimal risk as either 'a small chance of a reaction which itself is trivial, e.g. a mild headache or feeling of lethargy', or 'a very remote chance of serious injury or death'. The latest Royal College of Physicians guidelines (1996) state:

" 7.2 … Minimal risk could include everyday risks such as travelling on public transport or a private car (the latter having considerably higher risk) but would not include travel by pedal or motorcycle; in medicine, they would be no more likely and not greater than the risk attached to routine medical or psychological examination … Minimal risk is where the chance of serious injury or death is very remote and may be ignored. Minimal risk may also be used for the situation where the level of distress or clinical malaise is slight or where there may be a chance of a reaction which is itself trivial, e.g. a mild headache, a feeling of lethargy or a dry mouth. Attempts have been made to quantify minimal risk as a risk of death of <1 per million or of major adverse effect of <10 per million, and low risk as 1 to 100 per million for death and 10 to 1000 per million for major adverse event.

" 7.3 Benefit may be weighed against risk in two different ways. First and most obviously, the patient may benefit. This is typified in a therapeutic trial where at least one of the treatments offered may be beneficial to the patient … Second, society rather than the individual may benefit. In such situations, however large the benefit, to expose a participant to anything more than minimal risk needs very careful consideration and would rarely be ethical.

Therapeutic research refers to research with patients when treatment is given within a research protocol, for example as a part of a controlled trial. Non-therapeutic research involves participants, who may or may not be patients, when the research is not an integral part of clinical management. The question of non-therapeutic research is addressed elsewhere (Royal College of Physicians 1990b, Section 5.26):

" We have considered whether non-therapeutic research involving greater than minimal risk is ever permissible and conclude that, although the circumstances in which it is justifiable are likely to be very rare, they do exist. It seems possible that such research might satisfy a research ethics committee where the following conditions apply:

  i The risk of the research procedure is still small in comparison to the risks already incurred by the patient as a consequence of the disease itself;

  ii the disease under study is a serious one;

  iii there is great potential benefit in terms of the importance of the knowledge gained;

  iv there is no other means of obtaining the knowledge;

  v the subject understands well what is involved and wishes to participate.

The Royal College (Section 5.18) explicitly states that harm is to be interpreted widely to include discomfort and psychological harms.

These guidelines are interesting for at least two reasons. The first is that they markedly restrict the degree of risk that competent adults can take voluntarily, in contrast with many areas of life. The second is that, within the limits of risk allowed, some trade-off between risk and the value of research is envisaged. If the research is highly valuable, participants can be exposed to a greater degree of risk than in the case of less valuable research.

Consent, information and competent adults

The Declaration of Helsinki (Principle 22) states:

" … the physician should then obtain the subject's freely-given informed consent, preferably in writing' (World Medical Association 2004).

For consent to be valid, the person must be competent (have legal capacity) to give the consent, properly informed and free from coercion. The assessment of competence in the setting of research should presumably be approached in the same way as consent to treatment (see Chapter 6).

If the research involves the testing of medicines on human participants the Medicines for Human Use (Clinical Trials) Regulations 2004 govern the issue of consent. The regulations define consent as that which 'is given freely after that person is informed of the nature, significance, implications and risks of the trial'. Importantly, failure to provide sufficient information may also give rise to criminal liability. Furthermore the participant must have an interview with the researcher during which he must have been given 'the opportunity to understand the objectives, risks and inconveniences of the trial, and the conditions under which it is to be conducted. Normally consent must be formally recorded on a signed, written consent form. The signed consent form is, however, no guarantee that consent has been freely given. Consent once given can also, of course, be withdrawn at any time.

If the research does not involve medicines, the common law principles of consent apply (see Chapter 6). The relevant 'key information' would include the purpose of the research, what is involved in taking part, the risks and benefits, and its general methodology. Notwithstanding the common law, it would also seem the Clinical Trials Regulations 2004 governing consent may apply too. This is because the guidance on standard operating procedures issued by COREC in 2004 makes it clear that the policy of the Department of Health and COREC is to apply the research ethics review requirements of the Clinical Trials Regulations more generally. As such it would seem that all NHS research falling outside the Regulations should be governed and assessed by RECs as if it were covered by the Regulations.

Double standards in information provision

Several researchers (e.g. Chalmers & Lindley 2001) have argued that different standards are being applied without good reason to therapeutic research on the one hand, and to clinical practice on the other. This is particularly the case with regard to the amount of information provided to patients or participants. Contrast the following two situations.

Clinical case

Dr A sees patient B in the outpatient department. B is suffering from depression of a type likely to be helped by antidepressants. There are several slightly different antidepressants available. Dr A advises B to take a particular antidepressant (drug X) – the one with which he is most familiar and which is suitable for B. Dr A informs B about the likely benefits and the side-effects of drug X. However, he says nothing about the other antidepressants that might be prescribed.

Research case

A randomized controlled trial is under way to compare two antidepressants: drug X and drug Y. Although Dr A tends to prescribe drug X, on reflection she does not think that there is currently good evidence to prefer X to Y. It could be important to establish the relative effectiveness of each. Dr A therefore agrees to ask suitable patients whether they would be prepared to take part in the trial. Dr A sees B in the outpatient department. B is suffering from depression and would be a suitable candidate for the trial. In order to conform to the standards laid down by the research ethics committee, Dr A must obtain valid consent for B to enter the trial. She must inform B about the trial and its purpose. She must also inform B about both drugs X and Y, and tell B that a random process will be used to choose which will be prescribed.

In the research case, Dr A must inform B about both drugs, and about the method of choosing which to give. In the clinical case this standard of informing is not the norm. Is this difference justified? Box 14.4 summarizes some arguments for and against such 'double standards'.

Box 14.4   Some arguments for and against double standards in the provision of information

Arguments in defence of double standards
1. Double masters require double standards. Research trials and clinical practice are critically different because in the case of a trial the central purpose is to benefit people in the future (the research intention). There is a pressure on the doctors and those running the trial to make decisions that are good for the trial, in addition to considering the best interests of the patient. In the case of ordinary clinical practice the doctor has no double master. Her duty is simply to the best interests of the patient. The requirement for a more careful consent procedure arises from this difference.
2. Patients are likely to view the two situations differently. It is likely that, if patients were not informed that they had been entered into a trial and that their treatment had been chosen using a random process, they would be extremely angry. On the other hand, it seems much less likely that patients would be concerned if the doctor, within normal clinical practice, had selected 'in good faith' what he saw as the most appropriate treatment.
3. If people were to realize that trials were being conducted without full information then there would likely to be a loss of trust in doctors. This seems less likely in the case of patients realizing that doctors are influenced in their prescribing by industry-sponsored education – as long as the prescriptions are reasonable.

Arguments against such double standards
The three reasons given above can each be criticized:

1. It is naive to think that the fact that a doctor is acting in the best interests of her patient is sufficiently different from the doctor in the case of the clinical trial. In practice, the doctor is influenced in her prescribing by many factors. In fact, in the case of a randomized controlled trial there will have been much more careful scrutiny of the objective data regarding efficacy than would be normal in clinical practice. There have to be safeguards to ensure that patients are no longer entered into the trial when there is good reason to suppose that one drug is better than the other. But, if these safeguards are in place, there is no good reason to demand a high standard of consent in the case of research.
2. Points (2) and (3) above are both empirical claims that may or may not be true. If it is true that patients would like a different standard of consent in the case of a trial than for normal clinical practice, then this is irrational.

Incompetent adults

The legal position of research involving adults who lack capacity is now a complex combination of the Clinical Trial Regulations 2004 and the Mental Capacity Act 2005. The brief details of each are as follows:

Clinical Trial Regulations 2004

The Regulations govern trials of medicinal products involving human subjects. In addition to the provisions referred to above, the following key points should be noted. The Regulations:

- define adults as those aged 16 years and over
- define an 'incapacitated adult' as a person who is 'unable by virtue of physical or mental incapacity to give informed consent'
- allow an incapacitated adult to be entered into a clinical trial if informed consent is given on his behalf (in effect by a proxy) representing the adult's 'presumed will'
- the proxy must not be anyone who is connected with the trial
- the proxy is called a 'personal legal representative' (if she is a close friend or relative who is willing to act on the adult's behalf)
- if there is no such person, the proxy can be a 'professional legal representative' (e.g. the person's doctor)
- incapacitated adults can be involved only in therapeutic research only if it is not possible to recruit competent participants (but note that these regulations only cover the testing of medicinal products. The Mental Capacity Act 2005, and various guidelines, allow non-therapeutic research on incompetent patients in special situations; see below)
- research cannot be carried out with the incapacitated adult if he has previously made (when he had capacity) an advanced refusal indicating his wish not be involved in the trial
- if no such advanced refusal exists but the incapacitated adult objects to being a participant, her objections must be considered (but she can still be entered in to the project).

The Regulations also set out various conditions and principles that must be followed. These specify (amongst other things) that the trial has been designed to minimize pain, discomfort, fear and any other foreseeable risk, and that the incapacitated adult has received information according to his capacity of understanding regarding the trial, its risks and its benefits (see further Schedule 1 Part V).

Mental Capacity Act 2005 (MCA)

Sections 30–34 state that research in relation to a person who lacks capacity is unlawful unless a number of conditions are satisfied. However, because all research involving medicinal products is governed by the Clinical Trial Regulations, and research involving medical data is regulated by the Data Protection Act 1998 (see also the Human Tissue Act 2004), the Act's scope is limited to research that does not fall under these regulations and statutes. Examples of research for which the MCA is relevant include: the investigation of new surgical techniques; procedures that do not involve medicines such as brain imaging techniques or the analysis of blood samples; and psychological investigations. In brief the Act:

- applies to adults (those aged 16 years and over)
- covers 'intrusive' research, which means anything that involves touching the participant (unless consented to)

The Act states the following:

- The research must be connected with an 'impairing condition' affecting the adult (i.e. one that causes or contributes to the impairment of, or

disturbance in, the functioning of the mind or brain). For example, if the capacity of a participant is impaired as a result of dementia then the research must be aimed at helping our understanding of dementia.
- The research must be approved by a REC.
- The research can be either therapeutic or non-therapeutic.
- If the research is therapeutic, the benefits must justify the risks and the REC must have reasonable grounds for believing that the research cannot be carried out as effectively using those who have capacity to consent.
- If the research is non-therapeutic, the risks must be negligible and not interfere significantly with the participant's freedom or privacy, or be unduly invasive or restrictive.
- Nothing can be done in the course of the research to the participant that would be contrary to a valid advance decision (or other statement of which the researcher is aware).
- The research cannot be carried out if the participant appears to object, even if she is not able to understand the purpose of the research.

There are also detailed provisions in the Act that provide for proxy consent (in the Act this is called 'consulting carers'). Section 32 allows an incapacitated adult to be involved in research if a relevant person has been identified and consulted. This person (i.e. someone 'engaged in caring for or interested in the participant') must have no connection with the project, nor be acting either in a professional capacity or for money. The proxy must be consulted about whether the participant should take part in the research and what he thinks the participant's wishes and feelings would be (if she had capacity). If there is no such proxy a nominated person can be consulted.

The legal position with regard to medical treatment of incompetent adults is rather different in Scotland, mainly because of the Adults with Incapacity (Scotland) Act 2000 (see Chapter 6, especially Box 6.6). This Act specifically addresses the question of medical research involving the incompetent adult (defined for the purposes of the Act as a person who has attained the age of 16 years). According to the Act (Section 51), no surgical, medical, nursing, dental or psychological research shall be carried out on any adult who is incapable in relation to a decision about participation in the research unless certain conditions are met. These conditions are that: research of a similar nature cannot be carried out on an adult who is capable in relation to such a decision; the purpose of the research is to obtain knowledge of the causes, diagnosis, treatment or care of the adult's incapacity; or the effect of any treatment or care given which relates to that incapacity; and the research is likely to produce real and direct benefit to the adult. Furthermore, the participant must not indicate unwillingness to participate in the research; the research must be approved by the ethics committee; it must not entail any foreseeable risk, or only a minimal foreseeable risk, to the adult; and must not impose discomfort, or only minimal discomfort. Finally, consent must have been obtained from any guardian or welfare attorney who has power to consent to the adult's participation in research or, where there is no such guardian or welfare attorney, from the adult's nearest relative. The Act states: 'Where the research is not likely to produce real and direct benefit to the adult, it may nevertheless be carried out if it will contribute through significant improvement in the scientific understanding of the adult's incapacity to the attainment of real and direct benefit to the adult or to other persons having the same incapacity'. The other circumstances or conditions mentioned above must also be fulfilled.

Children and consent

The law regulating research on children is now a complex mix of common law, statute (the Family Law Act 1967, Mental Capacity Act 2005) and Regulations (the Clinical Trial Regulations 2004). For convenience, children and young people need to be divided in various age groups.

Children and young people aged 16 and 17 Years

Research involving medicinal products

If the research involves the testing of medicines then the Clinical Trial Regulations 2004 apply (see section above on *consent, information and competent adults* for regulations regarding competent participants, and the section on *incompetent adults* regarding incompetent participants).

Research that does not involve medicines

In research not involving medicines, e.g. the testing of a new surgical or diagnostic procedure, the position is more complicated. Although the Family Law Act 1969 (Section 8) allows competent 16–17-year-olds to consent to treatment, that section does not refer specifically to research. Common law principles therefore apply. Thus, if the young person is Gillick competent there is no good reason why researchers should not be able to rely on her sole consent. However, because there is no case that confirms this approach, the legal position remains unclear. It would thus be wise to obtain consent from someone with parental responsibility (in addition to the competent young person's consent). Unless the research is therapeutic, the risks should be minimal (see p. 222).

If a 16–17-year-old lacks capacity to consent, the provisions of the Mental Capacity Act apply (see p. 226). The provisions outlined in the section on incompetent adults should therefore be followed (see above). As we saw, these allow both therapeutic and non-therapeutic research to be carried out under certain conditions. As was noted in Chapter 10, however, there is an overlap between the Act and the common law in relation to incompetent 16–17-year-olds. It thus is arguably possible for researchers to use common law principles (which are not repudiated by the Act) and obtain consent from someone with parental responsibility. In practice, however, such a person would most likely be the same individual who would be consulted under the Mental Capacity Act 2005. Once again non-therapeutic research would be lawful under the common law only if the risks were minimal.

Children and young people aged under 16 years

Research involving medicinal products

If the research involves medicines, the Clinical Trial Regulations 2004 apply. There are, however, special provisions governing minors (i.e. those under

16 years of age). First the consent requirements must be met; namely, that informed consent (see above) be obtained from a person with parental responsibility, although in an emergency informed consent can be given by a legal representative (but not by anyone connected with the trial). It seems, therefore, that under the Regulations a minor cannot give sole consent even if Gillick competent. Second, the trial must be approved by a REC (with advice from a paediatric expert if no such person is on the committee). Other conditions include:

- the minor must have been given information (according to her capacity of understanding) about the trial, its risks and benefits
- prior to the trial the person giving consent (i.e. person with parental responsibility or legal representative) must be given the opportunity to understand the objectives, risks and inconveniences of the trial
- the trial must relate to a clinical condition suffered by the minor or be of such a nature that it can be carried out only on minors
- some direct benefit for the group of patients involved is to be obtained from the trial
- a minor can be involved in the trial even if he objects (but his objections must nevertheless be considered).

Research not involving medicines

Common law principles apply here. The legal position is much the same as in relation to competent 16–17-year-olds. Thus, in the absence of legislation on the issue, if the child is Gillick competent and the trial is therapeutic, researchers would be wise to obtain the consent both of the child and a person with parental responsibility. For non-therapeutic research to be lawful the risks must be minimal.

As to research involving those aged less than 16 years who lack capacity to consent, the legal position is governed by the common law and mirrors that of the incompetent 16–17-year age group (see above). The Mental Capacity Act 2005 does not apply to those under 16 years.

Current ethical guidance from the Royal College of Paediatrics and Child Health (2000), as well as from the MRC and the GMC, takes an approach that respects the autonomy of the minor to an extent greater than the law in that it endorses research relying on the sole consent of a competent young person (i.e. 'one with sufficient understanding and intelligence to understand what is proposed').

Consent by children to medical treatment has a different legal structure in Scotland from that in England and Wales (see Chapter 10). In the setting of medical research it may be the case that the Age of Legal Capacity (Scotland) Act 1991 allows 'mature' minors under the age of 16 years to consent to participation in research.

Coercion to take part

Researchers, and RECs, need to ensure that the recruitment method protects patients from pressures to take part in the research. In particular, it must be made clear that any medical treatment will not be affected by whether the patient takes part in the research, except to the extent that the research may involve treatment not available outside the research setting. In addition, ethics committees will be concerned that undue pressure may be brought to bear on patients to take part in the research if doctors receive payment for the research according to the number recruited. The International Conference on Harmonisation guidelines (1996) on good clinical practice in clinical trials specify that any payment to researchers should be stated in the patient information sheet.

The relationship between researcher and participant

Clearly it is unethical to use force to ensure that someone takes part in a research project. However, the idea of coercion is usually taken to cover much more than the use of force. One consideration is the relationship between researcher and the participant. The key question is whether the potential participant is in a special relationship with the researcher, so that it might be hard to refuse participation in the study. Examples of such special relationships are those between patient and doctor, and between student and teacher.

The payment of research participants

The Department of Health circular (1991) states:

> " Payment in cash or kind to volunteers should only be for expense, time, and inconvenience reasonably incurred. It should not be at a level of inducement which would encourage people to take part in studies against their better judgement, or which would encourage them to take part in multiple studies.

The courts would almost certainly take these guidelines seriously. This position, however, is open to ethical criticism. From the perspective of participant autonomy it might be asked why competent adults should not decide for themselves whether they wish to take risks, at a level that is accepted in other areas of life, for the sake of financial gain (Savulescu 2001). From the perspective of justice, the guidelines might justify paying an amount of money to a rich person that would not be justified for a poorer person. This is because a smaller amount might act as inducement for a poorer person.

Confidentiality

Most medical research involves collecting information concerning individuals that should be kept confidential. A researcher could be found negligent if reasonable precautions were not taken to ensure that information gained was stored in a secure manner. Furthermore, information should normally be passed to another person only with the explicit consent of the research participant.

Some clinical research requires access to patient details for recruitment purposes. For example, researchers may wish to contact all patients who were admitted to hospital with a particular disease. If the hospital gives the contact details of such patients to the researchers, then patients confidentiality will have been breached. This problem can usually be avoided by the hospital or relevant clinician contacting the patient directly to seek consent for contact details to be passed on to the researchers. More problematic is research that does not involve direct contact with patients but that is based on the collection and analysis of existing information in medical records. Seeking individual consent from each patient for access to health records may not be possible in the case of large studies or studies involving records from a long time ago. The GMC (2000, Section 31) guidelines state:

" Where research projects depend on using identifiable information or samples, and it is not practicable to contact patients to seek their consent, this fact should be drawn to the attention of a research ethics committee, so that it can consider whether the likely benefits of the research outweigh the loss of confidentiality.

The MRC (2007) gives guidance to researchers conducting research studies including those that involve access to confidential information. The Department of Health's guidance to local research ethics committees (Department of Health 1991, Section 3.12) states:

" Epidemiological research through studies of medical records can be extremely valuable. Patients are however entitled to regard their medical records as confidential to the NHS and should in principle be asked if they consent to their own records being released to research workers. However there will be occasions where a researcher would find it difficult or impossible to obtain such consent from every individual and the LREC will need to be satisfied that the value of such a project outweighs, in the public interest, the principle that individual consent should be obtained. Where a patient has previously indicated that he or she would *not* want their records released then this request should be respected.

RESEARCH IN THE THIRD WORLD

" The ethical implications of research involving human subjects are identical in principle wherever the work is undertaken; they relate to respect for the dignity of each individual subject as well as to respect for communities, and protection of the rights and welfare of human subjects' (Council for International Organizations of Medical Sciences 1993).

" Human subjects in any part of the world should be protected by an irreducible set of ethical standards (Angell 1988).

Case example: Controlled trials of interventions to reduce the perinatal transmission of HIV in developing countries

Research in the USA and France strongly suggests that a regimen of treatment with zidovudine (known as the ACTG 076 regimen) reduces the chance of vertical transmission of human immunodeficiency virus (HIV), i.e. from mother to child. The regimen involves oral doses for the mother while pregnant, intravenous doses during labour and further doses to the newborn infant. This regimen is too expensive to be generally available in the third world.

A cheaper, but effective, regimen would potentially prevent a very large number of babies in the third world from being infected with the HIV.

The ACTG 076 regimen was the standard in the USA because it was the only one that had been shown to be effective. The USA wished to sponsor research in the third world to find a cheaper regimen. It was thought possible that a cheaper regimen involving only oral zidovudine might be effective.

Two possible designs of study to be carried out in third world countries were considered. The first was to compare the cheaper regimen with placebo. The second was to compare the cheaper regimen with the expensive one (ACTG 076). The first design is aimed at answering the question: Is the cheap treatment better than nothing (placebo)? The second design is aimed at answering the question: Is the cheap regimen as effective as the expensive regimen?

It is generally accepted that the control group in a treatment trial should receive standard treatment (i.e. they should not be disadvantaged by taking part in the trial, compared with people who are not in the trial).

Arguments to the effect that it is unethical to conduct a placebo-controlled trial

1. It would be unethical in the sponsoring country (the USA) because standard treatment is the 'expensive' regimen. Thus the control group would be receiving placebo when there was an effective standard treatment. It is unethical for those in a third world country to have a lower standard than those in the sponsoring country: a double standard is operating.
2. Once we allow such double standards there is a danger that we will allow greater and greater exploitation of people in the third world – using them as 'research fodder'.
3. The Declaration of Helsinki states that controls in treatment studies should receive the best currently available treatment.
4. There is no scientific reason for preferring this placebo-controlled design to the alternative design, in which controls receive the expensive regimen.

Arguments to the effect that it is not necessarily unethical to conduct the placebo-controlled trial

1. If it were not for the trial, no-one in the third world trial would be receiving treatment. No-one, therefore, receives worse treatment as a result of the trial taking place than they would if the trial did not take place (in contrast to the situation if the trial were being carried out in the sponsoring country). There is no-one who has been harmed as a result of the trial.
2. Although it would be better to provide controls with the expensive regimen, this would cost the sponsoring country (or a pharmaceutical

company, or whomever) extra money. Certainly it might be right for a rich country, or a pharmaceutical company, to make expensive treatments available to poor countries. To some extent this takes place through aid programmes, etc. Certainly the rich countries may not be generous enough. But that is a different issue. If we do not think that the sponsoring country, or the pharmaceutical company, should be forced to provide the expensive treatment outside any trial, then why should it be forced to provide such treatment inside the trial?

3. The exploitation argument is wrong. Those who receive the (cheap) treatment as part of the trial are better off than they would be if the trial did not take place. It is in the interests of those in the third world for as many such trials to take place as possible. Some of those who take part in the trial are benefited; some are neither better off nor worse off. No-one is being exploited.

4. Some argue that from the scientific point of view there is something to be gained by using a placebo-controlled trial. Suppose that this is the case: that the placebo-controlled trial will establish whether the cheap treatment is effective more rapidly than the treatment-controlled trial. If this is true, then this provides an argument that the placebo-controlled trial is ethically preferable.

REFERENCES

Angell M 1988 Ethical imperialism? Ethics in international collaborative clinical research. New England Journal of Medicine 319:1081–1083

Chalmers I, Lindley R I 2001 Double standards on informed consent to treatment. In: Doyal L, Tobias J (eds) Informed consent in medical research. BMJ Books, London, pp. 266–276

Clinical Trial Regulations 2004 The Medicines for Human Use (Clinical Trials) Regulations. Statutory Instrument 2004, No. 1031. The Stationery Office, London. Online. Available: http://www.opsi.gov.uk/si/si2004/20041031.htm 20 Jun 2007

Council for International Organizations of Medical Sciences in collaboration with the World Health Organization 1993 International ethical guidelines for biomedical research involving human subjects. CIOMS, Geneva(www.cioms.ch)

Department of Health 1991 Local research ethics committees. HSG (91)5. DoH, London

Department of Health 2004 Standard operating procedures for research ethics committees. DoH, London

Department of Health 2005 Research governance framework for health and social care. DoH, London

General Medical Council 2000 Confidentiality: protecting and providing information. GMC, London

International Conference on Harmonisation of Technical Requirements for Registration of Pharmaceuticals for Human Use 1996 Good clinical practice: consolidated guideline. E6(R1) ICH, Geneva. Online. Available: http://www.ich.org/LOB/media/MEDIA482.pdf 20 Jun 2007

Medical Research Council 2007 Policy and guidance (Ethics and Research Governance). Online. Available: http://www.mrc.ac.uk

Nuremberg Code 1949. Online. Available: http://www.fuente.de/bioethik/nuremb.htm 20 Jun 2007

Royal College of Paediatrics and Child Health 2000 Guidelines for the ethical conduct of medical research involving children. Archives of Disease in Childhood 82:177–182

Royal College of Physicians 1990a Guidelines on the practice of ethics committees in medical research involving human subjects, 2nd edn. RCP, London

Royal College of Physicians 1990b Research involving patients. RCP, London

Royal College of Physicians 1996
Guidelines on the practice of ethics
committees in medical research involving
human subjects, 2nd edn. RCP, London
Savulescu J 2001 Taking the plunge. New
Scientist 169:50

World Medical Association 2004
Declaration of Helsinki: ethical principles
for medical research involving human
subjects. WMA, Edinburgh. Online.
Available: http://www.wma.net/e/
policy/b3.htm 20 Jun 2007

FURTHER READING

A useful website to guidelines about the ethical conduct of medical research with links
to other relevant sites is the Department of
Health site at: www.nres.npsa.nhs.uk Several
key guidelines and weblinks are given in the
references to this chapter.
The GMC guidelines to doctors taking part in
research (Research: the role and responsibilities of doctors) are available on the GMC
website at: http://www.gmc-uk.org/guidance/
current/library/research.asp(see also the list of
web resources on p. 253)
Annas G J, Grodin M A (eds) 1992 The Nazi
doctors and the Nuremberg Code: human
rights in human experimentation. Oxford
University Press, New York
Applebaum P S, Roth L H, Lidz C W,
Benson P, Winslade W 1987 False hopes
and best data: consent to research and
the therapeutic misconception. Hastings
Center Report 17:20–24
Brody B A 1998 The ethics of biomedical
research: an international perspective.
Oxford University Press, New York
Doyal L, Tobias J S (eds) Informed consent
in medical research. BMJ Books, London,
pp. 266–276.
A detailed examination of the ethical issues sur-
rounding consent to participate in medical
research.
Eckstein S 2003 Manual for research ethics
committees. Cambridge University Press,
Cambridge
Provides both background discussion of the
issues and practical materials relevant to eth-
ics committee members.
Elliot D, Stern J E (eds) 1997 Research eth-
ics: a reader. University of New England,
Hanover, NH
Deals with more general issues arising from
research, with several case studies.
Evans D, Evans M 1996 A decent proposal:
ethical review of clinical research. John
Wiley, Chichester

A very detailed and practical guide to the evaluation of clinical research.
Foster C 2001 The ethics of medical research
on humans. Cambridge University Press,
Cambridge
Looks at research from goal-based, duty-based
and right-based perspectives. Many case
studies.
Grayson L 2000 Animals in research: for
and against. British Library, London
This is a useful introduction and sourcebook to
further reading. Grayson's book addresses the
issue of animals used in research, a topic not
covered in this chapter.
Guiloff R J (ed.) 2000 Clinical trials in neurology. Springer, London
Macklin R 2004 Double standards in
medical research in developing countries. Cambridge University Press,
Cambridge
Mason S, Megone C (eds) 2001 European
neonatal research: consent, ethics committees and law. Ashgate, Aldershot
Murphy T F 2004 Case studies in biomedical
research ethics. MIT Press, Boston, MA
National Research Ethics Service, National
Patient Safety Agency 2000 Multi-centre
research ethics committees, guidance for
researchers. Online. Available: http://
www.nres.npsa.nhs.uk
Ross L F 2006 Children in medical research:
access versus production. Clarendon
Press, Oxford
Rothman D J 1982 Were Tuskegee and
Willowbrook 'studies in nature'?
Hastings Center Report 12:5–7
Smith T 1999 Ethics in medical research: a
handbook of good practice. Cambridge
University Press, Cambridge
A very detailed and practical guide to
evaluating all types of clinical research.
Useful for ethics committee members and
researchers.

RESEARCH

Disease, disability and human enhancement

15

Is apotemnophilia (Box 15.1) a disease? Is it right that doctors should treat it? Is it right that doctors should amputate healthy legs as part of treatment? And what are the connections between these three questions? In this chapter we discuss some fundamental concepts in medicine such as disease, illness and disability. Our interest, however, is not in semantics but in ethics. The question 'Is homosexuality a (mental) illness?' was being seriously discussed 50 years ago in the context of whether it should be removed from the major classifications of disease. This question, however, was not simply a semantic one, nor simply a scientific one: it also involved social and ethical values. Not far beneath the surface of this question lie issues such as: should doctors be involved in trying to change a person's sexual orientation, and should medical research aim at finding 'cures' for homosexuality? This particular question is now stale, but this type of question, and the closely connected broad issue of the goals of medicine, need to be reviewed frequently in the light of both social and scientific developments (for detailed discussion see Savulescu 2007).

In this chapter we raise some conceptual and ethical issues that arise in three contexts: what is disease; models of disability; and the use of medical interventions to enhance human abilities.

DISEASE

An apparently simple answer to the question of 'What is the goal of medicine?' is that it is the treatment and prevention of disease and disability. This, of course, raises questions about what constitutes disease and disability. Is apotemnophilia *really* a disease? Or is it a personal preference or fetish, more like the desire for body modification by plastic surgery for aesthetic or other reasons? If it is not a disease, is surgery warranted? Comparison can be made with gender identity disorder, and the same questions can be asked. And should the ethical question of whether it is right to amputate the healthy limb of a person with apotemnophilia, or the penis of a person with gender identity disorder, depend on the answer to whether these are diseases or not?

The *locus classicus* for the definition of disease is Christopher Boorse's biostatistical theory (for a detailed overview and response to all his critics,

Box 15.1   Amputation for 'apotemnophilia'

A Scottish surgeon, Mr Robert Smith, amputated a healthy leg from each of two patients suffering from apotemnophilia, a body dysmorphic disorder in which the patient feels incomplete with four limbs and wishes to have at least one limb removed. The patients had received psychiatric and psychological treatment prior to the operation, but had failed to respond to these methods. Both operations were carried out privately and not publicly funded, and the patients were satisfied with the results. The National Health Service Trust responsible for the hospital banned further amputations (Dyer 2000).

see Boorse 1997). It is a naturalistic account and based on the concept of *species-typical functioning*. There are four elements to Boorse's account:

1. The *reference class* is a natural class of organisms of uniform functional design; specifically, an age group of a sex of a species.
2. A *normal function* is a part or process within members of the reference class and is a statistically typical contribution by it to their individual survival and reproduction.
3. A *disease* is a type of internal state that is either an impairment of normal functional ability, i.e. a reduction of one or more functional abilities below typical efficiency, or a limitation on functional ability caused by environmental agents.
4. *Health* is the absence of disease (Boorse 1997).

This is a biological, evolutionary account of what pathologists classify as disease. Evolution aims at survival only long enough to enable reproduction or to confer reproductive advantages. It might appear that such a definition omits those areas of medical practice devoted solely to improving quality of life. For example, rheumatoid arthritis may not kill, but causes pain. Is it a disease on Boorse's account? It might be argued that it makes us less fit for survival. However, this argument faces the problem that, even if arthritis does not affect survival or reproduction, we would still want to consider it a disease because of the chronic pain it causes.

Boorse distinguishes disease from illness. *Illness* (or 'therapeutic abnormality') is a subclass of disease serious enough to have certain normative (that is, value-laden) features. A disease is an illness only if it is serious enough to be incapacitating, and therefore is:

- undesirable for its bearer
- a title to special treatment
- a valid excuse for normally criticizable behaviour.

Thus, disease is a value-free scientific concept and illness a value-laden (normative) concept. For Boorse, the fact that someone has a disease does not necessarily imply that she should receive treatment; the fact that someone has an illness, however, does have this implication. Boorse argues that many writers conflate disease with what doctors see as justifying treatment, but other goals may motivate doctors besides promoting health. He points out that doctors might legitimately prevent conception or perform abortion, without classifying pregnancy or fertility as diseases. It might be helpful, therefore, to distinguish between core, therapeutic medicine (involving the treatment of disease) and peripheral medicine, which could include contraception, circumcision, cosmetic surgery and even euthanasia.

There have been many objections to Boorse's account of disease. Boorse has claimed that his account is *naturalistic*. One objection is that it involves *covert normativism*, that is, the importing of value judgements about the goals of medicine (Fulford 1989). The values that are endorsed as the goals of medicine are those of survival and reproduction. Values that are rejected are those relating to reduced quality of life (such as chronic pain), where these do not affect survival and reproduction. Boorse's answer is that is just what the concept of disease is about. There are other values but these should not be packed into the concept of disease.

On Boorse's view everyone is diseased in that that they have scars, injuries and dead cells. To say that some part is diseased is to say nothing, however, about its significance. Ruse (1997) points out that, on Boorse's account, homosexuality is a disease, as is infertility. Boorse is happy to accept this, but claims that not all diseases warrant treatment, and that doctors rightly do things in addition to treating disease.

On Boorse's naturalistic account, identifying something as a disease or not is of only partial help in deciding when it is right or wrong for a doctor to intervene, and what interventions are appropriate. Both Boorse and his opponents might agree that doctors should not 'treat' homosexuality, even though Boorse believes it is a disease and his opponents do not. Thus, even though there is disagreement over whether the concept of disease is value free or not, all agree that values cannot be avoided in deciding when doctors should treat.

If doctors rightly do things in addition to treating disease it seems that we need a concept, such as well-being, to evaluate the impact of conditions on people's lives amenable to medical interventions. Aspects that decrease well-being include pain, disability, loss of freedom and loss of pleasure. Thus pregnancy, menopause, teething and menstruation can all impact negatively on well-being, for some people, and these negative impacts can, at least to some extent, be ameliorated by medical interventions.

Is apotemnophilia a disease?

Some argue that the request for amputation of a healthy limbs is a mental disorder, a form of psychosexual disorder involving sexual attraction to amputees (Elliott 2003). Bioethicists Bayne & Levy (2005) agree that it is a mental disorder, but of a different kind, representing 'a mismatch between their body and their body as they experience it', or body integrity identity disorder. They argue that this condition is poorly studied and treatments for it are typically ineffective. On Boorse's definition, it is a disease because these people's psychology causes them to harm themselves, rendering them less fit for survival. But is the question of whether this is, or is not, a disease (or disorder) relevant to the question of whether it is right for a surgeon to amputate a limb (or indeed right for the state to pay for it)? Bayne & Levy (2005) argue that individuals with this condition are often driven to destructive and dangerous practices (such as self-amputation by placing the limb over a rail track). When no other more effective treatments are available, surgeons ought to be permitted, they argue, to amputate such healthy limbs.

On this view doctors should perform surgery, not because it is necessarily in the person's medical interests, but because it is in his or her overall interests.

DISABILITY

The question of when are medical approaches to a problem appropriate has been a contentious issue, over the past 20 years or so, in the context of disability (see also Chapter 8 for discussion of disability in context of genetic testing and selection).

Naturalistic accounts of disability

The traditional approach to defining disability has been to see it as a property of an individual. As with the concept of disease, some have given a naturalistic account, defining disability in terms of a statistical deviation from a biological standard, appealing to the idea of species-typical functioning (see above, and Buchanan et al 2000). Although naturalistic accounts may account well for the concept of disease as described by pathology textbooks, they work less well as an account of disability (and indeed of mental illness; see Chapter 11). Deviation from the biologically or statistically normal does not have intrinsic normative significance. Loss of hearing with old age is certainly consonant with the biological and statistical norm, but hardly less disabling for that. Around 34% of all men aged 40–70 years have some erectile dysfunction, which is a part of normal ageing. As a result, 20 million men worldwide use Viagra (Cheitlin et al 1999). Quite reasonably, many men are not satisfied with species-typical normal functioning.

Evolution is not directly concerned with how well our lives have gone. What is normal for us as a species is what has, over human history, been conducive to our survival and reproduction. But, for us as rational beings capable of having good lives, deviation from such a standard matters only when it is likely to affect the quality of a life – by making it worse or, sometimes, better. The account of disability based on species-typical functioning offers us little assistance in answering normative questions.

Welfarist accounts of disability

As with the concept of disease, an alternative approach is to see disability as a normative, or value-laden, concept. One such approach is the welfarist account of disability, which links disability to a reduction in well-being, rather than to a statistical deviation from normal functioning. Kahane & Savulescu (in press) provide such a definition as follows: a disability is a relatively stable physical or psychological condition X of person P in circumstances C if X tends to reduce the amount of well-being that this person will enjoy in C.

This definition differs from that based on species-typical functioning in two important ways. First it relates disability to reduction in well-being rather than in terms of deviation from normal. Second, disability is relative to circumstances: it does not reside purely within an individual.

Social models of disability

The importance of circumstances are central to social models of disability (for a detailed account and critique of various models, see Shakespeare 2006). These models highlight, to various extents, the importance of social circumstances in defining disability.

The International Classification of Impairments, Disabilities and Handicaps (ICIDH) distinguishes three concepts and defines them as follows:

" Impairment is defined as deviation from a biomedical norm, and includes functional limitation. Disability is then defined as any restriction or lack, resulting from impairment, of ability to perform an activity in the manner or within the range considered normal. Finally handicap is 'a disadvantage for a given individual, resulting from an impairment or disability, that limits or prevents the fulfilment of a role that is normal (depending on age, sex, and social and cultural factors) for that individual' (World Health Organization 1980, quoted in Shakespeare 2006, p. 16).

Using these distinctions, impairment is the equivalent of the traditional naturalistic account of disability, and resides within the individual. But part of the purpose of these definitions was to move away from medical definitions and diagnoses 'and to create a framework which would make space for the social experience of disabled people' (see Shakespeare 2006, p. 16). One of those involved in the development of this classification (Bury) wrote (quoted in Shakespeare 2006, p. 16): 'Our aim was to bring handicap onto the healthcare agenda. That is, we were pressing for greater recognition of (what came to be called) social exclusion in response to disablement'.

The British social model of disability uses two concepts: impairment and disability, where impairment is similar to the above definition. Disability on this model, however, combines two things; it refers to 'the disadvantage or restriction of activity' (which by implication is related to the impairment), but also includes a further causal component: that the disadvantage or restriction of activity is caused by 'contemporary social organisation which takes little or no account of people who have physical impairments and then excludes them from participation in the mainstream of social activities' (Paul Hunt, quoted in Shakespeare 2006, p. 13).

The political purpose of these definitions is to focus attention on eliminating the disadvantages to people with impairment through social changes rather than through 'curing' the impairment. For example, rather than treating (or preventing) dwarfism, the focus, on this model, should be on changing society, both attitudes and environments, so that people with very short stature suffer no disadvantages as a result.

It can be difficult to get clear precisely what the points at issue are in the rather polarized area of disability studies, and where there are areas of agreement. Most agree that there are physical impairments, such as severe brain damage, that are undesirable for the person who suffers them. Most also agree that the degree to which (and even whether) a person with an impairment suffers any disadvantage depends on features of society, such as social attitudes and physical environment. It is this disadvantage that is being referred to by the term disability as defined in the social models. So what are the disagreements? They are of three types.

Conceptual disagreements

There are disagreements as to what should count as an impairment (using the above definition). For example, there is dispute over whether deafness is an impairment (see below), or very short stature.

Ethical disagreements

The main areas of disagreement are over issues that are ethical in nature, and in particular the extent to which disability should be reduced (or eliminated) through changes in society, or the extent to which they should be reduced through treating or preventing impairment. At one end of the spectrum (the extreme social model) is the view that society should change – through adapting the environment, work practices, payments and attitudes, so that no one with an impairment is disadvantaged compared with anyone else. On the extreme version of this view medical science and medical research should not be used to tackle impairments, or disabilities. At the other end of the spectrum (the extreme medical model) is the view that disabilities should be reduced entirely through tackling impairments (treating or preventing the impairment) and that society should not be expected to change in order to accommodate people with impairment. Between these extremes there is a spectrum of views as to how much is it reasonable for society to change, and in what ways; and what medical interventions to reduce both impairments and disabilities should be developed and used.

Factual disagreements

Some of the disputes appear to involve factual disagreements, for example whether there is in fact a possible society in which a person with a particular impairment (blindness, for example) suffered no disadvantages (disabilities) compared with those without the impairment. There might be further disagreements about whether, even if there is theoretically such a possible society, it is achievable politically.

Is deafness an impairment?

Using the terms outlined above, there is dispute over the question of whether deafness is an impairment. Some people in the deaf community claim that deafness does not reduce the quality of life, nor does it necessarily make it more difficult to interact with others, because signing is a unique form of communication that creates its own world of advantages. Such people often claim, further, that deafness represents a unique culture that can be fostered only by being deaf (Lane 2002). On a naturalistic account of impairment (species-typical functioning), deafness is an impairment and the ethical implication is that it should be treated or prevented (although it is logically possible to hold a naturalistic account of impairment whilst also believing that impairment should not be treated). On a welfarist account, the key issue is whether deafness is likely to increase or decrease the chances of having a good life. It is arguable that deafness reduces welfare in two ways. First, it prevents access to the world of sound. In a world without sound, deafness would not be bad. It is the *exercise* of the capacity to hear that is valuable, not the capacity itself. But the capacity to hear is, obviously, a necessary condition for enjoying those intrinsic goods that are necessarily auditory. Second, deafness reduces the chances of realizing a good life because it makes it harder to live, to achieve one's goals, to engage with others in a world that is based on the spoken word. Being able to hear is not a necessary condition for such activities and goods. But it is nevertheless significantly harder to get a job, harder to move in the world, harder to respond to emergencies where the alarm is aural, and so on.

The quality of life of a deaf child may depend on whether her parents are themselves deaf. Some argue that children of deaf parents would be better off deaf because they would then share with their parents being part of the deaf community. The argument against this position is that nothing prevents the hearing children of deaf people from learning to sign and communicate with their deaf parents, just as children of English parents brought up in China can learn Chinese as well as English. Is it not better to have the capacity to speak two languages rather than one, to understand two cultures rather than one? It would be disabling for a child of English parents living in China if the child spoke only English, even though it might be easier for her parents to communicate with her. Even if a condition is an advantage in the narrow context of the child's home, it may still be a significant disadvantage in the larger world.

Is it ever right to increase a person's impairment?

On both the welfarist definition of disability and the species-typical functioning view, Ashley was born with a severe disability (Box 15.2). But the implications of these views radically diverge when we turn to the effect in Ashley of the treatment devised by her doctors. On the species-typical functioning view, the treatment would increase Ashley's disability – driving her even further from the human norm. On the welfarist account, in the *context* of Ashley's brain impairment, and assuming that the claims made for the effects of the treatment on Ashley's well-being are correct, the treatment would be not disabling but enhancing. On the social models of disability, Ashley has a significant impairment that leads to socially caused disability. An implication of the extreme social model is that the 'Ashley treatment' is wrong: society should adapt to ensure she suffers no disability. Even less extreme social models would focus on enabling Ashley to live as good a life as possible through social rather than physical changes (for more discussion see Liao et al 2007).

Whenever there is a mismatch between biology, psychology, and social or natural environment resulting in a bad life, or even a life that is not as good as it could be, we have a choice (Kahane & Savulescu, in press): we can alter our biology, our psychology or our environment. This is occurring in medical practice when doctors advise diets that are low in fat and high in fibre and antioxidants, that is, diets that mimic the diet which our bodies are adapted to tolerate. But another approach is not to change our environment but to change our biology through drugs. The 'polypill' is designed to allow the body to

Box 15.2 The case of Ashley

In 2004 Ashley was a 7-year old girl from Seattle who was born with a condition called static encephalopathy, a severe brain impairment that leaves her unable to walk, talk, eat, sit up or roll over. According to her doctors, Ashley has reached, and will remain at, the developmental level of a 3-month-old baby (Gunther & Diekema 2006). Ashley can be given the best care if she can be lifted, cuddled, and fed by her parents – treated in other words as a young baby. Ashley, however, was growing. Ashley's parents and the doctors at Seattle's children's hospital devised what they called the 'Ashley Treatment', which included high-dose oestrogen therapy to stunt her growth, the removal of her uterus via hysterectomy to prevent menstrual discomfort, and the removal of her breast buds to limit the growth of her breasts. Ashley's parents argue that the Ashley Treatment was intended 'to improve our daughter's quality of life and not to convenience her caregivers' (http://ashleytreatment.spaces.live.com/).

tolerate a modern diet by chemically lowering our cholesterol levels, blood pressure, etc. We can, of course, alter both biology *and* environment, and try to make judgements in each situation as to what is, overall, the best way to reduce particular disabilities. That judgement, and the balance between making biological, psychological, environmental and social changes, will depend on the view we have on the different models of disability.

HUMAN ENHANCEMENT

Should medicine be used only for the treatment and prevention of disease and impairment, or should it also be used for human enhancement?

Medicine is already, to a some extent, being used for enhancement. Cosmetic surgery is used to 'beautify' people with no abnormality in the first place. Viagra, originally developed as an antihypertensive treatment, was found to be of use in diabetics with impotence. Now, millions of healthy men worldwide use Viagra to enhance erectile function beyond age-related norms. The potential over the next decades for medical technologies to be used radically to alter healthy people's lives goes far beyond current practice. Is this to be welcomed?

Definitions of enhancement

What is meant by 'enhancement'? There are three main definitions that parallel those of disease, impairment and disability (for a more detailed discussion, see Savulescu 2006a).

1. Naturalistic accounts

Naturalistic approaches define enhancement in terms of going beyond health-restoring treatment or health, based on a distinction contrasting *treatment versus enhancement*. Juengst (1998, p. 29) writes: 'The term *enhancement* is usually used in bioethics to characterize interventions designed to improve human form or functioning beyond what is necessary to sustain or restore good health'. Pellegrino (2004) uses a similar definition for the purpose of arguing against enhancement on the grounds that it is beyond medicine as a healing enterprise:

" … my operating definition of enhancement will be grounded in its general etymological meaning, i.e., to increase, intensify, raise up, exalt, heighten, or magnify. Each of these terms carries the connotation of going "beyond" what exists at some moment, whether it is a certain state of affairs, a bodily function or trait, or a general limitation built into human nature … For this discussion, enhancement will signify an intervention that goes beyond the ends of medicine as they traditionally have been held.

Daniels, following Boorse (see above), has argued for the use of 'species-typical functioning' as the definition of normality (Daniels 2000, Sabin & Daniels 1994). A complementary account of enhancement could, presumably, be given.

2. Social constructivist accounts

According to normativist accounts, enhancement is improved functioning that we value. One type of normativist account is based on social values.

Wolpe claims that enhancement is a slippery 'socially constructed' concept: 'Yet, ultimately, any exclusive enhancement definition must fail, in part because concepts such as disease, normalcy, and health are significantly culturally and historically bound, and thus the result of negotiated values' (Wolpe 2002, p. 389).

Canton (2003, p. 78) also claims that enhancement is a socially relative concept: 'The future may hold different definitions of human enhancement that affect culture, intelligence, memory, physical performance, even longevity. Different cultures will define human performance based on their social and political values. It is for our nation to define these values and chart the future of human performance'.

3. Welfarist accounts

Another type of normativist account is based on the value of improving human welfare. On this account, when we are considering human enhancement, we are considering improvement of the person's life. The improvement is some change in the state of the person – biological or psychological – that is good. Which changes are good depends on the value we are seeking to promote or maximize. In the context of human enhancement, the value in question is the goodness of a person's life, and for welfarists this is well-being. On this welfarist view, human enhancement can be defined as any change in the biology or psychology of a person that increases the chances of leading a good life in circumstances C.

The naturalistic and welfarist accounts may diverge. For example, on the naturalist account very low intelligence (for example an IQ below 70) is seen as a disease, or impairment. An intervention raising IQ from 60 to 70 would be seen as treatment; raising IQ from 100 to 110 as enhancement. On the welfarist definition, any increase in IQ is an enhancement in so far as it tends to increase well-being.

On the welfarist account, enhancements include a family of different kinds of improvements, including:

- medical treatment of disease
- increasing natural human potential, e.g. increasing a person's own natural endowments of capabilities within the range typical of the species *Homo sapiens*, such as raising a person's IQ from 100 to 140.
- superhuman enhancements (sometimes called posthuman or transhuman) – increasing a person's capabilities beyond the range typical for the species, e.g. giving humans bat sonar or an IQ above 200.

Future prospects for radical modification of humans

There is great public interest in enhancement of people. Some women employ cosmetic surgery to make their nose smaller, or their breasts larger. Some men pump their bodies with steroids to increase muscle bulk. Modern professional sport is often said to be corrupted by widespread use of performance-enhancing drugs, such as human erythropoietin, anabolic steroids and growth hormone. Many people attempt to improve their cognitive powers through the use of nicotine, caffeine and drugs such as Ritalin and Modavigil. People use psychological 'self-help', Prozac, recreational drugs and alcohol to feel more relaxed, socialize better and feel happier (for more discussion, see Savulescu 2006b).

Much more radical biological modification of human beings is possible. It has been possible since about the 1980s to transfer genes from one species into another. ANDi is a rhesus monkey who has had a jellyfish gene incorporated into his DNA: he glows fluorescent green. Genes from other species could be transferred to human beings, creating transgenic humans – fluorescent humans, for example (Savulescu 2003).

It has been hypothesized that ageing in human beings is related to the degradation of telomeres, the regions on the end of our chromosomes (Blasco 2005, Rudolph et al 1999). We may well discover genetic sequences that reduce the rate of telomere degradation. Transfer of these sequences into the human genome might radically increase lifespan. Stem cell science may also have the potential to extend human lifespan still further, by replacing aging tissue with healthy tissue (Harris 2000, 2002, 2004).

Increased amount of brain growth factors (Routtenberg et al 2000) and the signal transduction protein adenylyl cyclase (Wang et al 2004) have also produced memory improvements. Neural stem cells have also been identified that could potentially be induced to proliferate and differentiate (Rietze et al 2001), mediated through nerve growth factors and other factors (Palma et al 2005). In principle, human beings could be biologically modified to have significantly greater cognitive powers.

Other psychological characteristics besides cognitive power can perhaps also be altered. Gene therapy has been used to turn lazy monkeys into workaholics by altering the reward centre in the brain (Liu et al 2004). Genetically modified meadow voles, a species that is normally polygamous, have become monogamous (Lim et al 2004).

Physical abilities might also be altered far beyond current possibilities. 'Schwarzenegger mice' of immense strength have been produced through genetic modification so that myostatin is not produced (Lee 2004). Genetic manipulation to stop myostatin production, or the administration of blockers, would be expected significantly to increase strength in athletes and is likely to offer real potential for doping in the future (Savulescu et al 2004).

Although at present genetic technology is most efficient at selecting among different embryos, in the future it will be possible genetically to alter existing embryos. Considerable progress is being made in the use of this technology for permanent gene therapy of disease (Urnov et al 2005). It is likely that such technology could be used to alter non-disease genes in the future.

The ethics of enhancement

Technologies developed for medical treatments will increasingly be able to be used for human enhancement, and research aimed purely at enhancement might be funded. But is this right? What are the arguments on each side? (See Savulescu [2006b] for more detailed discussion.)

Arguments in favour of enhancement

1. Choosing not to enhance is wrong

Consider the case of the Neglectful Parents. The Neglectful Parents give birth to a child with a special condition. The child has a stunning intellect but requires a simple, readily available, cheap dietary supplement to sustain his intellect. The parents neglect the diet of this child and this results in a child with a stunning intellect becoming normal. This is clearly wrong.

Now consider the case of the Lazy Parents. They have a child who has a normal intellect but, were they to introduce the same dietary supplement, the child's intellect would rise to the stunning level that the child of the Neglectful Parent initially had. These parents cannot be bothered with improving the child's diet, so the child remains with a normal intellect. The inaction of the Lazy Parents is as wrong as the inaction of the Neglectful Parents. It has exactly the same consequence: a child exists who could have had a stunning intellect but is instead normal.

If we substitute 'biological intervention' for 'diet', we see that in order not to wrong our children, we should enhance them if that is possible. Unless there is something special and optimal about our children's physical, psychological or cognitive abilities, or something different about other biological interventions, it would be wrong not to enhance them.

Responses

There is a moral difference between failing to maintain a state of affairs and failing to bring about a better state of affairs.

There is a difference between interventions such as diet, and interventions that require sophisticated medical technologies or drugs.

2. Consistency

Education, diet and training are all used to make our children better people and increase their opportunities in life. We train children to be well behaved, cooperative and intelligent. Indeed, researchers are looking at ways to make the environment more stimulating for young children in order to maximize their intellectual development. These environmental manipulations do not act mysteriously. They alter our biology.

The work of Meaney and colleagues on the effects of different levels of mothering in rats has shown that early experience can modify the molecular interactions that regulate gene expression (Meaney 2001). Furthermore, maternal care and stress have been associated with abnormal brain (hippocampal) development, involving altered nerve growth factors and cognitive, psychological and immune deficits later in life.

Some argue that genetic manipulations are different because they are irreversible. But environmental interventions can equally be irreversible. It may be impossible to unlearn the skill of playing the piano or riding a bike, once learnt. One may be wobbly, but one is a novice only once. The example of the mothering of rats shows that environmental interventions can cause biological changes that are not only irreversible but are passed on to the next generation. To be consistent, if we believe that it is right to enhance people through education and diet then it is right to do so through biological means.

Response

Environmental enhancement *is* different from biological enhancement. Consider altering someone's political beliefs through argument compared with doing so through administration of a drug. The first, although it may be effective, still respects the person and her autonomy, and her political views remain her own. The second method is a biological form of brainwashing and fails to respect her autonomy.

3. Enhancement is no different ethically from treating disease

If we accept the treatment and prevention of disease, we should accept enhancement. The goodness of health is what drives a moral obligation to treat or prevent disease. But health is not what ultimately matters. Health enables us to live well. Disease prevents us from doing what we want and what is good. Health is instrumentally valuable – valuable as a resource that allows us to do what really matters: to lead a good life.

Disease is important because it causes pain, is not what we want, and stops us engaging in those activities that give meaning to life. Sometimes people trade health for well-being – mountain climbers take on risk to achieve, smokers sometimes believe that the pleasures outweigh the risks of smoking, and so on. Life is about managing risk to health and life to promote well-being.

The moral obligation to benefit people that provides the grounds for treating disease also provides grounds to enhance people in so far as this increases their chance of having a better life.

Can biological enhancements increase people's opportunities for well-being? There are reasons to believe they might. Buchanan and colleagues (2000) have discussed the value of 'all purpose goods'. These are traits that are valuable regardless of which kind of life a person chooses to live. They give us greater all-round capacities to live a vast array of lives. Examples include intelligence, memory, self-discipline, patience, empathy, a sense of humour, optimism and just having a sunny temperament. All of these characteristics may have some biological and psychological basis capable of manipulation with technology.

Response

Treatment and prevention of disease typically have a more significant impact on well-being than other enhancements and so should have priority. And the moral importance of treating disease is not simply that of improving individual well-being but also of restoring people to normal functioning. Commitment to this ideal does not entail commitment to enhancement.

Arguments against enhancement

1. The precautionary principle

We are unwise to assume we can have sufficient knowledge to meddle biologically with human nature. To attempt to enhance one characteristic may have other unknown, unforeseen and deleterious effects. Unforeseen effects are particularly likely for genetic manipulations because genes are pleiotropic, which means they have different effects in different environments. The gene or genes that predispose to manic depression may also be responsible for heightened creativity and productivity. There is a special value in the balance and diversity that natural variation affords, and enhancement will reduce this.

Responses

Such precaution is misplaced. The proper response to these concerns is to do adequate research before intervening. And because the benefits may be less than when we treat or prevent disease, we may require the standards of safety to be higher than for medical interventions. But we must weigh the risks against the benefits. If confidence is justifiably high, and benefits outweigh harms, we should enhance. Risks will always be present. We must consider whether the expected benefits outweigh the expected harms.

Natural variation is the product of evolution; we are merely random chance variations of genetic traits selected for our capacity to survive long enough to reproduce. There is no design to evolution. Medicine has changed evolution: we can now select individuals who experience less pain and disease. The next stage of human evolution will be rational evolution, where we select children who not only have the greatest chance of surviving, reproducing and being free from disease, but who have the greatest opportunities to have the best lives. Evolution was indifferent to how well our lives went. We are not. There is therefore no special value in the balance and diversity of natural variation.

2. Inequity: genetic discrimination

Enhancement will create a two-class society of the enhanced and the unenhanced, where the inferior unenhanced are discriminated against and disadvantaged all through life.

Response

Nature is inequitable. There are, for example, naturally 'gifted' children. Allowing choice to change our biology will, if anything, be more egalitarian – allowing the ungifted to approach the gifted.

In any case, how well the lives of those who are disadvantaged go depends not on whether enhancement is permitted, but on the social institutions we have in place to protect the least well off. There is no necessary connection between enhancement and discrimination.

3. Enhancements are self-defeating

Enhancements are often self-defeating. A typical example is increase in height. If height is socially desired, then everyone will try to enhance the height of their children at some cost to themselves, but no one in the end will have benefited: 'If everyone stands on tiptoe no one sees any further'. Economists have coined the term 'positional goods'. These are goods we value principally because they are markers of our success compared with others. Many enhancements will be for positional goods and will start a 'rat race', which will end in no improvement in well-being.

Response

Many enhancements will have significant non-positional qualities. Intelligence, for example, is not only a positional good; it enables an individual to process information more rapidly in her own life, and to develop greater understanding of herself and others.

Even with regard to positional goods, there is an issue of consistency. We allow individuals in society to pursue their own self-interest at some (positional) cost to others. This applies to education, health care, and virtually all areas of life.

4. Enhancement is playing God or against nature

Children are a gift, of God or of nature. We should not interfere with human nature.

Enhancement is tampering with our nature or an affront to human dignity.

Response

Most people implicitly reject this view – we screen embryos and fetuses for diseases, even mild correctible diseases. We interfere with 'nature' or 'God's will' when we vaccinate, provide pain relief to women in labour, treat cancer, or give antibiotics.

Indeed, when we make decisions to improve our lives by biological and other manipulations, we express our rationality and express what is fundamentally important about our nature. Far from being against the human spirit, such improvements express the human spirit. To be human is to be better.

THE FUTURE OF MEDICINE

Medicine in the 20th century made huge advances in the treatment and prevention of disease. Medicine in the 21st century will continue to make significant inroads into treating and preventing disease, but it may move beyond these traditional goals. Doctors may have to take increasing account of patients' autonomous wishes and broader conceptions of human well-being.

To make decisions about the use of medicine beyond the treatment and prevention of disease requires robust conceptions of disease, well-being, autonomy, disability and what actually constitutes enhancement. It will also require decisions about distributive justice.

As medical interventions multiply and their use extends beyond traditional roles, the next generation of doctors will face more complex decisions, have more responsibility, and require greater wisdom than any doctors before them.

REFERENCES

Bayne T, Levy N 2005 Amputees by choice: body integrity disorder and the ethics of amputation. Journal of Applied Philosophy 22(1):75–86

Buchanan A, Brock D W, Daniels N, Wikler D 2000 From chance to choice. Cambridge University Press, Cambridge

Blasco M A 2005 Telomeres and human disease: ageing, cancer and beyond. Nature Reviews. Genetics 6:611–622

Boorse C 1997 A rebuttal on health. In: Humber J M, Almeder R F (eds) What is disease? Humana Press, Totowa, NJ, pp. 3–134

Canton J 2003 The impact of convergent technologies and the future of business and the economy. In: Rocco M C, Bainbridge W S (eds) Converging technologies for improving human performance: nanotechnology, biotechnology, information technology and cognitive science. Kluwer Academic, Dordrecht, pp. 71–78

Cheitlin M D, Hutter A M, Brindis R G et al 1999 'ACC/AHA expert consensus document. Use of sildenafil (Viagra) in patients with cardiovascular disease. American College of Cardiology/American Heart Association. Journal of the American College of Cardiology 33(1):273–282

Daniels N 2000 Normal functioning and the treatment-enhancement distinction. Cambridge Quarterly 9(3):309–322

Dyer C 2000 Surgeon amputated healthy legs. British Medical Journal 320–332

Elliott C 2003 Better than well: American medicine meets the American dream. W W Norton, New York

Fulford K W M 1989 Moral theory and medical practice. Cambridge University Press, Cambridge

Gunther D F, Diekema D S 2006 Attenuating growth in children with profound developmental disability: a new approach to an old dilemma. Archives of Pediatrics & Adolescent Medicine 160(10):1013–1017

Harris J 2000 Essays on science and society: intimations of immortality. Science 288:59

Harris J 2002 Intimations of immortality – the ethics and justice of life extending therapies. In: Freeman M (ed.) Current legal problems. Oxford University Press, Oxford, p. 65–95

Harris J 2004 Immortal ethics. Annals of the New York Academy of Sciences 1019:527–534

Juengst E T 1998 What does enhancement mean? In: Parens E (ed.) Enhancing human traits: ethical and social implications. Georgetown University Press, Washington, DC, pp. 1–28

Kahane G, Savulescu J (in press)

Lane H 2002 Do deaf people have a disability? Sign Language Studies 2(4):356–379

Liao S M, Savulescu J, Sheehan M 2007 The Ashley Treatment: best interests, convenience, and parental decision-making. Hastings Center Report 37(2):16–20

Lee S J 2004 Regulation of muscle mass by myostatin. Annual Review of Cell and Developmental Biology 20:61–86

Lim M M, Wang Z, Olazabal D E, et al 2004 Enhanced partner preference in a promiscuous species by manipulating the expression of a single gene. Nature 429:754–757

Liu Z, Richmond B J, Murray E A, et al 2004 DNA targeting of rhinal cortex D2 receptor protein reversibly blocks learning of cues that predict reward. Proceedings of the National Academy of Sciences of the USA 101(33):12336–12341

Meaney M J 2001 Maternal care, gene expression, and the transmission of individual differences in stress reactivity across generations. Annual Review of Neuroscience 24:1161–1192

Palma V, Lim D, Dahmane N, et al 2005 Sonic hedgehog controls stem cell behaviour in the postnatal and adult brain. Development 132:335–344

Pellegrino E D 2004 Biotechnology, human enhancement, and the ends of medicine. The Center for Bioethics and Human Dignity Website. Online. Available:http://www.cbhd.org/resources/biotech/pellegrino2004-11-30.htmOct 2006

Rietze R, Valcanis H, Brooker G, Thomas T, Voss A, Bartlett P 2001 Purification of a pluripotent neural stem cell from the adult mouse brain. Nature 412:736–739

Disease, disability and human enhancement

Routtenberg A, Cantallops I, Zaffuto S, Serrano P, Namgung U 2000 Enhanced learning after genetic overexpression of a brain growth protein. Proceedings of the National Academy of Sciences of the USA 97(13):7657–7662

Rudolph K L, Chang S, Lee H W et al 1999 Longevity, stress response, and cancer in aging telomerase-deficient mice. Cell 96:701–712

Ruse M 1997 Defining disease: the question of sexual orientation. In: Humber J, Almeder R (eds) What is disease? Humana Press, Totowa, NJ, pp. 137–171

Sabin J E, Daniels N 1994 Determining medical necessity in mental health practice. Hastings Center Report 24(6):5–13

Savulescu J 2003 Human–animal transgenesis and chimeras might be an expression of our humanity. American Journal of Bioethics 3(3):22–25

Savulescu J 2006a Justice, fairness and enhancement. Annals of the New York Academy of Sciences 1093:321–339

Savulescu J 2006b Genetic interventions and the ethics of enhancement of human beings. In: Steinbock B (ed.) The Oxford handbook on bioethics. Oxford University Press, Oxford, pp. 516–536

Savulescu J 2007 Autonomy, the good life and controversial choices. In: Rhodes R (ed.) The Blackwell guide to medical ethics. Blackwell, Oxford, pp. 17–37

Savulescu J, Foddy B, Clayton M 2004 Why we should allow performance enhancing drugs in sport. British Journal of Sports Medicine 38(6):666–670

Shakespeare T 2006 Disability rights and wrongs. Routledge, London

Urnov F D, Miller J C, Lee Y L et al 2005 Highly efficient endogenous human gene correction using designed zinc-finger nucleases. Nature 435:646–651

Wang H, Ferguson G D, Pineda V V, Cundiff P E, Storm D R 2004 Overexpression of type-1 adenylyl cyclase in mouse forebrain enhances recognition memory and LTP. Nature Neuroscience 7(6):635–642

Wolpe P R 2002 Treatment, enhancement, and the ethics of neurotherapeutics. Brain and Cognition 50:387–395

FURTHER READING

Annas G 2000 The man on the moon, immortality and other millennial myths: the prospects and perils of human genetic engineering. Emory Law Journal 49(3):753–782

Annas G, Andrews L B, Isasi R M 2002 Protecting the endangered human: toward an international treaty prohibiting cloning and inheritable alterations. American Journal of Law and Medicine 28:151–178

Bickenback J 1993 Physical disability and social policy. University of Toronto Press, Toronto

Boorse C 1981 On the distinction between disease and illness. In: Cohen M, Nagel T, Scanlon T (eds) Medicine and moral philosophy. Princeton University Press, Princeton, NJ, pp. 49–68

Brock D W 1995 Justice and the ADA: does prioritizing and rationing health care discriminate against the disabled? Social Philosophy & Policy 12(2):159–185

Buchanan A E 1996 Choosing who will be disabled: genetic intervention and the morality of inclusion. Social Philosophy & Policy 13:18–46

Daniels N 2000 Normal functioning and the treatment/enhancement distinction. Cambridge Quarterly of Healthcare Ethics 9:309–322

De Grazia D 2005 Enhancement technologies and human identity. Journal of Medicine and Philosophy 30:261–283

Edwards S D 2001 Prevention of disability on grounds of suffering. Journal of Medical Ethics 27:380–382

Elliott C 2003 Better than well: American medicine meets the American dream. W W Norton, New York

Francis L P, Silvers A 2000 Americans with disabilities: exploring implications of the law for individuals and institutions. Routledge, New York

Fukuyama F 2002 Our posthuman future: consequences of the biotechnology revolution. Profile Books, London

Gillott J 2001 Screening for disability: a eugenic pursuit? Journal of Medical Ethics 27(Suppl II):ii21–ii23

Habermas J 2003 The future of human nature. Polity Press, Cambridge

Harris J 1992 Wonderwoman and Superman: the ethics of human biotechnology. Oxford University Press, Oxford

Harris J 2001 One principle and three fallacies of disability studies. Journal of Medical Ethics 27:383–387

Harris J 2005 Reproductive liberty, disease and disability. Reproductive Medicine Online 10(Suppl 1):13–16

Hull R 1998 Defining disability – a philosophical approach. Res Publica IV(2):199–210

Humber J M, Almeder R F (eds) What is disease? Humana Press, Totowa, NJ

Jones R B 2001 Impairment, disability and handicap – old fashioned concepts? Journal of Medical Ethics 27:377–379

Kamm F 2005 Is there a problem with enhancement? American Journal of Bioethics 5(3):5–14

Kass L R 2002 Life, liberty and the defense of dignity: the challenge for bioethics. Encounter Books, San Francisco, CA

Kass L R 2003 Beyond therapy: biotechnology and the pursuit of human improvement. Paper presented to The President's Council on Bioethics. Online. Available:http://bioethicsprint.bioethics.gov/background/kasspaper.html 25 Jun 2007

Kass L R 2003 Ageless bodies, happy souls: biotechnology and the pursuit of perfection. New Atlantis 1:9–28

Koch T 2001 Disability and difference: balancing social and physical constructions. Journal of Medical Ethics 27:370–376

Levy N 2002 Reconsidering cochlear implants: the lessons of Martha's Vineyard. Bioethics 16:134–135

McMahan J 1996 Cognitive disability, misfortune, and justice. Philosophy and Public Affairs 25(1):3–35

Miller P, Wilsdon J (eds) 2006 Better humans? The politics of human enhancement and life extension. Demos, London

Parens E (ed.) Enhancing human traits: ethical and social implications. Georgetown University Press, Washington, DC

Parens E, Asch A 1999 The disability rights critique of prenatal genetic testing. Reflections and recommendations. Hastings Center Report 29(5):S1–S22

Parens E, Asch A (eds) 2000 Prenatal testing and disability rights. Georgetown University Press, Washington, DC

President's Council on Bioethics 2003 Beyond therapy: biotechnology and the pursuit of happiness. Dana Press, New York

Reindal S M 2000 Disability, gene therapy and eugenics – a challenge to John Harris. Journal of Medical Ethics 26:89–94

Sandel M 2004 The case against perfection. Atlantic Monthly April 51–62

Sandel M 2007 The case against perfection: ethics in the age of genetic engineering. Belknap Press of Harvard University Press, Cambridge, MA

Savulescu J 2002 Deaf lesbians, 'designer disability' and the future of medicine. British Medical Journal 325:771–773

Savulescu J 2007 Genetic interventions and the ethics of enhancement of human beings. In: Steinbock B, London A J, Arras J D (eds) Ethical issues in modern medicine. McGraw-Hill, New York, pp. 516–535

Savulescu J, Foddy B 2007 Performance enhancement and the spirit of sport: is there good reason to allow doping? In: Ashcroft R, Draper H, Dawson A, McMillan J (eds) Gillon's principles of healthcare ethics. John Wiley, Chichester, pp. 511–535

Savulescu J, Hemsley M, Newson A, Foddy B 2006 Behavioural genetics: why eugenic selection is preferable to enhancement. Journal of Applied Philosophy 23(2):157–171

Shakespeare T (ed.) 1998 The disability reader. Cassell, London

Shakespeare T 2006 Disability rights and wrongs. Routledge, London

Silver L M 1999 Remaking Eden. Phoenix Giant, London

Silvers A, Wasserman D, Mahowald M B 1998 Disability, difference, discrimination. Rowman & Littlefield, New York

Sparrow R 2005 Defending deaf culture: the case of cochlear implants. Journal of Political Philosophy 13(2):135–152

Spriggs M 2002 Lesbian couple create a child who is deaf like them. Journal of Medical Ethics 28(5):283

Stock G 2002 Redesigning humans. Profile Books, London

Tong R 1999 Dealing with difference justly: perspectives on disability. Social Theory and Practice 25(3):519–530

Wasserman D 2005 The nonidentity problem, disability, the role morality of prospective parents. Ethics 116:132–152

Wasserman D, Bickenbach J, Wachbroit R (eds) 2005 Quality of life and human difference: genetic testing, healthcare, and disability. Cambridge University Press, Cambridge

Disease, disability and human enhancement

Useful web resources in medical ethics and law

GATEWAYS TO RESOURCES

Journal of Medical Ethics: http://jme.bmj.com/

Provides a useful list of classified websites, as well as a good selection of articles from the journal and abstracts for most articles published since 1990. There is also a link on this website to the journal *Medical Humanities*.

UK Clinical Ethics Network: http://www.ethics-network.org.uk

The first national network of clinical ethics committees in the world. This site provides educational resources in clinical ethics as well as information on individual committees.

The Ethox Centre: http://www.ethox.org.uk

A research and teaching centre in medical ethics at the University of Oxford. The site provides teaching materials used in medical student education.

Oxford Uehiro Centre for Practical Ethics: http://www.practical-ethics.ox.ac.uk

A University of Oxford research centre not only in medical ethics but also other areas of practical ethics.

Program on Ethics of the New Biosciences, James Martin 21st Century School (BEP): http://www.bep.ox.ac.uk

This University of Oxford research centre website is particularly strong on ethical issues that are likely to arise in the future, including issues arising from likely future medical technologies.

Canadian Bioethics Society: http://www.bioethics.ca

Useful web links as well as educational material in medical ethics.

253

Kennedy Institute of Ethics: http://www11.georgetown.edu/research/nrcbl/

This Georgetown University website for the largest library in medical ethics contains links to the National Reference Center for Bioethics Literature and other sites for accessing useful bibliographies, search tools and educational material.

Social science information gateway: http://www.intute.ac.uk

A comprehensive and well classified gateway to web resources in social sciences including ethics and law.

JOURNALS AND REPORTS

Journal of Medical Ethics

See above.

Bioethics: http://www.blackwellpublishing.com

Then follow links to journal *Bioethics*.

Nuffield Trust Bioethics Reports: http://nuffieldbioethics.org

Full text of these significant reports available online.

Other journals

See the *Journal of Medical Ethics* and Canadian Bioethics Society sites for links to other key journals.

PROFESSIONAL BODIES

General Medical Council: http://www.gmc-uk.org

Contains GMC guidelines covering many areas of medical practice and includes draft guidelines for comment and feedback.

British Medical Association: http://www.bma.org.uk

Some of the BMA's reports and codes of practice (such as that about advance directives) are available online.

Royal College of Obstetricians and Gynaecologists: http://www.rcog.org.uk

Online guidelines available.

WEB RESOURCES

UK government reports: http://www.lawcom.gov.uk

Law Commission reports are available as well as some government-sponsored educational documents, such as that on consent.

National Research Ethics Service (formerly UK Central Office for Research Ethics Committees): http://www.nres.npsa.nhs.uk

Useful links to sites relevant to the ethics of medical research.

American Medical Association: http://www.ama-assn.org

Some medical ethics learning resources, including case histories, available.

PHILOSOPHY ENCYCLOPAEDIAS

Stanford Encyclopedia of Philosophy: http://plato.stanford.edu

A gradually growing online encyclopaedia of philosophy.

The Internet Encyclopedia of Philosophy: http://www.iep.utm.edu

An alphabetical index of philosophical subjects.

LAW

The British and Irish Legal Information Institute (BAILII) database: http://www.bailii.org

An excellent database of recent legal cases, available free online.

Office of Pubic Sector Information: http://www.opsi.gov.uk

UK statutes from 1988.

Scottish legislation: http://www.opsi.gov.uk/legislation/scotland/about.htm

Provides links to Acts passed by the Scottish Parliament, such as The Adults with Incapacity (Scotland) Act 2000.

Other sites

See Social science information gateway (above) for many more websites relevant to law.

These resources were prepared with the assistance of Merle Spriggs and Ainsley Newson.

Index

Guardianship order, 170, 173
Gut reactions, 8, 9

H

Halsbury's Statutes of England, 57
Handicap, 239
Hanson v Airdale Hospital NHS Trust
    [2003], 52
Head injury, 80
Health care
    definitions/boundaries, 211
    goals of medicine, 235–238, 248
    treatment in Europe to avoid delay, 214
Health expenditure, 202, 203
Health professionals' rights, 43
Healthy-years equivalents (HYEs),
    202, 204
Heart attack, 127
Hedonic utilitarianism, 24
Hedonism, 34
    quantitative, 37
Hierarchy of desires, 42
Hierarchy of duties, 25
Hills v Potter [1984], 51
HIV/AIDS
    confidentiality issues, 101
    perinatal transmission, 231–233
HLA typing, 119
Homicide Act (1957), 177
House of Lords, 48
Human Fertilization and Embryology Act
    (1990), 103, 149–150, 158
Human Fertilization and Embryology
    Authority, 149
    register, 103
Human Fertilization and Embryology
    (Disclosure of Information) Act
    (1992), 103
Human Organ Transplants Act (1989),
    193
Human Reproductive Cloning Act (2001),
    129
Human Rights Act (1998), 43, 55–56, 104,
    114, 143, 181, 217
    access to health care, 213–214
    confidentiality issues, 104–105
Human Tissue Act (1961), 193
Human Tissue Act (2004), 118, 193, 195,
    196, 197, 199, 217, 226
Human Tissue Authority, 193, 198
    Codes of Practice, 193, 194, 195, 196,
    197
Human tissue removal/storage, 193
    consent, 194
Human Tissue (Scotland) Act (2004), 193
Hunter v Hanley [1955], 53–54
Huntington's disease, 121

Hydration, 182, 183, 184
Hypoglycaemic attack, 166
Hypothetical imperatives, 25

I

Ideal utilitarianism, 24
Identifiable patient data, 97
Identity of individual, 137, 138
    genetic, 132
Identity-altering interventions, 145
    assisted reproduction, 147–148
Identity-preserving interventions, 145
Illness, definitions, 236
Immunities, 44
Impairment, 239, 240
Implicit knowledge, 3
Implied consent, 73–74
In-vitro fertilization, 146, 148.
        See also Assisted reproduction
Incidental findings at surgery, 75–76
Incompetent adults, 82–91, 166
    advance directives, 83–84, 85
    best interests approach to health care,
        40, 70, 82, 84, 85–86, 90
    family involvement, 91
    caesarian section without consent,
        144
    confidentiality, 108–109
    end-of-life decisions, 182–183
    genetic testing, 117–118
    legal aspects, 84–86
    organ donation, 196, 197
    proxy decision-making, 82
    refusal of treatment, 166, 167
    research participation, 219, 225–228
    restraint, 85
    Scottish law, 86
    substituted judgement, 82–83, 85
Individual liberty, 26, 29, 40–41
Infants, conferred moral status, 138–139
Infertility, 147.
        See also Assisted reproduction
Information provision
    assisted reproduction, 148
    competent decision-making, 77, 80
    consent validity, 69, 70, 71
    nature of procedure, 72, 74
    research participants, 219, 223–224
        double standard, 224, 225
    resuscitation status, 192
    risks/benefits, 72–73
Informative model of doctor–patient
    relationship, 62–63
Informed consent. *See* Consent
Insanity, 176
Instituitional review boards, 217
Instruction directive, 83

Index

INDEX

Index